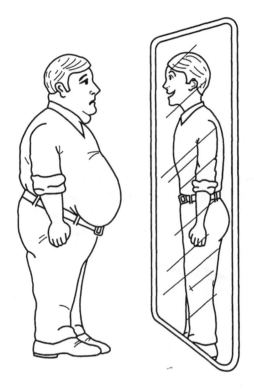

LOSE THE WEIGHT YOU HATE!

RITCHIE C. SHOEMAKER, M.D.

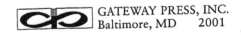
GATEWAY PRESS, INC.
Baltimore, MD   2001

Please direct all correspondence and book orders to:
Ritchie C. Shoemaker
1604 Market St.
Pocomoke City, MD 21851

Library of Congress Control Number 2001 097439
ISBN 0-9665535-2-7

Cover design by Janet Kratfel
Cover drawing by Bruce Rydell

Published for the author by
Gateway Press, Inc.
1001 N. Calvert Street
Baltimore, MD 21202

Printed in the United States of America

Dedication

This book is dedicated to the concept of living life fully. My life is filled with love of family and profession.

I believe that eating should bring pleasure to daily life with fresh, good tasting foods prepared and served attractively. I believe that the greatest pleasure for overweight patients comes from successful weight loss and maintenance. Learning the basic concepts of the chemistry of fat provides the understanding of how and why my weight loss program works so well.

This book is dedicated to enjoying life, food and nutrition without undue fear or guilt about weight.

TABLE OF CONTENTS

FOREWORD

Losing weight doesn't seem to be too hard to do. My patients tell me that they have lost hundreds of pounds before they began my program. Keeping the weight off has been the big problem. Everyone regains it seems, **until** they try a science-based approach to weight loss.

There are many plans people use to lose weight. The teachings I use have not been published previously. I focus my programs on the biochemical mechanisms that the body uses to make fat. By eating to defeat those mechanisms, the maintenance rate for my patients is quite high.

The successful maintenance of my patients' weight loss contributes to my enthusiasm about the program that I will outline for you. My main reason for writing this book is to show you how the sadness and frustration of failed weight loss attempts are easily replaced by the happiness and satisfaction that come from successful slimming, followed by maintenance of weight loss. You can have success, too. Try it my way for a while. My way works.

The style of writing I use is the same style that I use in talking. As they say on the Eastern Shore, "if my doctor won't talk to me, then I don't need to talk to him again." I want the medical terms I use to come alive to you, like they are to me. I want you to know how the body works. If the medical words sound too technical, read the passage again—the glossary will help. I believe that you, the reader, want to know what happens, why it happens, with enough detail to make your own decisions. Here are the facts, mixed in with a few opinions.

I want you to learn how and why my way works.

INTRODUCTION

Sooner or later, it happens to most of us.

Maybe it happens in a hotel bathroom—on the night before your long-anticipated high school reunion—when you gaze into the full-length mirror, gasp with sudden shock, and then blurt at your startled spouse: "Honey, I can't face them ... I'm too *fat!*"

Or maybe the awful realization takes place at a seaside resort, during that awful moment when you attempt to climb into your favorite bathing suit from summers past ... only to discover that the shrunken garment will no longer stretch itself to accommodate your expanded hips! (Or maybe it's your spouse who inadvertently triggers your fat-crisis, by waxing nostalgic about how good you *used* to look.)

Let's face it: Waking up to the knowledge that you've joined the ranks of the "overweight" has to be one of life's most dismal and depressing experiences. Of course, you knew all along that you were drifting toward Fat City ... but the final realization is upon you now, and it hurts. Why? Because if you're honest, you'll quickly admit the obvious: You *hate* that fat. And you hate your failure to keep it off ... even though you counted every last calorie in the "Cambridge Diet," and the "Beverly Hills Diet" ... before becoming a dedicated foot-soldier in the "Atkins Diet Revolution."

"Eating less fat and exercising more" is the answer, according to so many of the nutrition experts. But you've *tried* that already, haven't you? And it didn't work, did it? Sure, you lost a few pounds. Maybe you even shed *twenty* pounds, over the course of a few months. But then what happened?

It all came back, that's what. Within a matter of a few months, every pound returned to you ... until you wound up in your present plight—unable to wear your own clothes and gasping like a winded fire horse each time you climb the basement stairs. And what about your self-esteem?

Say, Katherine ... haven't you gained some weight since I saw you last?

Painful? You bet. But at least you're in good company.

For millions of Amerians these days, "being overweight"—even to the point of health-threatening obesity—simply goes with the territory. Increasingly, it's part of our national identity, as the Affluent Society rapidly becomes the Fat Society. Whether we blame this fast-spreading health condition on television, lack of exercise or the fastfood industry (they're less responsible for the problem than you probably think), the shocking fact remains: More than one-third of the U.S. population is now officially classified as "obese" by the U.S. Centers for Disease Control and Prevention (CDC).

The grim fact is that there are millions of other struggling souls out there right now who can't face *their* former high school classmates or get into *their* old bathing suits, either!

So why don't they just decide to get rid of that unnecessary baggage—and *do* it?

The answer to that question can be found in some recent statistics from the American Medical Association. According to the nation's doctors, only ten percent of the millions of people who set out to lose 30 or more pounds actually manage to accomplish the feat. And among that tiny fraction of successful dieters, only five percent—one in 20—are able to maintain the new, lower weight for more than a few months.

The bottom line: 99 percent of those who set out to lose 30 pounds or more and keep it off ultimately fail at the task. When the best advice of recognized experts results in dismal failure of weight loss and maintenance, what is the overweight patient supposed to do to defeat his weight problem?

They're stuck being fat. And they hate it.

Just like you hate it.

Question: Does anybody really feel good about the thick, oozy layer of flab that so often rides the belt-lines of 40-something men?

And what about those ballooning hip-bulges that can be found on the majority of women past the age of 40? What about their sadly sagging abdomens and their puffy thighs ... not to mention those drooping upper arms with their Jello-wobbly triceps?

Make no mistake: The models in the magazine ads didn't get there because they were able to show off bra lines straining against vast expanses of dimpled cellulite!

It hurts, doesn't it? It hurts to be stuck with at least 30 pounds you never asked for. And you *hate* it. Because it isn't fair! Not after you've sweated through all of those "miracle diets." Not after you listened so hard to the experts, and tried so hard to lose that weight. Remember how you switched to low-fat cream cheese on your whole-wheat bagel for breakfast? Remember all those "healthy, Mediterranean-style" lunches you endured, where your plate crawled with various kinds of pasta and the nearest red meat was located at least two counties away from the table?

And exercise? Don't even talk about it. Remember the Marathon Man? He had nothing on you, did he? (Even though you had to cram it all into the last remaining 30 minutes of daily "free time" in your insanely busy life.) How much did your "personal trainer" cost you last month? And how many dollars did you spend on membership fees at that health club you could never fit into your schedule?

How many thousands of sit-ups or hours of aerobics or miles on the treadmill did you actually manage to complete—before collapsing in an exhausted heap and then discovering that you'd worn out a cartilage in your knee?

Unfair! You ate what they told you to eat, and you took the stairs instead of the elevator at work, and you exercised until you developed mat-burns on your poor hindquarters ... *and what was the result?*

You stayed overweight, that's what.

You continued to struggle in a threatening world where your own clothes—all those size-12 and size-14 outfits still hanging there at the back of the closet—began to silently reproach you for having lost control of your waistline. (And now you face buying a new, expanded-size wardrobe.)

And right here is where yet another tragic aspect of failed dieting programs often makes itself known ... as weight-loss hucksters prey on the unhappiness and desperation of patients who can only maintain their *over*-weight bodies. Barraged by infomercials, full-page Sunday newspaper ads and nutriceutical-pushers, these frustrated patients are pursued relentlessly, for a single reason: their money.

Sad, isn't it? Unsightly and demoralizing, those excess pounds have been making you psychologically miserable. And they aren't helping your physical health any, either. Like most people today, you're reasonably well educated about the health risks associated with obesity. You've read the scare-stories about diabetes, high cholesterol, elevated blood pressure, gallstones, gout, degenerative arthritis and cancer. They are true. And you've noticed—indeed, how could you *miss* it?—that all of these ailments seem to turn up far more often in overweight folks than in their skinny neighbors.

Really, now: Aren't those bouncy folks in their Spandex exercise-suits enough to make you sick?

It's a depressing prospect, you must admit. And what about "quality of life?" Who wants to stand around gasping for breath —just because you bent over to tie your shoes, or to retrieve the *Daily Banner* from the front lawn? Are you really sure the problem is "deconditioning" and not your heart? And who wants to put up with all those fat-related sleep problems (the muscle cramps and the tossing and turning and the out-of-control snoring) that so often combine to keep overweight people and their worried partners awake half the night?

Misery! No matter how you analyze the problem, the answer always comes up the same: *Being overweight is bad for you.* Chronic obesity will take years off your life, and even if doesn't kill you right away, deep down it will eventually make you wish you were someone else.

But here's the good news for overweight people everywhere.

You don't have to live this way.

And the solution is so utterly simple. By using the chapters of this book as your daily guide, you *can* "lose the weight you hate." Even better, you can begin building a new, far more rewarding and satisfying lifestyle ... even as you discover a new way to think about eating and about the many different kinds of food you put into your body each day.

As you'll soon discover in these pages, I've been prescribing this unique, no-amylose diet for overweight patients for more than two decades. (As a matter of fact, my *first* weight-loss book—*Weight Loss and Maintenance: My Way Works*—quickly sold out its first two editions.) Along the way, I've made frequent presentations on the topic to this country's leading group of M.D. specialists in obesity (the American Society of Bariatric Physicians), and my lectures on the physiology of nutrition and dieting have been recorded on Audio Digest, then listened to by thousands of practicing physicians around the country.

At the same time, my current findings in clinical research on obesity have shown the fantastic promise contained in a newly developed medication, Avandia. Only recently, the U.S. Food and Drug Administration approved my study of this gene-modifying substance—manufactured by Glaxo SmithKline—showing that it can be safe and effective, without worrisome side-effects, when used in a weight-loss program that uses the diet that you will read about in this book.

The results of my Avandia study are simply astonishing. Avandia —when combined with my special "No-Amylose Diet"—usually burns off inches of fat (and dozens of pounds) within 12 weeks. Even the most difficult-to-slim-down dieters lose weight on this program, while also lowering their cholesterol levels (and especially LDL cholesterol). In most cases, they manage to burn at least 1.5 inches from their waists and 2.5 inches from their hips during the 12-week dieting period.

My approach to helping patients lose weight was recently presented to the Eighty-Third Annual Meeting of the U.S. Endocrine Society (*Endo 2001*), held in Denver, Colo. That paper, entitled "The Use of Rosiglitazone in Treatment of Hyperinsulinemic Obesity in Non-Diabetics," will also be submitted for publication in the journal *Endocrinology*.

So how does the "Shoemaker Plan" for rapid weight reduction and maintenance actually work?

It's simple. Instead of listening to experts tout programs that don't work (or counting calories until your mind goes numb), you merely follow a few basic steps, including these:

First, eliminate the foods that make your blood sugar rise quickly.

Second, don't put insulin on your fat-cell receptors. (I'll explain these words in Chapter 3.)

Third, don't "burn" protein (here's the biggest reason why most diets fail). Remember that lean body mass is controlled genetically.

Fourth, learn how to shut down your "binge-eating" behavior before it starts.

Fifth, get a handle on the basic "chemistry of fat" ... because understanding how the body manufactures and stores this stuff is the first step in dumping it.

Sixth, relax and begin enjoying the process of losing the weight you hate! (The original recipes included in this book will show you how.) That's right: I said you're going to *enjoy the process* ... once I start showing you how to prepare a huge array of mouth-watering dishes that will make you ask yourself: "Is this delightful meal really part of a *diet?*"

Seventh, look forward to the "glow of health," as you throw away diabetes pills and cholesterol medications you don't need anymore.

o   o   o

Another word to the dieting-wise: Don't be put off, in the pages that follow, by the fancy scientific jargon that occasionally creeps into the discussion. Sure, we're going to be talking a bit here and there about such entities as "insulin receptors," "amylose" and the "Glycemic Index." We'll also briefly discuss such fat-related lingo as "leptin," "tumor necrosis factor alpha," the "thiazolidinediones" and "uncoupling protein." No, you don't have to become an expert in "differential gene activation" resulting from environmental acquisition of obesity ... but I want you to know obesity as I do.

To paraphrase General Colin Powell (while referring to the Iraqi Army): "We are going to find the cause of your weight problem —and then we are going to kill it!"

The rock-solid scientific concepts in this book are there only to help you understand the reasons behind the Shoemaker Plan.

Once you grasp the principles involved, you'll be able to see for yourself just how logical, simple and easy-to-implement this diet really is. The science is there to help you know that my weight program is based on fact.

You're going to enjoy this book! As you read, you'll probably find yourself sending up an old-fashioned Bronx cheer at times for such traditionally sacred (and false!) dieting truisms as:

- O "Eat less and exercise more!"

- O "The key to good nutrition is the Food Pyramid!" (Eating six to 11 servings of complex carbohydrates—including amylose—is healthy and helps weight loss!)

- O "To stay thin, you must speed up your metabolism, because fat is always triggered by a *slow* metabolism!"

- O "The best gauge of ideal weight is the Body Mass Index!"

Remember, above all, as we begin the exciting adventure of shedding and then keeping off all that unsightly flab: the crucial step in understanding is "casting out false knowledge" ... and most weight-loss books are jam-packed with it. (Yes, you're about to meet a "cast-out of thousands," so buckle up!)

Maintenance is quite simple, as well, once you understand fat. And this book will also serve as your supportive guide to maintenance.

The bottom line: If you're like most people, the key reason you're still overweight is that you have never really *understood* the weight you hate.

But that's about to change. Together, we're going to launch an incredible journey through some fascinating information about hormone interactions and the biochemistry of fat cells.

We're going to savor the task of learning about fat, even as we savor the foods we eat on this diet. (Why not take a peek right now at the recipes in the Maintenance Guide? I want you to enjoy life, while enjoying good food that's prepared and served well.

Introduction

Eating is about to become a daily pleasure—especially when your fat doesn't come back.

We're also going to meet—and listen to—some remarkable weight-loss patients, each one of whom has a marvelous story to tell about his or her successful struggle to melt away pounds and pounds of fat, and then keep it off.

Practical, safe and healthy, my no-amylose diet is going to help you lose the weight you hate ... *forever.*

All set? Good. Grab your pencil. In Chapter One, while remembering Lao-Tze's immortal advice to travelers—*the longest journey begins with a single step!*—we're going to take a simplified, up-close look at how sugar and amylose get digested and then stored in the human body as fat.

CASE STUDY NO. 1: NURSE PATTY

Her name was Patty, she was 35 years old, and she weighed 220 pounds.

When I first met this struggling Registered Nurse—back in the summer of 1993—she was at the point of total despair. And no wonder: While struggling with her obesity for more than a decade, she had sweated through more than a dozen different diets without success.

In a word, Patty was *fat*. Hopelessly, uncontrollably *fat*. Lonely and afraid of encountering strangers, she had become increasingly isolated in recent years. Her idea of a good time? "Oh, I'll just go for a walk by myself," she told me, "or maybe sit in my apartment and watch TV." As she described her solitary lifestyle, I could see the tears gathering in her eyes.

Patty jumped at the chance to participate in my No-Amylose Diet. (As she told me later: "I did everything you asked me to, because I figured this was my last chance!")

This hard-working and dedicated medical professional was enormously encouraged when I explained that her obesity was not the result of gluttony or "lack of willpower." Her eyes lit up with understanding, as I pointed out that the key factor in her obesity—insulin resistance—was actually the result of genetic programming that lay completely beyond her control.

Once she understood the revolutionary weight-loss strategy

1

behind my diet—prevent "fat storage" by staying away from foods that contain the two major "fat triggers" (glucose and amylose)— Nurse Patty embraced my "Enjoy-Your-Diet!" lifestyle with determination and gusto.

During the next nine months, she shed more than 70 pounds.

Even more importantly, she has *kept* that 70 pounds of flab off ever since.

Not long ago, Patty told me a wonderful story about a family reunion she recently attended, here in Maryland. Her smile topped 10,000 kilowatts as she described how she'd been the "life of the party." Feeling self-assured and confident, she had danced the night away … before rising at 9 A.M. to enjoy a lively gala breakfast full of good foods (but without the toast and the hash-browns!).

As she told me later: "These days, I've got more energy than I ever thought possible. I follow the 'Weight-Maintenance' guidelines in your diet carefully—and they always encourage me to eat plenty of tasty, nourishing food prepared in ways that are endlessly creative. And yet I haven't gained back a single pound of the weight I lost.

"Thanks for showing me that staying thin can be part of an enjoyable, energetic lifestyle … and a lifestyle that *doesn't* require endlessly counting calories or measuring out food-portions!"

○   ○   ○

In this book, you're going to read several "Real Stories of Real People" … stories about successful dieters like Nurse Patty, who proved that you can LOSE THE WEIGHT YOU HATE!—provided only that you follow the simple guidelines in this revolutionary new approach to dieting.

My way works! Why not give it a try, and see for yourself?

INTRODUCING ...
THE DIET THAT ISN'T A DIET!

Flip on the TV set these days, and the odds are high that you'll soon find yourself listening to a late-breaking news report about how "more than one-third of all Americans have been officially declared 'obese' by the U.S. Surgeon General—and obesity can kill you!"

Spin that dial again, and all at once you're watching a talk-show guest rave about the "Miracle Diet" that helped her shed 40 pounds—even as it solved her marriage problems and made her a million bucks on the stock market.

Let's face it: In recent years, the desire to shed those extra pounds and trim up those flabby thighs has become nothing less than a national obsession ... as well as a multibillion-dollar-a-year industry peddling everything from high-octane "diet suppression" herbs and pills to the latest $400 "exercise bike" from a super-slim TV huckster.

Say what you will about the "Weight-Loss Boom" in America today, there's no getting around one basic fact: People care about how they look, and they also care about the health hazards (both psychological and physical) associated with obesity.

All of which brings us straight back to you, the reader who just picked up this book.

Question: Are you one of the tens of millions of Americans today who've become sick and tired of being 20 or 30 (or even more) pounds overweight?

Ask yourself: Have you ever dreamed of dumping all that unsightly flab, quickly and painlessly?

Have you ever fantasized about how great it would feel to melt away those 20 or 30 pounds you can't stand ... and to do it without counting calories, or worrying about "fat grams," or turning into one of those compulsive exercisers who spends his entire life jogging back and forth across the neighborhood? (And who has that much free time, anyway?)

In other words: Would you love to LOSE THE WEIGHT YOU HATE?

UNDERSTANDING FAT

You aren't going to believe me, not at first.

Nobody believes me at first ... not unless they've already watched other people succeed on my diet!

But before I tell you about the secret behind the astonishingly successful system for losing weight (and *keeping* it off) that I've developed over the past 20 years, let's pause for a moment to ask a crucially important question:

How much do you know about how the body makes and stores fat?

One way to answer that question is to take my Fat Quiz. Got your pencil? Great. Just answer the following questions "True" or "False."

THE FAT QUIZ

1. Losing weight and keeping it off successfully requires enormous will power and self-denial, and you aren't allowed to

enjoy savory foods prepared with style and pizazz.

FALSE. Although few people realize it, losing weight has almost nothing to do with "will power." Instead, you need to understand how the body stores fat—and then eat in such a way that you defeat the internal storage mechanism.

2. People become overweight because they're basically self-indulgent weaklings who don't know how to push away from the table before gulping down a triple-serving of mashed potatoes and three or four desserts.

FALSE. Most overweight people are subject to the exaggerated effects of powerful hormones (especially insulin) which lie beyond their control. In most cases, they do not eat to excess. Their weight problem is a function of where their metabolic machinery directs the storage of sugar—and has little to do with their character or attitude.

3. If you decide to really get serious about losing weight, you'll have to reconcile yourself to eating nothing but "rabbit food" such as lettuce, celery and carrots.

FALSE. The good news for dieters who adopt my program is that most of the foods you love to cook and eat are still allowed. The only off-limits foods are the relatively few that contain large amounts of fat-triggering amylose and glucose. (Amylose, by the way, is by far the most important "carbohydrate" for dieters to be concerned about—and diets that simply lump all carbohydrates together are not nearly focused enough to get the job done. Stand by for more info on the vital importance of avoiding amylose later in this chapter!)

I want my patients to live well and eat well ... and this book contains 50 of my own original, mouth-watering recipes! Each one has its own story to tell.

Unlike most of the "crash diets" floating around out there, my program celebrates the joys of good eating and embraces a lifestyle full of happiness about food. Maintenance begins with feeling good about yourself and your diet.

4. Jogging several miles each day is a good way to kick off a weight-loss program, because it burns off fat at a high rate of speed.

   FALSE. "Jogging" and other forms of aerobic exercise actually burn relatively few calories (unless you do them all day long). And you'll probably wind up trading those calories for a bottle of aspirin and a heating pad—after you come down with the all-too-predictable shin splints, ankle sprains, swollen knees and lower-back pain that so frequently accompany the exercise craze. I'll tell you how to stretch right and get into shape before beginning a vigorous exercise program. Exercise will often leave you feeling great—but don't expect life-changing benefits unless you work out 12 hours or more per week.

5. Starting your day off in the morning by drinking a cup of coffee and then skipping breakfast will help you lose pounds in a hurry.

   FALSE. Believe it or not, such "compulsive fasting" as skipping breakfast will only serve to turn on your brain's "hunger center," so that you'll store twice as many calories as fat from your next meal. The net result: You'll actually gain weight by skipping breakfast!

6. Your "lean body mass," which plays a vital part in the dynamics of fat storage, is controlled by your genes, and you cannot change its biochemistry or its role in fat storage.

   TRUE. You and I are going to be talking a lot about the importance of lean body mass during the next few chapters, because managing it correctly is crucial to both weight loss and maintenance.

7. As we consume food, the conversion and storage of blood sugar in "glycogen" for later use by the cells takes place at

the same rapid rate in all human beings.

FALSE. The process occurs rapidly only in those people who have low levels of the food-storage hormone "insulin." And this is an important fact to know, because learning your own body chemistry—and then learning how to "turn off" your insulin—is a key step, if you wish to neutralize the production of fat by your body.

8. Insulin is the "friend" of overweight people, since its primary function is to open cell membranes, so that they can receive and then harmlessly store blood sugar, thus preventing the eater from becoming fat.

    FALSE. Sure, insulin helps the cells to take in sugar ... but the moment the glycogen stores in cells become saturated, that same insulin hustles any additional sugar straight to the liver, where it's quickly transformed first to fatty acids and then to fat!

9. Medical doctors who have been forced to struggle with their own tendency to become overweight are often more understanding and empathetic about fat than skinny doctors who have "never been there."

    TRUE, TRUE, TRUE! The candid fact is that I rode the "dieting yo-yo" for several years, myself, before finally devising and then following the successful weight-reduction and maintenance program that you're reading about right now.

10. The more complicated and technical-sounding a weight-loss program the better, because that kind of overwhelming complexity proves that the doc knows what he's talking about.

    FALSE ... and ridiculous! I've coached thousands of patients through this successful system during the past two decades. The science I'm going to tell you about makes sense and the *words* also make sense—once you know how to think about how fat is made.

I am going to show you how to defeat fat manufacture. Most of my patients soon catch on to the few basic scientific principles on which the LOSE THE WEIGHT YOU HATE! program is based, and putting the program into action at mealtimes is a snap.

Forget about counting "points," "food exchanges" and "calories"—and start using your new understanding of fat and fat storage to defeat your weight problem!

O   O   O

So how did you do on the "FAT 101" Quiz?

If you're like most people, you probably had some difficulty coming up with the right answers to these basic questions about body metabolism and fat storage.

But that's okay—because this book is going to teach you (in simple, down-to-earth English) just how the human body converts the food you eat into the flab you hate ... and how you can ditch those unsightly pounds, while feeling good about yourself and your life in the process.

Yes, I'm going to show you how to melt away every last pound of that excess baggage you've been carrying around all these years, and I'll show you how to do it painlessly, almost effortlessly, without feeling starved and miserable. I should also point out that keeping that weight *off* is what my patients do best. And I've coached thousands of them through the process!

But the opportunity to lose weight, lots and lots of weight, quickly and painlessly is only part of the good news in this book.

That's because getting rid of all that extra physical poundage is actually the *easy* part of bringing obesity under control.

The tough part is keeping it from coming back!

Ask yourself: Do you know of any other highly touted activity in life that has a 99-percent failure-rate? Note well, however: My

9

carefully documented "maintenance rate" with patients is well over 70 percent!

Make no mistake: The most exciting and revolutionary aspect of the LOSE THE WEIGHT YOU HATE! approach to effective weight-management is Maintenance.

The best thing about this method of staying thin is that it's based on using your own body chemistry to guarantee successful maintenance.

As a matter of fact, you're about to discover that the "Dr. Shoe System" for achieving lifelong slimness is based mostly on achieving successful *Maintenance* ... and not on "quick and easy" dieting gimmicks aimed at erasing fat overnight.

The problem with the gimmicks, of course, is that they simply fail to meet the test of time. Sure, you can lose 20 pounds in six months with the grapefruit-at-every-meal approach (provided that you don't eat the meal!), or by starving yourself for several weeks and gobbling appetite-suppressants, while doing your best to ignore the risks of stimulant-medications and body protein-burning diets.

But guess what? Within a few months of dumping your "spare tire," you'll have gained back every one of those pounds that cost you so much torture to lose. Take my word for it: The failure of maintenance is the end result of the "eat-low-fat, count calories and exercise for 20 minutes, four times a week" approach to staying slender.

Take that wrong-headed approach and you'll end up as a "dieting yo-yo"—a thoroughly miserable creature who goes back up the weight-chart faster than the express elevator at the World Trade Center.

If you're like millions of other fat-battling people today, you've probably been through the "yo-yo cycle" several times. Like the others, you've hung on grimly through the dull, dreary days of near-starvation meals. (Let's face it, burning up your body's protein in this way causes bad things to happen: You look sick, feel bad, and soon get overwhelmed by constipation or fatigue or reflux or depression, or all of them at once!)

Like many of the other sufferers, you've tasted the sweet—if momentary—triumph of watching the needle on the bathroom scales dip lower by ten or 20 pounds, after several months of grueling effort.

But then, just like all the others, you've watched helplessly, powerlessly, while you gained back every one of those pounds (and maybe a few more) during the next six months or so.

Sounds familiar, you say?

Of course it does. Ask yourself: How in the world did the "Dieting Industry" become a $1 trillion-a-year business in the United States during the past two decades? The cause of the sales boom, of course, is that 99-percent failure-rate that will never change as long as patients listen to the opinions of "experts" who harp away about calories and exercise.

Ask yourself: Why are the women's magazines and the drug-store paperback racks all crammed to bursting, day in and day out, with headlines so bold and brazen that they take your breath away: "FANTASTIC MIRACLE-DIET LETS YOU LOSE TEN POUNDS OVER THE WEEKEND AND NEVER GAIN IT BACK!"?

Answer: Up until quite recently, nobody really understood the hidden scientific principles behind the process that triggers the manufacture of fat and the management of fat stores in the human body. Because of this widespread ignorance, absurd claims like the one above often went unchallenged.

Next question: How many times have you been told that "counting calories" and "limiting fat intake"—along with getting "at least 30 minutes of vigorous exercise per day"—are the keys to losing excess weight and keeping it off?

If you're like most people (including Ritchie Shoemaker, M.D., who used to struggle endlessly, himself, to keep his flab at bay!), you've probably been "propagandized" by self-proclaimed dieting experts whose pious pronouncements about "caloric intake" and "saturated fats" and "aerobic exercise" long ago became nothing less than cultural mantras.

Ladies and gentlemen, you are in for a surprise.

Those "dieting experts" were wrong.

Dead wrong.

As a matter of thoroughly startling fact, successful weight-management has very little to do with the number of calories you consume each day!

Nor does it depend that much on limiting the amount of fat —saturated or otherwise—that you take in during a meal. Sure, fat counts ... but aren't you already watching fat grams and hearing about eating "healthy Mediterranean diets" everywhere you go, these days?

As for exercise ... well, at the risk of outraging every Phys Ed instructor in the land, I'll give you the news as bluntly as I can: Although physical exercise certainly helps your stamina and your muscle tone (along with improving your cardiovascular fitness), it actually has very little to do with the complicated dynamics in which your body decides to create and store fat!

Shocking, isn't it?

But it's also true. According to the latest worldwide research on human physiology, the process of fat formation in humans is keyed not to the amount of food consumed ... but to the way in which the body stores food by converting it to fat.

That enlightening disclosure is only one of several insights to have been generated in recent years by complex biochemical studies that show how blood sugar ("glucose"), the basic energy-source we derive from the food we eat, is actually stored in the body, starting within a few minutes of beginning a meal.

In the coming chapters, I'll outline the program I've used with documented success in my medical practice over the past 20 years.

Thousands of patients, whether high school dropouts or Ph.D.s, have learned the medical terms I use and carried my weight-loss program through to successful completion.

But let me go back to the key "fat discovery" of recent years ... the discovery which serves as the scientific basis of my approach to weight-control. That research-breakthrough can be summarized as follows: *The amount of food you eat is actually far less important than the way in which your particular body-chemistry converts it into fat.*

That's the first big shocker that you and I are going to be talking about in this book. Together we're going to take a long, hard look at the reasons why some people can eat all they want and stay skinny, and others (like me) will gain two pounds merely by uttering the word "potato!"

Along with understanding your own particular "digestion chemistry," or "metabolism," we're going to explore the implications of the insight that the amount of exercise you get each day is also far less important (as a factor in controlling body weight) than your own body's genetically based fat-storing mechanism.

The bottom line is simply this: If you can understand how your own unique body chemistry operates to "store calories," you can quickly begin taking rapid, virtually painless steps to offset that "storage process" ... and thus prevent your body from creating the flab in the first place. Let your body burn fat and not store it!

As you might imagine, the physiological implications of the new scientific discoveries I'm describing are going to be of some real help to the nation's dieters during the next few years.

They're also going to dramatically change the way all of us go about the business of shedding extra poundage.

During the chapters that follow, I'm going to show you—in clear, simple, jargon-free English—exactly how the human body stores food-derived energy in the form of fat.

After that, I'm going to show you what happens when we eat certain foods that stimulate the body's digestive system to quickly "load up" each cell with as much glycogen as is genetically possible.

Next, I'm going to paint you an easy-to-read picture of what the body does with any *additional* glucose that suddenly arrives in the bloodstream. (Quick answer: That extra sugar gets shunted down to the liver, where it's quickly converted to the "fatty acids" that will fill up fat cells in your over-fed body!)

After only a few brief chapters of LOSE THE WEIGHT YOU HATE!, you're going to know all you need to know about the "physiology of fat"—and you're going to understand for yourself exactly why this dieting breakthrough offers astonishing hope to millions of Americans who have been playing the depressing "yo-go game" far too long.

I'm also going to tell you the truth about cholesterol, fiber, exercise, gout, weight-loss medications and other important aspects of nutrition. The exciting proof of the benefits of a gene-manipulation approach to weight loss using Avandia and the sobering truth of environmental acquisition of diabetes and obesity have never been published before. Once you understand the simple biochemistry involved in making and storing fat, you will know why traditional concepts like "eat less and exercise more" are of little value for those patients with genetic causes of obesity.

Before we take an up-close look at some of the chemistry involved in human metabolism, though, let's cut directly to the dieting chase.

I told you on Page 1 that I was going to show you how to lose your extra weight (I want women to have 20 percent of their total weight as fat, and men to have 15 percent), in order to feel better and look better and re-energize your life. And the best part is that my program will show you how to do this without counting calories, or worrying about "fat grams," or turning into a compulsive exerciser.

That's a mighty big claim, and you have every right to ask: "Oh, yeah? How's he going to do *that*? What will this new dietary regimen require of me, and how much will I be allowed to eat?"

Good questions. Here are some of the answers.

Under the LOSE THE WEIGHT YOU HATE! system of losing weight and keeping it off, you will:

O Never count calories or study those depressing "Calorie Charts" again. Stop counting and start living!

O Never count "fat grams" or worry about the "percentage of fats and especially saturated fats" in your dinner again. Your food should look good, taste good and be good for you.

O Never waste time by planning unrealistic and impossible-to-implement "exercise schedules" again. You can throw the dusty exercise bike away. If you have time and like to exercise, that's great; I will show you how to do it safely.

O Never starve yourself by nibbling dry crackers and celery sticks at mealtime, while your belly rages like some under-fed Godzilla and your energy level plunges toward the center of the earth. (Get ready to learn about "protein-sparing foods" and "positive-nitrogen balance.")

Dieter, your liberation is at hand!

Instead of trying to control the amount of food you eat, the LOSE THE WEIGHT YOU HATE! technique will show you how to control your body's metabolic response to that food with a few simple steps.

This is the radical discovery—the fact that getting fat is a function of food *storage* and not food *consumption*—that lies at the heart of my new, scientifically validated approach to both eating and health.

So innovative and original is the LOSE THE WEIGHT YOU HATE! system for healthy eating, in fact, that from this point on, I'm not even going to use the word "diet" in discussing it!

15

Throughout the chapters that follow, you'll notice that this depressing word, full of negative connotations (the first three letters of which spell ... what?) is rarely used ... and that such terms as "weight maintenance" and "metabolically healthy" are usually employed instead to describe this joyful and vitally healthy method for remaining forever slim.

In other words, I'm going to tell you about a *lifestyle* that keeps weight off, and not just a short-term diet.

So what's the key, exactly, to "Doc Shoe's" system of weight loss and permanent maintenance?

The key step, as you've probably gathered from the preceding paragraphs, is to avoid those foods that "tell" the body to rush glucose into every cell, and then, once glucose-saturation occurs, to begin converting the glucose into fatty acids (and ultimately into fat).

Instead of counting calories, charting fats, worrying about "junk carbohydrates" or becoming an exercise nut, the LOSE THE WEIGHT YOU HATE! approach asks you to accomplish a single, simple task: avoiding those foods that contain large amounts of fat-triggering glucose, along with its near-cousin, a powerhouse form of food-based complex carbohydrate known as "amylose."

The chemistry here is actually quite simple—and it tells us that amylose consists of many glucose molecules linked together to create starch. Amylose is quickly broken down, however (into the basic sugar known as "glucose") by an enzyme in our saliva called *amylase. (Of course there are many other sugars in addition to glucose and amylose—as you'll see in pages to come—but these two are by far the most important when it comes to the formation and storage of human fat.)*

In practical terms, my diet eliminates amylose. This means that you will be asked to avoid such high-amylose foods as breads, potatoes, rice, oats, barley, rye, bananas, and vegetables that "grow beneath the ground." (I'll show you why this is so important in a later chapter.)

By eliminating these "high-Glycemic Index" foods from your daily intake, you will shut down the mechanism that the body uses to convert amylose into glucose, sending it rushing into the cells. In this way, you will also shut down the "fat trigger" that goes off whenever your cells become sugar-saturated.

Remember: Except for these targeted foods (roots, tubers and above-ground grains such as wheat and rice), you will be allowed to eat what you want. You will never again face the daunting task of "measuring portions," and you will never again worry about taking a "second helping" of meat loaf or a third helping of "String Beans Almondine" (or a second glass of freshly squeezed juice with that morning cheese omelet).

That's right: The LOSE THE WEIGHT YOU HATE! method of weight-loss and maintenance doesn't require you to fret day and night about every little morsel you put in your mouth ... providing, of course, that the morsels aren't on the "forbidden list" of high-amylose and high-glucose foods. Don't eat foods you don't want to wear!

So what will you be "allowed" to eat, day in and day out, if you decide to have a go at the LOSE THE WEIGHT YOU HATE! approach to a slimmer lifestyle?

The answer to that one is easy: You can have anything you want (within reason, of course) ... provided only that it doesn't include one of the dietary culprits contained on the "high-Glycemic Index" *(see Appendix 2 for a list of high glycemic-targeted foods)*.

After you've gotten rid of the flab, the LOSE THE WEIGHT YOU HATE! maintenance program will allow you to consume amylose—but only within the parameters dictated by your genetically programmed starch-storage mechanism. You'll also be permitted to enjoy a thick steak now and then, or a heaping portion of green peas with melted butter ... or maybe a tumbler brimming with creamy whole milk, or even an occasional bowl of your favorite Mint Chocolate Chip ice cream. The maintenance program is not as restrictive as the weight-loss program. When

17

you're doing maintenance, you can safely consume not only that thick steak, but also an occasional sandwich or bowl of pasta.

And what *can't* you eat during the weight-loss phase? Answer: All of the above-ground, high-amylose cereals (no more bagel with low-fat cream cheese in the morning, and no more double-helping of Puffed Rice breakfast cereal). No more of Grandma's muffins, no more white bread from the supermarket, no more russet potatoes and no more bananas or spaghetti or honey dribbled over a slice of toast made from whole wheat bread.

On the other hand, you'll be allowed to eat all you want of fruits that taste good, such as apples, pears, peaches, plums, melons, oranges and grapes ... even as you feast on sizzling lamb chops with oregano, or charbroiled hamburgers topped with raw onion and blue cheese, or grilled trout in a tangy paprika-and-dill sauce.

Allowed, also, will be the entire vast array of "above-ground" vegetables, including such salad-favorites as cucumber, lettuce, tomato, pepper and artichoke hearts, along with peas and the rest of the bean family (pinto, navy, string, lima, soy and all their cousins). Add in the squash family, cruciferous vegetables like broccoli, cauliflower and cabbage, just look at the good foods you will eat every day. Don't leave out tomatoes, eggplant or okra either.

As you'll soon discover in these pages, LOSE THE WEIGHT YOU HATE! represents nothing less than a brand-new way of life for those of us who've endured too many years of misery as calorie- and fat-counting failures of the dinner table.

More than anything else, I want my program to be an enjoyable, exciting experience for everyone who decides to take on the challenge of living a healthier, more energetic life.

If you have a weight problem, LOSE THE WEIGHT YOU HATE! is a prescription for a healthy lifestyle that will defeat the chronic disease of obesity.

For that reason, you'll find this book jam-packed with dozens of original, mouth-watering and easy-to-prepare recipes designed to bring out the flavor and the excitement in the many healthy foods that you'll be encouraged to eat. Whether you're digging into an elegant platter of "Poached Salmon with Fiddlehead Ferns," or sinking your steak knife into a choice offering of "Beef Wellington with Goose Pate Sauce," you're going to find that this weight–loss book is very different from all the others you've seen.

And the biggest difference, of course, is that this program actually works!

While following the LOSE THE WEIGHT YOU HATE! program of weight loss and maintenance, you and I are going to "accentuate the positive" ... by cooking and sharing together some of the most savory and pleasing meals you'll ever eat.

We're also going to sit back occasionally and listen to some remarkable stories about some very remarkable people who proved that they were fully up to the task of losing the weight they hated!

2

*I*T'S ALL IN THE GENES!

You've heard it thousands of times before.

It's one of the most repeated—and outrageous—health-myths ever perpetrated on the U.S. Public:

> *Cutting back on calories—and especially calories*
> *from dietary fat—is the key to losing weight!*

Like several other "medical myths," the idea that obesity usually results from ingesting too many fat-grams has become part of the conventional wisdom about dieting and nutrition in recent years.

And yet—for most dieters—it's completely wrong.

As a matter of fact, the latest research *(see Appendix 4)* on weight loss shows convincingly that it has relatively little to do with fat intake ... and even *less* to do with the total number of calories we absorb each day.

Surprising? If you're like most American dieters, you've probably spent a great deal of time listening to (and believing) experts who intoned solemnly about the vital importance of "pushing away from the table," and "eating more slowly," and "being careful to leave something on your plate."

Sorry, but that's very bad advice for most folks who want to lose weight.

Don't believe me? Just take a look at what happens when well-intentioned, powerfully motivated dieters simply cut back on total calories—without thinking about how the different food sources of those calories produce some *very* different effects on fat manufacture and fat storage alike.

According to current medical opinion and the popular press, obesity almost always results from over-eating and lack of exercise. Example: The latest CDC study now blames "suburban living" and "use of the family car" (as opposed to walking) for the rise in obesity! Ask the "academic physicians" to explain today's surging fat epidemic, and they'll quickly start to huff and puff about the dangers of overindulging in the French fries from McDonald's or Burger King ... while stretched out full-length on the sofa watching other people play sports on television, or sitting for hours staring at a computer screen.

At first glance, their approach seems utterly convincing.

Remember when we thought that low-fat diets were the magic bullet that would gun down high cholesterol and heart disease? Back in the good old days of dieting, when our understanding of the dynamics of fat was dictated to us by the anti-cholesterol gurus at the American Heart Association (AHA), nobody dared to question the actual effects of adding corn syrup to "low-fat" foods so as to make them palatable.

And why were the gurus so surprised (given the high volume of sugar in the syrup) when low-fat dieters gained an average of eight pounds per year ... without significantly lowering their cholesterol?

My experience with thousands of successful dieters during the past two decades proves conclusively that the highly vaunted strategy for weight-loss (eat less, exercise more!) provides nothing more than a prescription for losing trivial amounts of weight, followed by a guaranteed and rapid re-gain of most of it within a year.

Let's face it: these universally espoused diets—all built around the concept of less food, more exercise—don't work because they fail to address the *real* cause of obesity in most people, which is genetic programming: genetically controlled insulin levels.

Now, I'm not denying the fact that some people simply eat too much. Nor do I question the medical soundness of that ancient Greek maxim: "Moderation in all things." For those folks with an out-of-control "starch tooth," cutting back on the chocolate cake and the butter-soaked garlic bread certainly makes good sense. As a matter of fact, there are many cases in which the frequent, almost ritualistic consumption of a single food—such as bagels and doughnuts during the office break, or ice cream after supper —becomes the major culprit responsible for weight gain. (If you guzzle the 100 calories in a soft drink three times a day, you can easily put on two pounds a month.)

But the over-eaters actually represent only a small minority of those who suffer from obesity. The truth is that most fat people get that way not because they're weak-willed sad sacks who can't drive past the Dairy Queen, but because their genes (the source of the biological "blueprint" that controls all bodily processes) manage fat digestion and storage in ways that leave them vulnerable to obesity.

In other words: the genes in most overweight people operate in such a way that dietary *starches* are stored with supreme efficiency in fat cells, where they are tucked away for future use. (*Note to the reader*: When you hear me talking about "high-insulin" people cursed with insulin-receptors that don't handle sugar efficiently, think "genetics!")

Skinny people are different genetically; it's that simple.

The ways in which their bodies handle that vitally important energy-compound—glucose—differ markedly from those found in overweight patients. As a result, the skinny types tend to store fewer of the starch grams they take in as fat.

That's the fundamental difference between fat and skinny—and it has much more to do with molecular proteins and hormonal interactions than with will power!

READING THE FUTURE IN YOUR GENES

Whenever I start thinking about the amazing power of genes, I'm reminded of a wise old teacher—Ted Dorman—who had a knack for bringing fancy ideas straight down to earth. A thoughtful philosopher and a shrewd observer of human behavior, Dorman helped me make sense of some tangled concepts in Genetics 101 by asking me a rather blunt question, back in the middle of my courting days.

"Ritchie, nobody can read the future. But have you ever wondered how that good-looking young woman sitting at the next table will look after 30 years of marriage?"

I stared at him. "I have no idea, Ted. How could I possibly determine *that?*"

Ted grinned. "Genetics," he said. "Introduce yourself, and ask to meet her mother. Then remind yourself: Physical features are the phenotype [expression of genes] of the genotype [genetic information].

"In other words, when you meet that good-looking young lady's mother, you'll actually be looking at the younger woman—about 30 years down the road!"

Dorman was right, of course, and his observation applies to weight-problems just as much as it does to physical features. And his insight—when applied to obesity—can help us understand the scientific basis for the no-amylose diet I'm telling you about.

It's All in the Genes!

Let's call it "Dorman's Principle," and let's put it in italics:

Fat on your body is nothing more than the expression of "fat instructions" contained in your genes.

It's true. After more than 20 years of practice as a family physician in Maryland, I can tell you that the vast majority of my obese patients got that way because of their genetic backgrounds—and not because they couldn't tear themselves away from the *All-You-Can-Eat Smorgasbord*. (In other words, their phenotype was simply the result of their genotype.)

Perhaps a fictional example can help us here. Let's take a tall, skinny guy (we'll call him "Stick"), who has an insulin level of 3, and a short, stocky guy ("Fireplug"), with an insulin level of 25.

Now let's weigh them both carefully.

Next step: let's invite both of them to a traditional, all-you-can-eat Chesapeake Bay Fourth of July cookout, where they'll be welcome to partake of tons of Maryland seafood (the steamed crabs are especially appealing) … along with corn on the cob, fried clams, french fries, homemade ice cream and gallons of beer.

Have at it, guys! And they do. And while stuffing himself *way* beyond full, each man takes in the same number of calories.

Next step: 24 hours after the dust has settled and the picnickers have all gone home, let's put Stick and Fireplug back on the scales.

And guess what?

The needle shows that Stick stayed skinny … but Fireplug picked up two pounds!

How can this be true? After all, if obesity obeyed the laws of thermodynamics (ah, but it doesn't), then total calorie consumption would be the only variable that mattered, in terms of weight-gain at the picnic. But since we know that Stick and Fireplug ingested the same number of calories, some other principle must be at work.

Indeed, it is. And that principle is at the heart of the *Lose The Weight You Hate!* approach to dieting. Call it "Shoemaker's Dictum," as follows:

When it comes to gene-based obesity, what matters isn't the number of calories you take in, but the number that get stored.

Is the picture becoming clear? Obviously, Fireplug's genetic programming went right to work on all those Chesapeake goodies he was eating … and it did a highly effective job of storing most of them as fat.

But Stick's genes weren't nearly as effective at processing and storing the calories he ate. As a result, he didn't gain a single ounce.

The dynamics of genetically programmed fat storage can be seen with even more clarity if we feed Stick and Fireplug a typical American breakfast (typically full of *starch*, that is), consisting of two pieces of toast, a stack of pancakes, a heaping order of "hash-browned" potatoes and a couple of scrambled eggs.

Next step: Once the skinny guy and the chubby guy have downed this hefty breakfast, let's send them off to *another* seafood feast.

Once again, the genes that control insulin's ability to move molecules of sugar into cells will prove decisive. Twenty-four hours after ingesting his "All-American Breakfast," before the seafood bash, the skinny Stick has gained no additional weight, because his body burned the sugar and amylose efficiently. And Fireplug? All too predictably, the amylose contained in his super-sugary meal set off a steep rise in blood sugar … leading to maximum fat storage and a net gain of more than one pound—on top of the two pounds he'd picked up from his later seafood gluttony. He will likely lose the temporarily gained weight, but if he keeps eating the forbidden amylose, the temporary weight gain isn't temporary any longer.

The bottom line here is quite simple: If you eat amylose before ingesting other foods (such as the crabs and the beer at that feast), you wind up gaining even more weight than you would have gained without first taking in this fat-triggering starch.

In other words, if your genes prevent your body from rapidly burning blood sugar (as in the case of Fireplug) and you eat a lot of starch, you're going to be overweight—and you will not be able to shed the flab and keep it off, no matter how hard you try. Even worse, if you eat starch before downing food that is "allowed" to you in a diet, your fat-storage mechanisms will have kicked into high gear before the first bite of Silver Queen sweet corn has vanished down your gullet.

No discussion of obesity and dieting should exclude the key significance of the brain's hunger and satiety center—the hypothalamus—and the way in which it so powerfully influences how much we eat.

Indeed, the often overlooked hypothalamus actually provides the basis for the huge U.S. "appetite-suppressant" industry, while also looming as the organic source of the "binge" eating behavior that torments so many obese Americans today.

BEWARE THE "YO-YO DIET!"

The Saga of Stick and Fireplug underscores the key strategy of this entire book, which is to teach you how to use your knowledge about "fat genes" and other interacting fat-storage variables as your major weapons in the battle against obesity.

Make no mistake, however: The genes come first. And the growing importance of genes in health care can be seen in all those recent, front-page stories about the "Human Genome Project"—a vast, international research effort which only a few months ago successfully produced the first-ever "map" of our genes. That map was a huge step forward for medicine, of course, because it will allow science to begin targeting—and then manipulating—genetic defects that contribute to disease.

Decoding the Genome promises to revolutionize our understanding of medicine, because it will allow us to actually change such flawed genetic instructions as those which trigger unhealthy obesity in human beings. Change the instruction and you change the *expression*, right? Now all we need is an effective method for repairing defective genes (by excising the flawed segments and splicing in healthy nucleotide sequences), and *voila!*, no more obesity problem!

Unfortunately, it's not quite that simple, however. To understand why we probably won't ever be able to "engineer skinny people" (if we even wanted to), let's back up a few steps … by reminding ourselves of the thoroughly interesting fact that *biology isn't physics*.

If you remember your Physics 101, you probably remember a fundamental principle: "For every action, there will be an equal and opposite reaction." But that old saw doesn't hold true in biology. In this much more complicated world, you get an entire cascade of reactions—and a cascade that quickly triggers an endless *series* of biochemical reactions and counter-reactions.

Although the biochemistry of fat storage isn't terribly difficult to understand, the blunt fact remains that many doctors haven't bothered to study it. And because they're not really familiar with the physiology involved in converting amylose and glucose to fatty acids, they often tend to simplify their approach to dieting by telling patients: "Just don't eat as much, and be sure to get plenty of exercise!"

All too often, that advice simply means that the dieter will go on to lose protein (the source of "lean body mass"), along with the hated fat. And what happens next? In most situations, the dieter will quickly regain that lean mass, as his or her body predictably responds to what it perceives as a life-threatening nutritional deficit.

The bottom-line result?

I call it the "Yo-Yo Diet"—an excruciatingly frustrating state of affairs in which the half-starved victim endures endless days of low-energy hunger ... only to watch his or her weight-loss gains evaporate within a few months, as lean body mass reasserts itself and the needle on the bathroom scale starts to soar again.

The problem with yo-yo dieting is that it so often leads to reduced self-esteem, and even to outright depression, as the disappointed dieter teeters on the edge of giving up the struggle against fat entirely. And to make matters even worse, riding that Perpetual Yo-Yo *also* sets you up for a host of physical health problems ... including such nasty conditions as reflux esophagitis, constipation, dry skin, and constant fatigue.

Who needs the misery of the yo-yo?

But my no-amylose diet works differently. Instead of asking the weight-loss candidate to cut back across-the-board on calories (a strategy that will soon trigger the yo-yo), I focus on those calories that are *stored most efficiently.*

Example: While some folks who eat 100 calories of a complex carbohydrate (whole wheat bread, let's say) will eventually store 90 of them as fat, others will end up with only 50 of those calories preserved inside fat cells.

And what happened to the missing calories, among this group of physiologically blessed carbo-eaters?

It's simple. Those calories were burned as energy in muscles, or perhaps converted to life sustaining glycogen reserves in the cells. (Or maybe they weren't absorbed at all, and wound being fermented by bacteria in the large bowel.)

So how can we help the *un*-lucky eaters—the ones whose body-chemistry turns out to be so highly efficient at converting the amylose to fat?

Once again, the concept is simple. We're going to turn off that storage mechanism ... by sharply limiting our intake of foods that are most readily stored as fat.

In other words: Instead of asking dieters to slash their calorie-intake overnight (an impossible quest, if you think about it), the Shoemaker Diet merely asks them to cut back on those fat-triggering foods which have what we call the "High Glycemic Index."

The good news for those who embrace my *Lose The Weight You Hate!* Approach to dieting is that tight control of these "starchy" foods (think bread, pasta, cereal) is relatively easy to accomplish. And once you've got a handle on your "high-glycemic" intake, you can eat your way to a healthier, slimmed-down life—without counting calories or measuring out portions or calculating fat grams day in and day out.

So how does the human body store fat, exactly, and why is this process so important to your own struggle against obesity?

The first step on the road to understanding the process of fat storage is to identify the key hormone—insulin—that regulates the management of glucose in the human bloodstream.

Next step: Let's remember our genetics lesson from a few pages above. If you're like millions of Americans today and struggle with "high insulin" because of your genetic makeup, you're going to find it almost impossible to avoid becoming overweight. Why? Because the insulin resistance that triggers your over-production of this key hormone will *also* prevent your body from "burning off" glucose ... which will then be converted to fat. (If you don't think that obesity is "all in the genes," ask yourself this amusing question from comedian Jerry Clower: "Did ya ever see a *mule* win the Kentucky Derby?")

So how does the process of fat storage actually work? Simply put, insulin operates as a pick-up and delivery system (think UPS or FedEx) that moves sugar molecules from the blood and then transports them to muscle or liver cells where they can be burned for energy or stored in glycogen for later use.

In most cases, the "FedEx delivery" of these sugar particles occurs at the outer wall (membrane) of a liver or muscle cell, where glucose-entry takes place. To picture the process clearly, imagine the FedEx man arriving at the membrane, then handing the "package" to a clerk—known as the "insulin receptor," whose job is to carry it through the membrane and into the cell.

Once inside, the glucose molecule is quickly converted into the human form of starch, known as "glycogen." This complex carbohydrate consists of many glucose molecules bonded together, and it serves as a kind of energy warehouse that can be broken down later, whenever the body requires a burst of energy.

As an aside, it should be noted that cellulose, manufactured by some plants, is a *different* type of "sugar warehouse," but the basic structure of plant starches—contained in amylose and cellulose—is almost exactly the same as that found in glycogen. The point is that in this case, clever Mother Nature simply linked the particular glucose molecules together a little differently. So be careful when you use the term "complex carbohydrate"—because glycogen, amylose and cellulose are all complex carbohydrates but are handled by the body *very* differently.

A key step in the process of sugar-digestion begins whenever a cell needs to burn sugar for fuel. When that happens, a group of specialized enzymes is dispatched (according to gene-regulated instructions) to break down the glycogen in the warehouse, thus converting it back to usable glucose. By keeping sugar carefully and precisely stored inside the cell, the body's metabolic machinery avoids the danger of being gummed up by free-flowing glucose, and thus maintains its efficiency.

Remember: glycogen supplies are controlled and managed genetically, and most people have anywhere from three to four pounds of the stuff (about 6,000 calories' worth) floating around in the cells of their bodies at any one time. Remember, also, that when these cellular glycogen-stores are saturated, they cannot absorb any more sugar. The surplus remains in the bloodstream. At this point, the "FedEx clerk" closes his window, and additional sugar will not be taken into the cell until some available glycogen has been burned, freeing up room for storage of the newly delivered glucose.

Don't try to describe this proven scenario to the "carbohydrate loaders," however, or those who believe in high-amylose diets—because they will not accept the scientifically demonstrated truth!

So what happens when the cells are sugar-saturated in this way … and then a new FedEx package is suddenly dispatched from the digestive system to the glucose-management system?

In that situation, the resourceful human body turns to a second sugar-storage process entirely, in order to prevent excess sugar from lingering in the bloodstream (the condition known medically as "diabetes").

What happens in this back-up system is that insulin now begins to stimulate special cells in the liver to break the glucose down and convert it into smaller molecular fragments—which are then linked together to form the long, straight chains that make up the "fatty acids."

Next step: the ever-resourceful FedEx insulin-delivery system goes to work to move the fatty acids into already existing fat cells, where they can be stored for future use, if ever needed. To use the medical terminology involved: the insulin now "binds to a receptor on a fat cell."

Once this occurs, and the insulin is "bound," the glucose and fatty acids that have been captured by the fat cell remains unavailable for mobilization back into the bloodstream for up to eight hours—as opposed to what happens in liver and muscle cells, where the period of insulin-binding is quite brief. But what if you aren't eating and you need a sudden burst of energy to mow the lawn, or study for a geometry final, or battle an opponent in a mid-summer tennis match?

Answer: No problem. You will burn some of the relatively few calories you have stored in glycogen. Don't forget that the body attempts to resupply the glycogen reserves or else the cell dies. Glycogen stores are controlled genetically. In that situation, the liver quickly reaches for its genetically controlled lean body mass (protein) and breaks it down into amino acids. The result is instant sugar that has been converted from amino acids in the wink of an eye. Unfortunately for the dieter, however, this process (gluconeogenesis) creates a protein-deficit that is guaranteed to be made up automatically, as soon as the miserable yo-yo weight-loss patient returns to normal eating habits. Protein stores never forget a debt.

Based on these physiological realities, then, the strategy for avoiding both excessive fat storage *and* protein-burning becomes simple enough: to lose weight and keep it off, you need to avoid those foods that will make your blood sugar rise quickly. In this way, you will prevent the insulin surge that always occurs with a rise in blood sugar … which means that you'll also prevent the rapid saturation of glycogen stores in cells *and* the resulting transformation of glucose into fatty acids. At the same time, you will prevent protein-burning by permitting fat cells to re-supply sugar whenever necessary.

How effective is the Shoemaker approach at interrupting the body's genetically programmed fat-management system—and thus helping the dieter to shed fat and keep it off? To answer that question, I always refer patients to my carefully maintained patient follow-up records … which show that 70 percent of those who lose 30 pounds or more on my diet will not gain back *a single pound* during the following year! The bottom line for a successful weight loss program is the maintenance rate at one-year follow-up.

WELCOME TO THE NO-AMYLOSE APPROACH

In order to understand the crucial importance of "strategic eating" (rather than merely counting calories) to achieve weight loss and maintenance, let's take a quick look at what actually happens to dieters who follow the conventional dieting wisdom so often dispensed by the news media.

According to the universally applauded weight-loss gurus, the ideal dieting breakfast might include such predictable fare as a whole wheat bagel smothered in low-fat cream cheese. Spread *butter* on that toasted bagel, says the CDW (Conventional Dieting Wisdom), and you can expect to be dead by nightfall from cholesterol-buildup or a massive fat attack.

Along with the bagel, of course, you will be encouraged to drink a big glass of unsweetened orange juice. *(Lots of Vitamin C and dietary fiber, hurray, hurray!)*

Sounds like a healthy, energy-packed breakfast so low on calories and fat that it's sure to give your diet a major-league boost, right?

Wrong. The flour in that bagel consists mainly of ground-up wheat seeds. These seeds contain lots of wheat germ, wheat bran and wheat starch (aka amylose), which is actually a storage-form of glucose ideally suited to the germinating wheat plant.

Too bad that the same amylose is *not* so well suited to human beings, most of whom will experience a rapid surge in blood sugar within minutes of ingesting it!

The surge takes place after our saliva mixes with the flour. When that happens, an important enzyme known as *amylase* quickly begins converting the *amylose* into its individual glucose building-blocks—so that it can be quickly stored in the cells as glycogen, or converted into fatty acids and steered toward fat cells for storage.

Highly efficient, the amylase does its work well, and your blood sugar is rising before the bagel even hits your stomach. To obtain a blood-sugar boost this rapid and powerful without the bagel, in fact, you'd have to swallow an entire tablespoonful of pure table sugar—since the two substances have the same Glycemic Index: 100.

The point here is that amylose provides a tremendous stimulus for insulin secretion—especially for those of us cursed with genes that direct us to digest amylose rapidly in saliva, only to then store it more slowly in liver and muscle cells.

So much for the wheat in the bagel. But what about that low-fat cream cheese? Take a close look at the label, and you'll discover that in most cases, the excised dairy fat was replaced by corn syrup … which turns out to be one of the most potent blood-sugar elevators in the entire kingdom of food!

By the time that ersatz cream cheese hits your stomach, you can be sure that your blood sugar-level is already crashing through the roof … and your insulin output is surging like Niagara.

As for that "unsweetened" orange juice … did you know that in most cases, the producers add glucose at the canning factory in order to sweeten the taste? Go ahead: squeeze a fresh orange and sample the sweetness. Now break out a commercial orange juice product … and ask your grade school-aged child to tell you which one contains less sugar, if you aren't able to make that determination for yourself.

You might also want to ask yourself: How does a diabetic usually respond to a low-sugar reaction? Answer: He or she quickly downs a pint of orange juice! Since fructose—the natural form of sugar found in oranges and other fruits—does not raise blood sugar levels rapidly, the quick boost has to come from factory-added glucose.

The key insight here is that not all carbohydrates produce the same effect.

But let's get back to that breakfast table. At this point, after your early repast of bagel-and-OJ, both sugar and insulin levels are surging. Responding, your body has begun to store starch calories as fat with maximum efficiency. At the same time, that insulin is turning on a group of enzymes in the intestine—the disacchari-dases—that specialize in digesting sugars such as sucrose, lactose, galactose and maltose.

This cascade of insulin effects (and there are any more of them)

35

is activated by any rapid rise in blood sugar. And we should note that these insulin responses are *not* related to the calories taken in; instead, they are controlled by the different effects produced by various foods on levels of blood sugar. This fact explains why we call insulin "the hormone of the fed state," and there's no doubt that it manages the storage of both sugar and fat with supreme efficiency. Insulin also affects protein metabolism, but indirectly, based on what is happening with glycogen and fatty acids.

To sum up the most important point in a few words: The impact of insulin on dietary protein is affected far more by what gets eaten *with* the protein than by the amount consumed.

When insulin is released rapidly—following a sudden rise in blood sugar—the level of sugar in the blood will soon begin to fall. Because human physiology depends on a complex system of checks and balances, the body cannot allow insulin to have free rein during digestion … and indeed, the activity of this key hormone is carefully controlled by counter-regulatory hormones that are operating at every moment to assure a chemical balance throughout the system.

One of those counter-regulatory hormones, glucagon, is manufactured in the pancreas by specialized cells operating near the Islets of Langerhans—the better-known pancreatic cells that make insulin.

Glucagon's major assignment is to trigger a quick rise in blood sugar—a step that opposes insulin by mobilizing sugar stores in liver and fat cells, along with stimulating the breakdown of protein. Rising glucagon levels often make diners feel "fuzzy," and perhaps even a bit nauseated. Anyone who's been given an injection of glucagon in order to dry up intestinal secretions during a gastrointestinal procedure (such as a colonoscopy) will remember what a "glucagon rush" feels like.

Another important glucose-elevator is epinephrine—aka as the "adrenalin" that plays such a major role in the "flight or fight" stress mechanism. Epinephrine accelerates blood flow and increases the heart-rate (sometimes erratically), while also triggering bouts of perspiration.

A third group of counter-regulators includes the steroid hormones, or glucocorticoids, such as cortisone. The adrenal gland is the source of much of our epinephrine and all of our glucocorticoids.

The physiology of these biochemical cascades is staggeringly complex ... but the major result is easy to describe. When these counter-regulatory hormones begin to mingle—and to trigger their *own* unfolding cascades—you can be sure that blood sugar will start to rise. Yet the human symptoms of the cascades seem far removed from the "sudden energy burst" associated with glucose-intake. In most cases, those symptoms leave patients feeling weak, woozy and wobbly, while also suffering from headaches, sweats, uneasiness, palpitations and nausea. And yet those symptoms are often misdiagnosed as hypoglycemia.

Question: What really causes the sleepiness and sluggishness that attacks you about an hour after that ten o'clock bagel?

Answer: The "sugar rush," of course. And what makes you feel so hungry again, usually within a few minutes of the rush? In most cases, that second round of hunger pangs is the work of the counter-regulatory team of sugar-elevators. Is it any wonder that most of us end up dozing in our chairs—after that yearly Thanksgiving dinner in which the turkey arrives surrounded by mashed potatoes, bread, stuffing, pumpkin pie (don't blame the pumpkin, it's the sugar, corn syrup and crust!) and banana pudding?

In a later chapter, I'm going to introduce you to yet another layer of "hunger control"—two specialized areas that regulate our feelings of hunger and satiety, located in the master neuro-endocrine gland of the brain, the hypothalamus.

At this point, however, all we need to understand is that rising blood sugar activates the satiety center in the ventral-medial section of the gland—whereas *falling* blood sugar activates its sidekick (the hunger center) in the ventral-lateral part of the same organ.

In recent years, a great deal of research has been performed on the bio-chemicals that turn off the hunger center and turn *on* the satiety center, and maybe some day will see physicians using these potentially helpful chemicals as therapeutic agents for obesity. But the good news is you don't have to earn a Ph.D. in chemistry in order to lose weight!

Rather than spending five years in the library examining the research, simply observe the following ultra-simple rule:

Don't eat foods that make your blood sugar rise quickly!

In other words, don't open the Pandora's Box of insulin responses by devouring that side-dish of spaghetti, or the pile of rice they just heaped on your plate ... or the freshly baked herb bread that looks as if it will surely melt in your mouth.

And it does, just as surely as amylose is quickly broken down to sugar.

EXERCISE AFTER HIGH-GLYCEMIC MEALS

So much for your "healthy" breakfast!

And now, at the risk of over-squashing the bagel-with-low-fat-cream-cheese-and-OJ-breakfast, I want to lay the "exercise myth" to rest—and quickly.

Ask yourself: What really happens when you bang out the push-ups or jog around the track? The answer, of course, is that your cell-stored glycogen begins to become depleted. How will you replenish it?

Since your fat stores are being protected by the insulin locked on your fat cell receptors, your body must resort to its protein supply, or lean body mass. And the result, known as "protein wasting," only guarantees that the lost lean body mass will have to be made up later, when you regain all those shed pounds.

And there's more. As you lose protein, several other negative scenarios begin to unfold. You feel exhausted, for starters. Your skin sags and hair goes dry and stringy. Your stomach sours and your increasing irritability encourages you to eat more than ever.

Unfortunately, you can't solve these problems simply by doing more exercise.

But many of my patients are convinced that working out more often is the key to successful weight-loss. Many of them work very hard at squeezing in an hour of "exercise time" right after breakfast, and before work. Or maybe they'll try to compress the workout into the lunch hour, after gulping down a turkey sandwich. Their philosophy is to "break a sweat and get that heart rate up —just in time for a quick shower and then back to work."

Sorry, but these mini-workouts simply aren't enough to keep the flab off.

Which is why I so often find myself counseling patients who wail in despair: "Doctor … I work out every day—but I just don't lose any weight. My trainer always says, 'Muscle weighs more than fat … you're just picking up more muscle!'"

Wrong. When it comes to weight control, only one equation matters: "One pound equals one pound!"

Then the patient moans: "But I always feel so *tired*. I'm getting more discouraged by the day!"

What's really happening here? It's simple. These frustrated patients are simply learning a basic nutritional fact: The consumption of amylose by *untrained* athletes will lead inevitably to protein-burning and re-gaining of lost weight.

Of course, it's also true that heavy exercise in excess of 12 hours per week—at 250 calories per hour (not just a slow "jog, mind you!")—can improve "insulin affinity" and reduce insulin resistance. And that's precisely why highly conditioned marathon runners can get away with eating bowls of pasta on the night before a 26-mile race.

But most of my patients don't have 12 hours extra per *month* to spend on exercise, let alone 12 per week. Yet it takes only a few hours to learn how to make my no-amylose diet work for you—as a successful lifestyle that will help you get rid of the weight you hate and keep it off, even as you enjoy good food that's attractively prepared and served with style.

All right, then: Time for 30-second chapter review.

Question: What's the secret to avoiding obesity?

Answer: Having low-insulin genes in your parents.

Question: For the rest of us, what's the secret to burning fat and then keeping it off?

Correct answer: The secret is to avoid burning off your protein stores by preventing amylose- and glucose-triggered surges in blood sugar.

In the next few chapters, you're going to discover that you can enjoy your mealtimes—while munching happily on dozens of different foods—without consuming the few kinds of sugars that will send your fatty acid stores through the roof and cause your weight to soar.

Welcome to the Shoemaker Approach To Dieting—a strategic plan for controlling the biochemical dynamics of dieting, even as you celebrate the joys of the dinner table.

Quick Example: Take a look at my savory, dill-scented recipe for "Beef Wellington" *(see the Recipe section in the back of the book)*, and then grab your apron for some *real* fun!

_G_ETTING BEHIND
THE GLYCEMIC INDEX

Who says the "biochemistry of fat storage" can't be dramatic and exciting?

Example: From out of the blue, just the other day, came a report in the Washington Post on the arcane and abstruse subject of ... fat storage!

Scientists have discovered a hormone that may explain the link between diabetes and obesity—a tantalizing finding that could someday lead to new treatments for the disease. Dubbed "resistin," the hormone is produced by fat cells and prompts tissues to resist insulin, the substance the body needs to process blood sugar. ...

When I read this front-page story—back in January of 2001— I nearly broke into a round of exuberant applause, myself. _Way to go, researchers!_ Why was I so pleased by the recent discovery of this "fat storage hormone" ... after a series of experiments in which scientists isolated the key substance while feeding sugar to mice?

Answer: I was delighted to hear the news about resistin because this scientific breakthrough underlines the results of my own recent research into the biochemistry of diabetes and obesity. During more than two decades of helping overweight people shed their flab and *keep* it shed, I've spent hundreds of hours studying the complex chemical interactions that that take place whenever the human body creates and stores fat.

The bottom line of my research dovetails nicely with the recent news about the discovery of resistin, including this key conclusion: *Mice given resistin were not able to process blood sugar as well as those that were not given the hormone.*

Described by the scientists who found it as "part of the missing link between obesity and diabetes," resistin now appears to be a key factor in the complicated—and genetically programmed—process by which insulin resistance prevents the swift and efficient transportation of glucose into muscle and liver cells, where it can be quickly burned off.

As I noted in the last chapter, insulin resistance is also the major culprit responsible for the rapid rise of blood sugar in people who unwisely load up on food starches such as bread, pasta and potatoes.

The new research on resistin seems highly promising because "defeating resistin" would possibly mean an end to insulin resistance, but practical application is years away. On the other hand, my tried-and-proven no-amylose diet provides an effective method—right here and now—for losing weight and keeping it off.

So let's turn away from the complicated chemistry for a while, and instead focus on the practical aspects of our rapidly expanding knowledge of fat manufacture and storage.

In other words, let's take a closer look at the guiding principle of LOSE THE WEIGHT YOU HATE!, which tells us: "It's not the number of calories you eat that counts—but the number of calories that get *stored*."

GETTING TO KNOW THE GLYCEMIC INDEX

Originally devised back in the 1950s as a method for helping to control the sugar-intake of diabetics, the Glycemic Index (GI) is a compilation of the effects of given foods on the rate of blood-sugar elevation in human beings.

Knowing the "rate of rise" is essential to managing fat-storage, of course, because the rate determines the insulin response ... which then determines how quickly (and efficiently) free fatty acids will be manufactured and how quickly the fat cell insulin-receptors will be saturated.

There's no doubt that the Index provides diabetics and weight-watchers with a powerful tool for monitoring the foods they eat, in order to gain pinpoint control over the process of fat formation and storage. So why hasn't this nifty system become part of our everyday nutritional vocabulary in America? And why did we all wind up talking so obsessively about "low fat" as the winning strategy for ditching our extra pounds and living leaner, healthier lifestyles, instead of focusing on the intricacies of the Glycemic Index?

Unfortunately for those of us with weight-control problems, the GI fell victim to what scientists call "incomparable results." That happened because some of the scientists who studied the GI asked their subjects to fast before testing, while others didn't. In addition, some of the subjects involved were struggling with diabetes, while others remained free of this increasingly common blood-sugar ailment. To complicate matters even further, some studies of the Glycemic Index focused on trained athletes, and some scrutinized the physiology of overweight, out-of-shape patients. Nor were male-female ratios consistently maintained in these various studies.

Is it any surprise—given all of these incomparable methods and incomparable results—that the American Diabetes Association (ADA) has chosen not to endorse the use of the Index?

Regardless of this unfortunate development, however, there's simply no doubt that the GI provides a valuable tool for measuring the impact of different foods on fat manufacture and storage.

Although many of the studies involved dissimilar methods (apples and oranges, instead of all apples), their findings remain reproducibly clear. And the key insight toward which they point now seems evident beyond a reasonable doubt.

That insight is the basis for the diet that I want you to use. It tells us that the rate of rise of blood sugar is highest for foods containing glucose ... or foods containing compounds that are quickly broken down into glucose. Those foods include certain identified plant starches, each one of which is loaded with the complex carbohydrate, amylose.

Let me be very clear: Not all starchy vegetables contain amylose. Lima beans and butternut squash are full of starches, for example, but amylose isn't among them.

The good news for dieters is that learning which foods contain this fat-triggering substance—and which ones *don't*—couldn't be simpler. (All you have to do is jump ahead a few paragraphs and look at my list of "No Mores.")

Mastering the list of "off-limits" foods is crucial—because research shows that there's no significant difference between glucose foods and amylose foods, in terms of their effect on fat storage. The bottom line is that restricting the intake of these two types of food will eliminate the inevitable "insulin protection" of fat stores that occurs with every surge of blood sugar.

But what does my GI-based approach to controlling fat storage actually require of those dieters who embrace it?

Simple. In order to dump their hated fat, they need to avoid high-Index foods.

In other words, they need to make up a list of "No Mores"— of foods they will carefully avoid during the weight-loss (as opposed to maintenance) portion of the no-amylose regimen.

THE "NO MORES": A COMPREHENSIVE LIST

In order to fend off insulin-resistance via soaring blood sugar, dieters should agree to eat:

- O No more roots or tubers, including white and sweet potatoes, beets or any other vegetables that grow beneath the surface of the earth (and yes, the list *does* include those two traditional favorites that dieters once depended on: carrots and peanuts, both of which will make you fat!);

- O No more bananas (the only fruit that's restricted);

- O No more products made from wheat, rice, oats, barley and rye.

- O No more foods laced with added sugar, sucrose, corn syrup or malto-dextrins (aka "fake sugar").

If this list of "No Mores" sounds too broad and sweeping to manage successfully (and I can hear many of you crying out in pain: "How can I live without *pasta*?"), don't despair. Wait until you read the long list of foods that you *will* be allowed to enjoy on *your new* diet!

Meanwhile, here's some more good news for those of you who were afraid that you'd be asked to starve yourselves on this diet. Under the Shoemaker Regimen, you'll be permitted to eat all the fruits, protein and above-ground vegetables that you want.

In addition, the LOSE THE WEIGHT YOU HATE! system frees you from ever having to count calories again. Nor will you be asked to measure fat grams or haggle over portion-sizes. (Although I do recommend that if you can *see* the fat on a piece of steak or on a lamb chop, don't eat it.) Under the rules of this diet, all you have to do is sit down at the table and start eating—as much as you want, whenever you want, provided that you do not gorge endlessly on the "safe" foods.

During 20 years of helping people lose weight, by the way, I've rarely encountered a patient who abused the "all you want" provision of this diet. And why would they? In most cases, eating medium-sized standard portions of the allowed foods will keep your hunger safely at bay.

Now, if you're like most of the thousands of folks I've counseled over the years, you're probably asking yourself at this very moment: *Wait a minute ... how can this be true? How can I eat all I want ... on a diet?*

Let me ease your anxiety and soothe your troubled mind.

Remember, please, the key principle we elucidated together in the last chapter—the principle that says most fat comes from storage of starch calories. Eliminate the amylose and *presto!*, you've eliminated most of the calories that turn into free fatty acids and later into cell-stored fat.

Common-sense question: Does eliminating the amylose in your diet mean that you're free to gorge on ten pounds of lima beans each day?

Common-sense answer: Of course not. If you're eating compulsively—and eating huge quantities of *anything*—you won't be able to lose weight, or to keep it off. Let common sense be your guide, and don't abuse your right to "eat all you want" of the no-amylose foods! Be honest with yourself, too. Losing weight does involve saying no.

Remember, also, that "fat counts." It's not the crucial factor in determining obesity ... but there's no denying that eating large quantities of the stuff will wreck any diet. Solution: If you can see the fat clinging to the edges of a steak (or clinging to *any* fried food), don't eat it.

READY FOR CHEMISTRY 101?

In order to understand why this diet is so effective, let's take a quick look at the biochemistry involved in converting amylose to sugar and then storing it as fat.

Let's start by dragging out that familiar term from your high school Chem textbook: "carbohydrate."

Simply defined, a carbohydrate is a chemical compound that includes carbon, hydrogen and oxygen. In fact, sugars such as glucose and sucrose and fructose are actually nothing more than molecules of carbohydrate arranged in a ring structure. (Remember, also, that modifications of that structure are what produce related compounds such as the sugar alcohols—mannitol, sorbitol and xylol, for example—and the syrups.)

Next step: Do you remember how that chemistry teacher in the 11th grade pointed out that "many simple sugars have six carbons?" If so, you may also recall that the most important of these simple sugars are galactose, fructose and glucose ... and that there are some other six-carbon sugars (and even a few of the five-carbon variety), as well.

So far, so good. But what happens if we start putting the sugars, themselves, together? Answer: If we link two simple sugars together, we come up with a disaccharide—such as sucrose, lactose and maltose. But we can also form chains of three sugars. Once we reach four sugars and beyond, however, our definition changes; we now call the resulting compound a "complex carbohydrate." (And don't forget that the complex carbohydrates we're most concerned about are glycogen, amylose and cellulose.)

So much for the basic chemical building-blocks involved in fat production.

To understand exactly how they work in concert to make people heftier than they want to be, let's step back and think about what goes on in the human body when you eat a tuna fish sandwich, or a slice of key lime pie.

Remember: The human body does not metabolize all complex carbohydrates in the same way. Example: The plant starch known as amylose is digested in a series of complicated steps that begin when a saliva-borne enzyme—amylase—begins to convert this complex sugar to glucose, even as you chew the amylose-bearing food (a slice of bread, maybe, or a ripe banana), prior to swallowing it.

But another complex carbohydrate (beloved of rabbits, by the way) isn't digested by humans at all. We call this substance "cellulose," and you can find tons of it in such green vegetables as lettuce. Because the human digestive system lacks the necessary enzyme—cellulase—we cannot process the sugar locked up in lettuce, cucumbers and celery, and we could in theory eat them all day long without ever gaining a single ounce.

Feed those same greens to a rabbit, however, and the animal will soon experience a sugar rush, then rapidly grow plump. That's because the rabbit's digestive system contains the cellulase necessary to handle the task of converting the cellulose back to good old glucose, where it soon becomes available for fat manufacture and storage.

All of this makes good sense, if you think about it. Because humans don't make cellulase, the Glycemic Index rating for cellulose-based foods remains very low. But since we *do* manufacture amylase and use it efficiently, the same GI rating for amylose-containing foods such as bread and pasta turns out to be quite high.

Fortunately for all of us, fruit sugar (fructose) and milk sugar (lactose) do not enjoy high GI ratings ... which means that, essentially, we can eat all we want of these foods. (Milk fat remains a secondary problem, however, so I'm not going to recommend unlimited dairy products.)

Next point: Although fructose doesn't provide a great deal of readily available sugar for energy, it can be converted to more useful glucose inside a cell. The process of converting fructose to glucose, and then back to fructose, in a cell takes place in a series of steps we call the "Futile Cycle." Along with releasing heat during each of those interconversions of simple sugars, the Futile Cycle also serves to regulate glucose levels within cells. (Remember how hot you get, right after eating a big meal? The heat spreads throughout your body as the Futile Cycle mops up those billions of excess glucose molecules).

For a quick look at how dieters can manipulate a much more important mechanism of heat production as yet another strategy in the war against obesity, see Chapter 13, which describes an exciting new drug, Avandia, and also explains how it can play a major role in slowing down the Biochemistry of Brown Fat.

As an aside, every time I hear a diet "expert" babble on about calories I think of a basic concept of science: Biology is not physics. The concepts in physics called thermodynamics just don't apply to calories. Just look what you have already learned about the different effects of the types of calories on their fate in the body. Now factor in heat production. Even if a calorie eaten meant a calorie stored, what happens when heat is released? While energy is not created or destroyed by our metabolism, what happens when we waste fuel in the form of heat? How does that affect our weight? Add one more confounder (there are many others, of course) to the nearly dead thermodynamic argument to blow it away once and for all. That confounder is gas, intestinal gas. How does that natural process occur *(see fiber, Chapter 15)*? Any sugar that isn't absorbed by the time it reaches the large bowel will be fermented, feeding the bacteria that live there. Calories in means calories out!

Because glycogen stores are controlled genetically (and also because there are many sugar and insulin receptors along the cell membrane), human cells must have a way of disposing of excess glucose, whenever large amounts of it are ingested during a meal. Of course, this process works with marked efficiency in those nutritionally lucky human beings whom we describe as "skinny." If you think about it, you'll soon realize that the extra layer of fat in a high–insulin patient serves an effective heat-insulator ... and an insulator that genetically skinny patients do *not* have.

Although the relevant studies are so far incomplete, the early evidence clearly suggests that the Futile Cycle is far more efficient among skinny patients than among the Fireplug-types. We can speculate how efficient storage of starch as fat might have helped our stocky ancestors survive times of nutritional deprivation in cold climates. The skinny, Futile Cycle using, glucose-wasting ancestor might have been better adapted for survival in warmer climates where food would likely be available year round.

To understand how the parts all fit together, take a quick look at the Sample Glycemic Index table *(Appendix 2)*. Notice anything that stands out? Well, for one thing, it's pretty obvious that the high-GI foods are either derived from plant seeds (wheat, for example, or rice, or oats, or barley, or rye) ... and also from vegetables that share a single defining characteristic: they all grow underground. Of course, bananas also contain lots of amylose, and thus earn a high GI rating.

The only exceptions here are corn and sorghum. But we don't have to worry about corn ... because although this supremely ubiquitous vegetable contains plenty of amylose, each kernel also houses a substance that serves as a natural inhibitor of amylase. The result is that corn doesn't rank very high on the GI list, because the inhibitor prevents rapid breakdown of corn amylose in humans.

SHOOTING DOWN THE "FOOD PYRAMID"

The research data that support this theory of fat storage are indisputable. Still, some people remain unconvinced—and troubled by some of the myths about "good nutrition" that they've absorbed over the years.

Example: Although most of my thousands of patients have had little trouble understanding—or accepting—the biochemistry of my no-amylose diet, many have found themselves fretting over the idea that they will be required to live without some of the "major food groups" contained in the U.S. Food and Drug Administration's famed "Food Pyramid."

The goal of the sacred Pyramid, you undoubtedly recall, is to make certain that consumers lower cholesterol (by reducing fat intake), while also achieving Nutritional Nirvana by wolfing down anywhere from six to eleven servings of complex carbohydrates each and every day.

Sorry ... but the Pyramid should be turned on its point immediately, because it's simply bad advice for millions of Americans (including me) who would gain 15–20 new pounds each year, if they downed all those servings of glucose and amylose!

Another frequent question from my patients focuses on vitamins, as they wonder out loud: "If I do manage to avoid the high-Glycemic Index foods, Dr. Shoemaker, won't I become vitamin-deficient?" The answer is "no," of course ... but I never object when they insist on taking extra vitamins. An over-the-counter, inexpensive vitamin is fine.

CONCLUSION: SIMPLICITY WORKS!

The best part of your new diet is that fact that it's so simple and easy to implement.

In order to lose the weight you hate, simply avoid rapid rises in blood sugar and blood insulin by avoiding glucose and amylose. Once you begin fending off those regular insulin surges, you'll discover that your body won't store starch calories efficiently as fat.

Be warned, however: The human metabolism never "forgets" how to store fat! As some of my patients who failed at maintenance soon discovered, the body will quickly rediscover its penchant for transforming starch calories to fat, should a successful dieter resume the habit of loading up on glucose and amylose at every meal.

Let me say it one more time: You new diet is a "lifestyle"—a program for maintaining your weight loss far into the future, by sticking to the rules of maintenance!

Let's face it: Many overweight patients are genetically programmed to struggle day in and day out with elevated insulin levels. These folks are all but certain to store their starches as fat—and to burn off protein whenever they attempt to lose weight by cutting back on food (and especially on fat).

Question for the scientists: Are all of these obese, non-diabetic patients also insulin-resistant?

Answer for the scientists: As we've seen in these first few chapters, their liver and muscle cells certainly are ... but their fat cells are *not*. (Otherwise, patients with high insulin levels would always exhibit low levels of blood sugar—a condition known as "hypoglycemia.")

Fair enough. But what are the actual *steps* involved in losing excess weight and then keeping it off? What do you have to do to get started on the diet, with fact as your ally and fear of dieting failure as just a bad memory?

Good questions. Here are the steps, presented in sequence:

First: Drop by the laboratory for a blood analysis test and a measurement of your insulin level. Make sure you fast for 14 hours first.

Second: Begin a dietary diary in which you chart what you eat at each meal and during "snack time." These data will help prepare biochemical and cultural profiles of your eating habits, and also to understand how they fit into your life.

Third: Sit down with your physician using this book as your guide to design a protein-sparing, fat-burning diet that will quickly begin to melt away the weight you hate.

Fourth: Having fully understood the relationship between the Glycemic Index and your own genetically programmed insulin level, settle back to enjoy the foods that are good for you (and also taste good) ... secure in the knowledge that as long as you follow Shoemaker's Rules for Maintenance, your jettisoned flab will never return!

4

*M*ELLY'S FIRST OFFICE VISIT: A MEDICAL DRAMA IN ONE ACT

Introduction

How can Ritchie Shoemaker's LOSE THE WEIGHT YOU HATE! program help you jettison that extra poundage (and keep it off forever!) — even as you feast on the foods you love and begin enjoying a more invigorating, active lifestyle?

To find out for yourself how easy it is to follow my custom-tailored diet, just settle back in your easychair, pour yourself a fresh cup of coffee ... and watch me take a typical patient through her "First Office Visit," during which I'll briefly review the basic metabolic and nutrition principles on which the LOSE THE WEIGHT YOU HATE! system is based.

Ladies and gentlemen, it's showtime!

THE SETTING

It's Tuesday morning in the modern, pleasantly furnished offices of DR. RITCHIE SHOEMAKER, a Family Practice physician in picturesque Pocomoke City, Maryland. The warmly furnished waiting room features framed originals of the doctor's various medical degrees and a few copies of his latest book, "Desperation Medicine" ... a controversial medical expose on how several commonly misdiagnosed illnesses—such as Sick Building Syndrome and chronic Lyme Disease—are actually caused by a newly discovered group of pathogens-biotoxins made by microorganisms.

Flanked by framed copies of his recently published articles in the Baltimore Sun and the Washington Post, a jumbo-sized notice in 42-point boldface underlines Dr. Shoemaker's philosophy of service to patients:

IF YOU'VE BEEN WAITING FOR MORE THAN 20 MINUTES, ASK THE RECEPTIONIST FOR AN EXPLANATION!

Standing in the doorway of his Consulting Room is 50-year-old RITCHIE SHOEMAKER, a 1977 graduate of Duke University Medical School and a veteran "family doc" who has been caring for this small Eastern Shore community for more than two decades.

A husky, broad-shouldered figure who wears a brightly colored sports shirt rather than the traditional white lab coat and stethoscope, Dr. Shoemaker has gained a few pounds since his days as a wrestler at Carlisle High in Pennsylvania. One look at his torso is enough to show the audience that he would be overweight, himself, if he didn't adhere closely to his own weight-management program!

Enter MELLY PATTERSON, a 55-year-old executive secretary in the local mega-corporation. MS. PATTERSON is wearing a stylish, tasteful but shapeless dress that hides some but not all of her extra weight. At 172 pounds, she's more than 30 pounds overweight. Her face shows the stress she's feeling; as she ENTERS the doctor's Consulting Room, her expression radiates anxiety and frustration. She seems depressed and exhausted.

MISS MELLY has already been weighed, measured and put at ease— as much as possible—by DR. SHOEMAKER'S loyal and super-efficient staff nurses, Joyce Harper and Debbie Hudson, who tell each and every patient the same thing: "Some of this will be new to you, but give it a chance. Don't fight the doctor's system, and you're in for a wonderful surprise!"

Now MISS MELLY steps into the doctor's simple, white-painted consulting room. The props include two chairs and an exam table. Here the decorative furnishings are highlighted by several "horse paintings" executed by Ritchie's 17-year-old daughter, SALLY, an ardent rider.

DR. SHOEMAKER:
> *(Bright, friendly)* Good morning. My name is Ritchie Shoemaker.

MELLY PATTERSON:
> *(Timid, still looking down)* Hello. I'm Ms. Patterson— Melly.

RITCHIE: *(Reaching out to shake her hand)*
> Good to meet you. *(Glancing down at her file)* You sure have traveled a long way to lose weight! What can I do to help you today?

MELLY: *(Already in tears; dabbing at her eyes with a Kleenex)*
> Doctor Shoe ... I mean, Ritchie, I have to tell you, I'm at my wit's end. I'm really running on empty! Really ... I just drove 50 miles because I heard you could help me from my friend Betty. She lost 60 pounds ... and she says she's kept it off, by using your system. I hope you can help me.

RITCHIE: *(Hands folded on the table; smiling patiently at her)*
> Of course I can. Once you learn the system, it's simply a matter of time.

MELLY: *(With a rueful laugh)*
> They told me my health insurance won't pay for this

55

visit, but I don't care. All I know is, I can't go on
this way.

RITCHIE: *(Still smiling; watching her intently)*
How much have you spent already trying to lose
weight, without success?

MELLY: *(Letting it all pour out in a rush)*
I've wasted thousands of dollars!

RITCHIE: *(Calm, thoughtful)*
I see. Well, let's do it the *right* way this time! Let's
save time, let's save money, and let's help you feel
good about yourself.

MELLY: *(Nodding eagerly)*
I need to have this weight *gone*, doctor. I really do.
I ... I don't want to look like my mother!

RITCHIE: *(Nodding empathetically; still watching her carefully)*
Well, the first step is to tell you the good news: Most
of what you've heard in the past about fat is incorrect.
Melly, the "conventional wisdom" on this subject is
simply wrong. Let me show you what I mean. May I
ask you a few questions?

MELLY: Sure, go right ahead.

RITCHIE: Have you talked to your internist about losing
weight?

MELLY: Of course I have! He told me to use "will power." He
said I should "keep pushing away from the table," and
that I shouldn't eat any fat.

RITCHIE: *(Nodding and smiling; he's heard all this before)*
How much do you weigh right now, Melly, and how
much would you *like* to weigh?

Melly's First Office Visit: A Medical Drama in One Act

MELLY: *(Looking away, as if ashamed)*

I'm at 172 pounds right now, and it's the most I've ever weighed. And I hate it! I used to be only 139 … but that seems like a long, long time ago.

RITCHIE: *(Nodding cheerfully)*

I know that feeling, Melly. How long ago was it, really, that you weighed 139? And what happened to you, that made your weight take off like that?

MELLY: *(Frowning; puzzled)*

Well, my weight was under control until about two years ago. Then something happened. I'm 55 years old … and I guess middle age caught up with me overnight! I've tried everything, and nothing works. I'm telling you, if I even *look* at a bag of doughnuts, I gain five pounds! *(Still dabbing at her eyes with the Kleenex.)*

I've tried every weight-loss program in the book, Ritchie, and I've exercised until I thought my legs were going to fall off! But nothing helped. I've been to one doctor after another, and they all told me the same thing: I've got to "learn how to push away from the table, consume fewer calories, eat less fat … and exercise more."

(Shaking her head woefully)

I went on the "cabbage soup" diet six months ago, and it nearly put me in the hospital! I'm sick of the "miracle diets" and I'm sick of the appetite suppressants. I went to this one doctor and he gave me a B–12 shot and some vitamins. He charged me $60 for a little bag of pills that kept me up all night, then he took off. I was left with no diet, no weight-loss, nothing more than a receipt for $60.

I've tried everything I could try without a prescription,

and I've come up with zilch.

(Looking him squarely in the eye)

Can you help me, Ritchie—or am I out of luck?

RITCHIE: *(Another big grin; this is obviously the part of the scene he enjoys most.)*

You bet I can help you, Melly! For starters, I want to give you some very good news.

MELLY: *(Eying him doubtfully)*

What's that?

RITCHIE: Usually, being overweight isn't your fault ... and it certainly didn't happen because you lacked "will power." Most of the time there are simple, metabolic reasons why people have trouble losing weight.

MELLY: *(Listening raptly, but still suspicious)*

What do you mean, Ritchie?

RITCHIE: I mean that in spite of what you've been told, your weight problem didn't occur because you were eating too much food.

MELLY: *(Eyes lighting up)*

Well, to tell you truth, I really *don't* overeat. I watch every calorie, and I do everything I've read in the newspaper that I'm supposed to do. It just burns me up that Jane, who works in the next office and is on my leadership team, can eat anything she wants, doesn't gain an ounce. If I have to listen to her talk about her nutrition ideas one more time, well, I don't know what I would do. She eats twice as much of the same food that I do, but I'm the one who gains.

RITCHIE: What you've read is wrong. *(Beaming now; he really gets a kick out of shooting down the "myths.")* And Jane clearly

58

doesn't understand anything about why you have a weight problem.

Melly, do you actually know how fat is made?

MELLY: *(Doubtful; hesitant)*

Well … I guess I've never really thought about it, doctor.

RITCHIE: Not many people have. But the answer to that question will tell you what a scientically based weight–loss program is all about! And here's the bottom line: You didn't become heavy because of what you ate … but because of the way your particular body–chemistry processes the food you take in.

Too bad you'll never find that fact in the newspaper, or on a talk show, or in your favorite magazine. Unfortunately, it seems that people are constantly being bombarded with bad advice.

MELLY: *(Blinking slowly, taking it all in)*

But … I don't get it. Doesn't everybody digest their food the same way?

RITCHIE: They sure don't! Tell me something, Melly; have you ever run into one of those "perpetually skinny people" … the kind who stay thin as a beanpole no matter how much they eat?

MELLY: I sure have. I've got a friend like that: Georgia Evans, out at the university. No matter what she eats, she never seems to gain a pound. She is always complaining that she would like to be a little fuller in her hips. Honestly, I'd like to see her choke on how much she eats! *(MELLY laughs for the first time during her visit.)*

RITCHIE: *(Laughing with her)*

That's exactly how I used to feel, Melly.

59

MELLY: *(Startled, peering at him)*

You?

RITCHIE: That's right. The fact is that people like you and me are very different than your friend, Georgia. We're different in terms of the way our bodies process fat.

(Leaning forward intently; this part is important)

You see, Melly, when Georgia eats a cinnamon bun with sugar frosting on her mid-morning coffee break, her body-chemistry goes right to work digesting all that flour and sugar in speedy, efficient fashion.

In a nutshell, what happens is that her insulin does a good job of transporting the sugar and flour from the bun through her cell membranes, where it's then stored away as "glycogen."

(Picking up the pace now; RITCHIE obviously loves to talk about this stuff)

If the process works efficiently, as in the case of Georgia, then the flour and sugar from the bun wind up tucked away safely inside her cells, where they can be burned off harmlessly and not later stored as fat.

But what if Georgia's system doesn't handle those nutrients efficiently, because of a genetic problem that interferes with the programmed functioning of her insulin ... and thus causes her sugar-storage system to produce far too much of this key digestive hormone, so that her metabolism is swamped by it?

What happens if, as a result, the over-produced hormone can't do its proper job of helping the cells to absorb all that flour and sugar from the cinnamon bun?

MELLY: *(Still puzzled; not yet "seeing the light")*

I ... I guess her digestive system would have to find

some other way of disposing of the sugar and flour.
Is that it?

RITCHIE: *(Getting excited now)*

Bingo! Unlike Georgia and her "perpetually skinny"
friends, you can't eat that cinnamon bun with impunity. Why not? Because the moment you do, the sugar
that's in the frosting and the amylose that's in the
flour will set off a sharp rise in your blood glucose
level.

When that happens, your insulin will kick in, ready to
do its job of transporting the glucose into the billions
of cells in your body for storage.

But remember: If you have what the doctors call
"insulin resistance," your system will work differently than skinny Georgia's. Normally, insulin helps
the body to store sugar in liver and muscle tissue,
where it's quickly burned as energy. But there are
some people for whom it doesn't work this way.
They have "high insulin" due to their insulin resistance ... and the higher the insulin, the worse the
weight problem.

So what happens, in your case? Simple. In a flash,
your body adjusts to the sudden surge in blood sugar
by "turning on" another metabolic process, entirely:
a process that transforms the flour and sugar into
"fatty acids," and then into plain old American fat!

MELLY: *(Nodding eagerly now; beginning to understand)*

So it's the rapid rise in blood sugar that causes the
"fat attack?"

RITCHIE: Exactly. For people like us, that cinnamon bun
works as a "fat trigger." It sends our blood sugar
levels through the roof ... and when our insulin
doesn't put sugar into liver and muscle, then we

start making fat. This is the reason I say it isn't how *many* calories you take in that counts—it's how quickly the calories are stored as fat.

(Grinning delightedly at her)

In other words, Melly, you've been blaming the wrong villain for your fat problem. You didn't gain all that extra weight because of how much you ate ... but because of *what* you ate!

Tell me: What's your favorite breakfast food?

MELLY: *(Startled; stammering a little)*

Why ... I always have a plain bagel with low-fat cream cheese in the morning. I'd always been told—

RITCHIE: *(Chuckling; he's "been through this before")*

You've been told over and over again that a bagel is good for a weight-loss program, right?

MELLY: Sure.

RITCHIE: But that bagel is full of amylose, Melly. Within a couple of minutes of starting to eat it, your blood sugar is climbing like an Apollo moon shot. And a few minutes later, you've already started making fat.

I'll bet you've also been told that you can eat pasta whenever you want, provided only that you don't smother it in a high-calorie sauce.

MELLY: *(Startled again)*

How did you guess? I was raised on pasta! Geez ... I spend half my life trying to find new ways to prepare *spaghettini* and *penne*. I thought pasta was good for me!

RITCHIE: *(Still chuckling)*

Sorry, Melly. Those pasta products are pure amylose ... which is simply the basic form of starch you find in all cereal grains and plants that grow below the ground. I'm talking about tubers, like potatoes, and cereal grains, like the wheat and other cereals you find in *macaroni* and *rigatoni* and all the other pastas.

Eat that harmless-looking bowl of *linguine* with clams, and your blood sugar will skyrocket. Trust me: You'll be making fat within minutes.

But if you stay away from the glucose and the amylose, your "sugar-trigger" will never go off. You can eat your fill of other foods—hundreds of different foods—and they won't be converted instantly into fat.

MELLY: *(Puzzled, frowning)*

Can you back up a step, Ritchie? What *is* this amylose-stuff, anyway?

RITCHIE: No problem. Amylose is simply a whole bunch of glucose molecules, linked together to form a complex carbohydrate. But the key thing to remember for our purposes is that the "linkage" is quickly broken down by an enzyme found in saliva, called amylase, which rapidly begins to convert the amylose to glucose.

In other words: to prevent blood sugar–surges (and resulting fat storage), all you have to do is avoid foods that contain amylose. You can eat most *other* foods to your heart's content.

MELLY: Are you telling me I won't have to starve myself in order to shed this fat?

RITCHIE: *(Nodding happily)*

That's exactly what I'm telling you. I've helped thousands of patients like you during the past 20 years. They've lost 30, 40, 50 pounds each. As for your friend, Betty … you already know how well

63

she's done. She lost 60 pounds and maintained that weight for over five years!

That kind of success is what usually happens within a few months of going on my program. Most of my patents keep the weight off. I'm not bragging when I tell you that my "maintenance rate" with my patients is more than 70 percent.

My patients prevent that excess poundage from ever returning, Melly ... not by controlling how much they eat, but by being careful about *what* they eat.

Wait until I show you the huge list of foods you can still enjoy, and in larger quantities than you'd expect! And wait until you see the dozens of delicious recipes I've worked out over the years, so that you'll actually enjoy the process of losing the weight you hate!

MELLY: *(Brightening; hope has begun to return)*

I can hardly believe my ears, Ritchie. Are you telling me I don't have to count calories at every meal? I don't have to avoid "saturated fats" like the plague? I don't have to exercise like a maniac?

All I have to do is stick to the "approved" foods on your list? Oh, what about onions? They grow below the ground and it says here that I can have onions and garlic.

RITCHIE: *(Rising to his feet; he's "all business" now)*

You bet! Melly, I took a long, careful look at the detailed medical history and the blood test-results you sent me last week, and at first glance they were just as normal as you could ever want. But there's a lot more chemistry to look at, if we're going to solve your problem.

We need a blood test to show your insulin level, because that particular test, more than any other, will determine your maintenance-regimen, after my program helps you lose the weight you need to lose.

We'll get started on all that lab stuff in a minute. But you've already accomplished the first step. Right now, you understand all you need to know about the program. And the good news for you today is this: My system isn't about starving yourself, or sitting around scribbling on "calorie charts" all day long, or taking a bunch of pills!

This is a lifestyle, Melly, not a diet.

I'm talking about a program that celebrates all the good things in life, and especially food. You're going to find that you enjoy preparing these meals, and that you enjoy eating them even more. From now on, you're going to worry far less about "quantity" than "quality." As matter of fact, you'll be encouraged to eat as much as you want of many different delicious foods … not just lettuce and cucumber, as so often happens in a weight-loss program. And, yes, onions are OK. They don't have amylose.

MELLY: *(Rising to her own feet now and shaking his hand; her eyes are shining with recovered hope.)*

I can't wait to get started! What should I do first?

RITCHIE: I'll be back in a few minutes to conduct your physical exam. We're going to do a heart-tracing (EKG) and then we'll schedule the rest of the blood tests that your doctor didn't order. After we get done today, I want you to start reading about my program. I'll be talking in more detail, in those materials, about some of the scientific nuts and bolts involved in weight-loss … such as "receptor-binding sites," and "enzymes making and breaking cholesterol," and "brain centers of satiety and hunger."

Before we're done, you'll know the chemistry of weight-loss inside-out!

(With a bright, upbeat smile at her)

I also want you to take a look at some of the daily menus for my program—just look at the delicious foods that are involved.

I think you're in for a terrific surprise ... when you see just what you're going to be eating in the days ahead!

EXIT MELLY PATTERSON

Epilogue (A Soliloquy By Dr. Shoemaker)

RITCHIE: *(Directly to audience)*

Like the thoroughly delighted Melly Patterson, those who sign on for the LOSE THE WEIGHT YOU HATE! weight-loss and maintenance program will be pleasantly surprised to discover that my approach to "eating smarter" still allows them plenty of choices —and plenty of *food*—*each* time they sit down to the family table at meal times.

I base the weight-loss segment of my program on a simple mathematical formula I've worked out over the years.

It's called "00-2-3."

The numbers in the formula provide a handy short-hand that tells you exactly what you have to do each day, in order to follow the LOSE THE WEIGHT YOU HATE! guidelines, as follows:

O   The daily regimen calls for 0 sugars (glucose or sucrose) each day. (Cheer up: Later, after you've lost the weight and gone on "Maintenance," you'll be allowed an occasional ice cream cone or slice of cake!)

O   Under the LOSE THE WEIGHT YOU HATE! system,

you will take in 0 amylose each day, as well. After you reach Maintenance, however, you can enjoy a bowl of spaghetti or other pasta once in a while. And remember: Once you reach the "Maintenance" phase of my diet program, you still won't have to worry about calories and you will be allowed a calculated number of servings of amylose per week.

○ The weight-loss portion of Lose the Weight You Hate! Mandates that you get two daily servings of protein, totaling at least 6–8 ounces. … which means you'll get to sink your teeth into seasoned rotisseried chicken, or savor sliced smoked turkey, or sit down to a plate-sized grilled hamburger topped with blue cheese, for example, each and every day.

○ The program allows you three full servings of "low-Glycemic Index," or "above ground" vegetables each day. Included on the expansive list are such favorites as cucumber, lettuce, tomato, zucchini, eggplant, asparagus, brussel sprouts, peppers, lentils, peas and all of the bean family—pinto, navy, string, lima, soy and all the rest. And the good news here is that you can eat as much of these veggies as you wish!

○ Finally, under my weight-loss schedule, you will also be permitted three tasty fruits each day. The fare will include such as apples, pears, peaches, plums, oranges and grapes … along with glass after glass of most of the freshly squeezed fruit juices. With the rise in the number of super-stores, with their vast fresh fruit sections, this is the time to develop a taste for mangoes, papaya, kiwi fruit and year round strawberries. And remember, you will eat lots of these no-amylose fruits on my diet!

○ ○ ○

EXIT DR. SHOEMAKER AND ... CURTAIN

Question: How hard is it to meet the daily food consumption-goals of the LOSE THE WEIGHT YOU HATE! program?

Answer: As thousands of my patients over the past two decades will attest, it's not hard at all! As a matter of fact, you'll soon discover that the foods on the "permitted list" (whether for weight-loss or Maintenance) will allow you to prepare some marvelously appetizing and visually pleasing menus each day.

Here's a typical "Wednesday menu" to show you what I mean.

FROM:

"A Day in the LOSE THE WEIGHT YOU HATE! Life"
Wednesday, April 22nd

If You're on Weight-Loss ...

Breakfast

> tomato juice
> cantaloupe slices
> coffee the way you like it
> *Huevos Rancheros*

Lunch

> *Salad:*
> chick peas
> olives
> artichoke hearts
> extra turkey chunks
> green peppers
>
> sugar-free lemonade

Dinner

Garden salad:
tomatoes
blue cheese
mushroom
avocado

Sweet Sausage Casserole:
zucchini
cheese
sweet Italian sausage

peaches and pears
sugar-free iced tea

If You're on Weight-Maintenance (Insulin 10, 1 Amylose per Day) ...

Breakfast

tomato juice
cantaloupe slices
coffee the way you like it
Huevos Rancheros
2 slices of toast

Lunch

Salad:
chick peas
olives
turkey chunks
green peppers
artichoke hearts

lemonade

Snack

Tostidos with salsa

Dinner

Sweet Sausage Casserole:
zucchini
cheese
sweet Italian sausage

buttered garden peas
peaches and pears
artificially sweetened iced tea

Tasty!

To find out just what you can do with these ingredients, take a look at the recipes I've included at the back of the book. There you'll find the instructions for making your *Huevos Rancheros* along with some thoughts about the health-value of the food you're eating today.

Just to get you started, here is the recipe for that great casserole served on Wednesday.

RECIPES

Sweet Sausage Casserole with Zucchini

My wife, JoAnn, is the cook tonight—and once again she's enjoying herself thoroughly.

Fresh yellow squash and zucchini were pretty and plentiful in the grocery store today, so JoAnn will make her zesty zucchini and sausage casserole. Even our daughter, Sally, who consistently avoids green vegetables, loves this casserole!

Brown one pound sweet Italian sausage and cut into small

70

chunks. Let simmer to help drain off fat. Pat dry with a paper towel and toss with one tablespoon flour. Make six cups of thin sliced zucchini and chop one cup of onions. Saute in butter until tender. Do not brown. Remove from heat and coat with three tbsp. flour with four twists of black pepper.

To make the casserole, mix in 16 oz. of cottage cheese and ¼ cup of parmesan. Stir in two well beaten eggs. Bake 30 minutes at 325 degrees. When the casserole is bubbly hot and the zucchini tender, take the casserole out of the oven and top with 4 oz. of cheddar cheese. In two minutes this casserole is ready.

The dish is so good it serves four the first time ... and three the next!

5

INTRODUCING "DOUBLE-0-2-3" ... THE SECRET CODE FOR WEIGHT LOSS!

If you're a James Bond fan (and who isn't?), you probably remember that the famed British secret agent was known throughout the world of espionage by a second "code name" that soon became a glittering legend: "Agent 007."

Sorry, Mr. Bond, but I couldn't resist borrowing a piece of your famous code name for my no-amylose diet!

And welcome, ladies and gentlemen, to the fascinating, celebration-of-food lifestyle that goes by the name of "00-2-3" ... which turns out to be the not-so-secret code that tells my dieters precisely what they're allowed to eat (and *not* to eat) during the weight-loss segment of my program.

Like Agent 007, who overcame enormous odds in order to bring down such arch-villains as Goldfinger, Odd Job and Dr. No (Just Say No To Amylose!), my "00-2-3 Plan" never fails to accomplish its mission—provided that the dieter who follows it is careful to observe the simple nutritional guidelines upon which the program is based. (Hang on: I'll tell you what each number in the code means in a minute.)

That dieting mission—should you choose to accept it—is to lose your extra pounds to reach your ideal percentage body fat, and then to keep the weight off forever by following a few simple and easy-to-manage dietary restrictions from "Dr. Shoe."

For overweight citizens everywhere, the good news is that you're virtually guaranteed to lose at least 30 Big Ones, if you stay on the program. Even better, more than 70 percent of my weight-losers succeed in keeping the discarded flab off for at least a year. Compare that to the one percent maintenance-success rate to be found in the typical weight-loss program!

In order to prepare for the 00-2-3 Lifestyle, I ask my patients to take a few simple steps, as follows:

O   First, I want you to keep a "diet diary" for two weeks. Write down everything you eat and drink—and don't leave anything out. (This means you must include the cookies you took from the Break Room when you thought no one was looking, and the three Budweisers you drank while bowling—and even that succulent chicken dumpling Grandma made you sample when you went over there to install her storm windows!)

O   Second, I'm going to ask you obtain a comprehensive laboratory blood analysis, including a fasting blood test to determine your insulin level.

Why do I insist on these preliminary steps? It's simple: When I went back and examined the records of the 30 percent of my patients who failed to maintain their weight-loss, I discovered that they had all failed to complete either one—or both—of these two steps. My way works—so please give it a chance!

WORKING THE 0-0-2-3 PROGRAM

As you'll see in a moment, my Secret Code instructions for losing weight are based on a couple of key nutritional concepts. For starters, the Shoemaker system recognizes one often ignored fact: Most diets force their adherents to "burn" protein by locking up sugar as fat and throwing away the "insulin key." But my system avoids this danger by making sure that the dieter eats extra protein each day. At the same time, the no-amylose diet prevents rapid rises in blood sugar and keeps insulin from making fat.

Now for those numbers.

First of all, you should understand that the four digits in the code refer only to the weight-loss phase of my program. Maintenance, using the low glycemic index diet 0-1-2-3, *(see Chapter Seven)* is virtually guaranteed, once you adopt my enjoyable new "Eating Lifestyle." With that in mind, here's a number-by-number breakdown of the elements in the program:

00-2-3: GETTING BEHIND THE NUMBERS

○ The first "0" in the sequence tells us that the weight-loss dieter will eat "0" sugars (glucose or sucrose) each day. And that restriction includes the corn syrup (yes, that includes the high-fructose corn syrups, too) and maltodextrins that are often added to so-called "low-fat foods."

○ The second "0" announces that dieters will be permitted no servings of amylose each day during the weight-loss phase. They will also learn exactly what amylose *is*, and what it does.

○ The "2" in the sequence means that dieters will be asked to eat two servings of protein per day.

○ The final "3" in the series describes two different serving-amounts. It tells us that dieters will be allowed three servings of vegetables that grow above the ground *and* three servings of fruit per day.

75

Could anything be simpler than this four-digit code for defining and limiting food intake to healthy, attractively served meals during weight-loss?

But wait a moment ... did I hear someone out there in the audience wailing that familiar question: "What about the Food Pyramid? How can we know we're eating healthily—if we aren't *eating the recommended allowances from all the food groups?*"

Glad you asked, my friend!

Because your question gives me one more chance to hammer at a key insight in this book: the heretical-but-accurate observation that the dietary guidelines of the FDA Food Pyramid should *not* be applied to those who are trying to lose weight ... or to those who are trying to keep it off in order to achieve successful weight maintenance! Imagine telling someone to eat 6 to 11 servings of sugar to help lose weight and stay healthy. That is exactly what the Food Pyramid is. The only thing worse than eating the Food Pyramid is believing that complex carbohydrates like amylose have magical health benefits.

So much for the Pyramid. And while I'm at it, let me try answer another question that often occurs to patients who sign on for the Shoemaker diet:

"Doctor Shoe, everyone knows that most animal protein contains at least some saturated fat. Won't those extra servings of protein that you recommend cause my cholesterol to go up?"

Surprisingly, the answer to this very insightful questions turns out to be "no." As numerous studies have shown in recent years, attaining the proper body weight—while also reducing insulin surges—usually serves to lower cholesterol all the way down to the patient's genetically determined baseline-level *(see Chapters 10 and 11)*.

The next question seems rather obvious: How much protein should a dieter eat?

The answer is ... "enough!"

Of course, that answer does fly in the face of the CDW (Conventional Dieting Wisdom) on this issue. According to the U.S. Medical Establishment, most people should eat precisely 0.7 mg per kilogram of their body weight in protein each day. Translation: If you weigh 200 pounds, about 90 kilograms, you should be eating no more than 63 grams of protein daily—or two ounces of chicken or hamburger or lake trout each day.

Can you see why I so often find myself arguing with dietitians about protein? Two ounces of protein a *day*? (Don't ask for proof —there isn't any.)

My program differs significantly, as you might expect. During the weight-loss phase, my patients are urged to consume at least six ounces—and hopefully, eight ounces of meat (that's final, cooked weight, by the way).

A word to the wise, here: Although going beyond these recommended protein levels won't sabotage your weight loss, you will have to worry about the possible effect on your kidneys of filtering this much protein—and you probably shouldn't attempt it, if you suffer from kidney stones or significant renal disease. (That's one of the reasons for obtaining a comprehensive blood analysis before setting out on this diet.)

For obvious reasons, you should consult with a physician who knows about you and your kidneys before launching this weight-loss program.

When it comes to deciding how much protein to eat, common sense should be our guide. And the same principle applies to consumption of saturated fat (SF). Although poor SF has been "demonized" in recent years by the "eat less and exercise more" crowd, this form of fat isn't nearly as hard on your system as most people think. Still, why push it? The best way to deal with the "fat issue" is to avoid eating any fat that you can *see*, along with any fat that turns solid at room temperature.

The bottom line about these food choices is that protein (usually from animals such as cows, pigs, chickens, sheep and shellfish,

77

but vegetarians can use this diet approach, too) always ranks as an acceptable option, when selecting a snack or transition food on this diet.

Next question: How can vegetarians be sure of getting enough of this daily protein? Answer: Those who eat milk or eggs or both —and many vegetarians belong to this category—should have no trouble. There's no denying, however, that pure vegetarians will have to work hard to consume this much daily protein from legumes and other substitutes for meat.

But don't make the mistake of thinking that eliminating all animal protein will prevent obesity! Surprisingly enough, I've treated dozens of dedicated vegetarians who were also high-insulin, overweight patients over the edge of obesity ... and these folks faced a formidable challenge in order to be sure of eating enough protein, while also avoiding amylose.

UNDERSTAND THE "STARVATION RESPONSE"

Another key aspect of successful dieting—and one that usually gets far too little attention in the typical "eat less" diet—is the "starvation response" that sets in whenever we skip meals or eat significantly less than our usual amount at any given meal.

Although our grandmothers warned us sternly against it, most of us skip meals now and then, especially breakfast. Well, it turns out that Grandma was correct ... because skipping a meal invariably produces what the professional dietitians refer to as an "artificial fasting state." And when *that* happens, you can be sure of one thing: The next calories that are consumed by the "starvee," say, at lunch time, when breakfast was a cup of coffee, will be absorbed and then stored much more efficiently.

The starvation response is controlled by—you guessed it—our old friend insulin, aka the "hormone of the fed state." Following a fast, insulin boosts the biochemical efficiency of the enzymes (disaccharidases) that break down lactose, sucrose, maltose and other sugars into simple sugars.

Skip a meal, and your body will adjust by making sure that you retain many more nutrients (especially including fat) from the next one you eat. Simply put, the lesson to be learned here is: Skipping meals won't help you lose weight!

That insight is absolutely crucial, when it comes to losing weight. It also helps to remember that the starvation response is linked to the feeding center in the hypothalamus. Did you know that the mere act of chewing without swallowing (gum, for example), or swallowing without chewing (including water), is enough to turn on the feeding center? For that reason, simply eating a handful of grapes or an apple or a piece of ham on the way in to the office each morning is a good way to blunt the insulin-controlled starvation response. There aren't many calories in that piece of leftover ham, but look what happens when you tell your brain that you aren't starving.

Let me say it one last time in this chapter: the foods that must be avoided are those containing significant amounts of glucose or amylose. But I strongly urge my dieters to enjoy all other foods to the max—and that includes dozens of different carbohydrates, proteins and fruits. (To help you enjoy, I've assembled a series of mouth-watering recipes that feature the approved foods on my list. These can be found in the recipe section at the end of the book.)

If you're like most dieters, you're in for a very pleasant surprise ... once you understand how short my list of "taboo" foods really is. Example: When it comes to fruits, only one (the common banana) contains enough amylose to disqualify it from your dining room table.

The list of prohibited veggies is somewhat longer, however. Any vegetable that grows beneath the ground (whether defined as a "root" or as a "tuber") will contain enough amylose to be a problem. For our purposes, such "healthy foods" as peanuts, carrots

79

and radishes—all underground-dwellers—don't differ in the least from potatoes, sweet potatoes and sugar beets. Since all six of these offenders are loaded with amylose, they are hereby stricken from your "permitted" list!

Because the fat-making propensities of these rapidly digested complex carbohydrates seem so obvious, it's hard to understand why the U.S. Food and Drug Administration (FDA) continues to insist that Americans should consume so many of them. But that's precisely what the FDA Food Pyramid recommends … while advising the citizenry to eat six to eleven servings of cereal grain or bread products (including pasta) each and every day. (Surely the FDA "consensus panel" that came up with this wrong-headed approach understands that amylase in saliva breaks amylose down into glucose even faster than Flash can run!)

For people interested in weight-control, the Food Pyramid simply makes no sense. And that's why I'm careful to .insist that my dieting patients eat nothing made from wheat, rice, oats, barley or rye during the weight-loss portion of my program. Once the maintenance stage has been reached, however, my slimmed-down patients can enjoy a controlled number of these servings per week—with the actual number of servings depending on the individual's particular metabolism and insulin level.

I don't deny that many people look at me strangely, when I first explain to them that such healthy, "no fat" foods as pasta and bananas are actually helping to make them overweight! But those incredulous looks usually turn to pleased smiles after five or six weeks, as the benefits of the "LOSE THE WEIGHT YOU HATE" approach begin to make themselves felt. After treating thousands of overweight patients in recent years, I can tell you flatly that eating my way makes you look younger and feel better. It also leaves you with energy to burn as it helps you mobilize fat stores for daily living!

With this outcome in mind, I suggest that you take a picture of yourself before, during and after my program. The picture is for you, no one else. (Just look at that jaw line emerging from the extra chin.) That way, you'll get an up–close look at the "glow of health" that I observe routinely in my weight-loss patients!

But enough of the "No Mores."

Because it's a lot more fun to talk about all the foods (and eat them too!) that you *can* enjoy while participating in the weight-loss segment of my program.

It's also quite gratifying to realize that you won't be counting calories or measuring out portion-sizes under my tutelage. (No more adding up fat grams, either!) But remember to be reasonable—why try to wipe out the profit margin at your local *smorgasbord* restaurant? Just eat until you're full ... and then stop!

Here are a few basic mealtime suggestions to help you visualize the hours of eating enjoyment that lie ahead:

- O To start your day off right, I suggest that you enjoy as much fruit at breakfast as you wish. And why not include some protein (scrambled eggs with melted cheddar?) ... while also planning some protein-containing foods for lunch?

- O For a satisfying lunchtime, I recommend a large salad (underline that word *large*!), but without the croutons or the "low-fat" dressing, which usually turns out to be loaded with sugary corn syrup or crammed with the stealth sugar bomber, maltodextrins. Instead of the low-fat poisons, add some sliced ham, turkey, roast beef or tuna to that salad ... or wax creative in another way by whipping up a "Chicken Caesar" salad.

- O To make that luncheon even more satisfying, heat up a cup of savory soup ... but stay away from the amylose-heavy noodle- or potato-based versions, while also avoiding any vegetable-beef soups that include carrots, potatoes or barley.

- O An afternoon snack each day will help to keep both your energy and your spirits elevated. Fresh fruit will usually give you a pronounced lift: Why not spice up the trip home from work by munching on a juicy Golden Delicious apple or a melt-in-your-mouth Bartlett pear? For snacking variety, try butter-free popcorn or baked *tortilla* chips on other occasions. Melt some real cheddar cheese (no, cheese food isn't real cheese) on the tortilla chips to make a quick, safe, taste treat.

O The main meal of the day (usually the evening meal, in this culture) should include a serving of protein (a New York strip steak or broiled salmon or a boneless chicken breast), along with two different kinds of above-ground vegetables (lima beans and butternut squash, let's say, or maybe stewed tomatoes and fresh corn on the cob).

O My diet places no restrictions on spices or condiments. But I do ask my patients to use good judgment when experimenting with yogurt or cheese as flavor-enhancers, because of the concentrated amounts of milk fat, sugar, corn syrup and maltodextrins to be found in these products. (Yes, be sure to read the label on that low-fat, high-fructose corn syrup-laced yogurt!)

O What about alcohol? Although I'm pleased to report that booze is *not* banned under my dieting regimen, I do ask patients to remember that there are a surprisingly large number of calories in a glass of beer. Nor should we forget that such harmless-seeming beverages as tonic water are actually crawling with sugar ... or that alcohol, itself, carries seven calories per gram.

(It's a curious metabolic fact that for many people, drinking alcohol actually causes blood sugar levels to *drop*. If you don't believe me, just ask a Type I diabetic or an alcoholic to describe their low-sugar reactions!)

I don't recommend overindulgence in alcohol, of course, but drinking in moderation can add to the quality of life. Patients in my 00-2-3 program are permitted up to two mixed drinks (no sugar, please!) or three four-ounce glasses of wine or four bottles of beer per day. (And no ... you are *not* allowed to drink more than the limit in order to "catch up," if you drank less than the max allowed on the previous night!)

O Remember that the "diet diary" is a powerful tool for monitoring your progress on the 00-2-3 program. By reviewing this log that records everything you consumed during the previous two weeks, I can keep a close eye on your eating patterns and ensure your healthy nutrition. I don't deny that keeping a food diary can be a hassle at times ... but it's worth the trouble, because research shows that a high percentage of people who don't maintain the diary for two weeks will fail to achieve their weight-loss goals.

IT'S ALL A MATTER OF "ATTITUDE"

So there you have it: Shoemaker's Secret Agent Code (Double-0-2-3!) for weight loss and successful maintenance. Time now for a final question:

Q. What's the biggest stumbling-block en route to losing at least 30 pounds and then keeping it off?

A. Your attitude!

During my many years of experience as a family practitioner, I've found that many people sill cling to the "Major Dieting Myth" —the misguided idea that losing weight simply means cutting back on fats and total calories, while being careful to exercise more.

Again and again over the years, I've found myself struggling to help patients who repeatedly kid themselves by declaring: "How can a couple of slices of wheat bread hurt my diet? Hey, this stuff is supposed to be *good* for you!"

These patients need to work on their "dieting attitude" ... by recognizing once and for all that such high-glycemic foods as wheat bread and bananas and linguine aren't "harmless" at all … and that if we eat them while trying to lose weight (or keep it off), we are going to fail!

6

LIVING THE NO-AMYLOSE DIET MEANS WEIGHT LOSS

LIVING THE LOW-GLYCEMIC INDEX DIET MEANS MAINTENANCE

OR "LIVING WELL IS THE BEST REVENGE —AGAINST FAT!"

Here are three questions for would-be dieters, as they contemplate the possibility of embracing Dr. Shoe's "Double-0-2-3" program for losing weight and keeping it off using the 0-1-2-3 low-Glycemic Index diet:

First: Are you ready to enjoy a much more exciting lifestyle than anything you've ever known in the past?

Second: Are you prepared to begin eating some of the best-tasting (and healthiest) meals you've ever sunk a fork into, once I show you how to prepare gourmet-style dishes with the "approved" foods on my list?

Third: How are you going to use all of the extra energy and vitality that will soon be flowing your way ... as your re-vitalized system begins to shuck off the listlessness and fatigue so often triggered by obesity?

Those are exciting questions—especially when you realize that the answers are going to change your life!

But before I begin showing you just how rewarding and satisfying a "Day in the Low-Glycemic Life" can really be, let's quickly review the three or four basic scientific principles on which my entire weight-loss system is based.

CONTROLLING FAT STORAGE IS THE KEY

Principle #1: The calories that are most efficiently stored as fat come from a particular type of complex carbohydrate (amylose) which the body quickly breaks down into simple glucose.

Principle #2: This process of storing calories as fat works with even greater efficiency in those of us who struggle with genetically programmed hyperinsulinemia (also known as "insulin resistance").

Principle #3: By avoiding those foods that trigger sudden rises in blood sugar—foods high in amylose and other sugars—we can reduce the efficiency of fat storage.

Principle #4: As the body begins to create less fat from complex carbohydrates and as it protects its protein stores, it will be forced to mobilize "fat stores" for energy ... a process that will soon result in weight loss.

Principle #5: By preventing surges in blood sugar, my diet short-circuits the "starvation response" and thus inhibits "protein wasting" ... which is the major culprit responsible for re-gaining lost weight.

Principle #6: Eating low-Glycemic Index foods will also prevent over-production of cholesterol, while helping to reduce blood pressure and control diabetes in many patients.

INTRODUCING ... A DAY IN THE LOW-GLYCEMIC LIFE!

Grandma was right, ladies and gentlemen: Eating a "healthy, nutritious breakfast" really *is* an important step on the road to physical and mental well-being.

All too often, however, our well-intentioned grandmothers were sadly mistaken about the *content* of that All-America breakfast that so many of us were required to consume before departing for school each morning.

If you're like most folks of middle-age or older, you probably remember the heaping, sugar-laced bowls of Corn Flakes and Rice Krispies ... along with the stacks of pancakes, waffles, doughnuts and biscuits that so often appeared on the family breakfast table in years gone by.

Do you also remember the pitchers of frothy orange juice that were usually "made from concentrate" ... and also marked with that telltale warning from the wily manufacturer: "Sugar added?"

And how about all those steaming mounds of "hashed-brown potatoes" that we all enjoyed so much, while also devouring *Mark Trail* or *The Katzenjammer Kids* in the Sunday comics section of the newspaper? (Younger breakfasters might want to think about those delicious "sausage biscuits" now available at almost every "drive-through" carryout—and whether or not they're going to make you look any better in a bathing suit next summer.)

Ah, the joys of the traditional American breakfast!

But guess what?

Although Norman Rockwell did a terrific job of painting the Sunday morning breakfast-scene, the inescapable fact remains that all those butter pancakes and all those sizzling mounds of hashed-browns were actually causing significant nutritional problems for millions of Americans!

They were making us *fat*, for starters. By triggering high-speed surges in human blood sugar, such high-amylose goodies as the toasted cinnamon bagel and the sugar-sprinkled French toast were causing many of us to quickly convert sugar to fatty acids ... en route to the rapidly expanding pot bellies and the bulging hips that would prove impervious to all ensuing efforts at dieting and exercising.

Nostalgia aside, it's high time that we all understood: Eating 14 pounds of sugary starch at breakfast each morning is simply not a good idea ... not unless you're planning to make a living by doing side-splitting imitations of the Goodyear Blimp!

So what *should* we all be eating for breakfast, instead of the jelly-doughnuts and the buttermilk biscuits dredged in molasses?

Here are a few choice selections from the Shoemaker Breakfast Bar ... all of which have been chosen to provide healthy, start-off-your-day nourishment—but without triggering a Sudden Fat Attack.

DR. SHOEMAKER'S OK BREAKFAST: THE LINEUP

(Remember: You can combine these approved breakfast foods in any way you wish.)

O Fresh Fruit Cup: Try slicing some peaches, melons, apples and pears the night before, then toss them with some concentrated lemon juice in order keep them fresh.

O Freshly squeezed fruit juices: Yes, you can have all you want ... but you *cannot* have the "commercial" juices, most of which are loaded with added sugar.

O Elegantly presented strawberries: Line them up in a circle, along with some fresh cantaloupe chunks, and your breakfast will win raves for being colorful *and* tasty.

O Sizzling omelets, with two eggs and lots of green peppers or onion or tomato slices or mushrooms or any other "approved vegetable." Did you know that the typical omelet takes less than three minutes to make? Be creative, because the possibilities here are literally endless.

○ The McDonald's "All-America Sausage Biscuit Breakfast": You think I'm kidding, right? "He's actually gonna let me eat a McDonald's Sausage Biscuit on a *diet*?" Sure, I am! Go ahead and enjoy the sausage and the cheese ... but make sure that biscuit goes straight into the trash can! Or better yet, give it to someone you're not real fond of who is on a standard "diet."

And while I'm at it ... here's a side-note about the best way to cut down on the fats contained in such traditional sources of breakfast protein as sausage, bacon and scrapple. To get rid of most of their saturated fat, try browning these meats in a frying pan. Now add water to the pan ... turn the heat down, and gently steam the fat out of the sausage or bacon. Then simply pour off the fatty water and brown the meat again. (Your breakfasts guests will never even notice that you've slashed their saturated fat-intake at least in half, as they rave about how good your crispy bacon tastes.)

Next question: Even as that early morning cheese-omelet sizzles in the pan, I can hear a nation of worry-warts asking themselves: "Do I really dare to eat an egg? What about the cholesterol? I'll be dead before sundown!"

Not really.

You know, I never cease to be amazed by the panic-in-the-streets reaction that sets in among Americans, whenever you serve them an egg!

I don't blame them, however. Instead, I put the responsibility for this needless anxiety squarely on some folks who ought to know better—namely, the "Medical Establishment" gurus at such high-toned U.S. institutions as the Food and Drug Administration and the National Institutes of Health, who have been frightening all of us for years with their scary pronouncements about eggs, cholesterol and "related risk factors" for heart disease *(see Chapter Ten)*.

Although you won't be reading any bulletins from the U.S. Heart, Lung and Blood Institute on this topic, the latest research shows clearly that eating three or four eggs a week does not pose a significant health hazard.

If you still need convincing on this touchy subject, go visit one of those hotel "breakfast buffets" on a Sunday morning. Belly up to the serving-bar, and what do you find? You find lots of sliced fruits … lots of sausage and bacon … and a chef in a paper hat standing by to crack some eggs and make you an omelet!

Why not take a lesson from these geniuses of the breakfast buffet and learn how to make the same pleasing—and nutritious—foods at home?

But enjoying your breakfast more is only one of the benefits you'll gain from the Double-0 Lifestyle. Another payoff will occur around 11 o'clock, when you discover that you're not suddenly desperate for a pre-lunch snack! (If the urge to nibble on something sweet does show up, try substituting a juicy peach or a handful of glossy-skinned grapes for that frosting-smeared jelly doughnut. You have to buy the fruit first and have it readily available, however.)

Another advantage of the Shoemaker approach to breakfast is the way it makes life so much simpler for the business traveler or vacationer. If you're out there on the road, why not enjoy a breakfast of fresh fruit, raisins, apricots or prunes, and eat them "right out of the box?" (Remember that cashews, almonds and pistachios are also nutritionally safe for you and don't require a refrigerator, a fork or even a slice of bread! You may even come to enjoy pistachios for a quick breakfast on the way to the airport in the hotel van. I guarantee you that the guy in the seat behind you will suddenly be interested in sharing your pistashio stash.)

LUNCH TIME: AIN'T NOTHIN' LIKE THE REAL THING!

When it comes to the business of eating lunch, Thomas Babing-ton Macauley, the famed British historian, said it best: "As civilization advances, poetry declines!"

If you're like most workers in the harried America of the New Millennium, you've probably noticed that the phrase "enjoying a leisurely lunch" has all but vanished from the modern lexicon. These days, the "poetry" of cooking and serving fine food has been replaced—especially at lunchtime—by the gustatory horror of the "drive-through meal" ... whether that meal consists of a hastily assembled burger-with-fries or a basket of ersatz Mexican tacos with *jalapeno* biscuits. I remember the time, some years ago, I took my daughter, Sally, for a quick snack of French fries (that was what she wanted) at the local McDonald's.

"Yes, one small order of fries, please."

"OK, would you like some fries with that?"

Is it me—or is there something truly grotesque about a society that doesn't take time to stop and eat a decent lunch?

Take heart, however, because there *are* some things you can do to make your mid-day meal more pleasing to both the palate and the eye. For starters, why not begin preparing your healthy, nourishing lunch on the evening before you eat it? Try whipping up a fresh garden salad (you can even add some slices of ham, turkey or cheese), then wrapping it securely and hiding it in your lunch box.

Remember, also, that leftovers from dinner can often be micro-waved successfully. Or you might want to prepare soup the night before lunch, then resurrect it the next day via microwave or stove. Another clever strategy: Visit a deli over the weekend, then refrigerate some choice cuts of ham, turkey or roast beef for lunchtimes in the days ahead. (Remember, though, that if your lunchtime fare includes pastrami, bologna or salami, you'll be in-gesting a fair amount of saturated fat, so proceed judiciously.)

Next step: Go ahead and slosh plenty of ketchup, mayonnaise

91

and/or mustard on your lunchtime meats. You can enjoy these condiments without fretting—because you're *not* going to be eating any bread with them! As a matter of fact, I always recommend against the "low-fat" spreads and condiments, which often contain nothing more sophisticated than corn syrup as a substitute for fat. Go ahead and enjoy the good stuff because the odds are much higher that you'll stick to a diet if you like the way the food tastes!

And while we're on the subject of abused American foods: What about soup?

Ever found yourself wondering: What happened to the thick and hearty black bean soup of days gone by ... or to the nourishing and somehow comforting lentil soup that dear old Grandmother used to simmer all day long? Instead of these old-fashioned favorites, we have inherited the Campbell Soup Company's "chicken noodle" and "sugar-added tomato" varieties ... the kind of thin, watered down lunchtime fare guaranteed to leave poor Macauley rolling in his grave.

Here are a few soup suggestions that should allow you to leave Campbell & Co. in your fast-vanishing wake:

O Although clam chowder does contain a few potatoes, you'll benefit if you can find a good one. And the starch in those potatoes won't affect your blood sugar nearly as much as the sandwich and the crackers that you won't be eating with this tasty soup *(see Recipe).*

O You can go right ahead and enjoy a bowl of cream of mushroom or asparagus soup, because these milk-based concoctions are perfectly harmless, in terms of blood sugar rates. (Ditto for tomato soup—provided that you can find one without added sugar.)

O For summertime dining, you can't beat *gazpacho*, which ranks as my personal favorite. Served cold and tomato-based, this crowd-pleaser contains lots of healthy vegetables, all of which grow above the ground.

BEWARE OF "GRAZING"

Although many dieters don't realize it, one of the most dangerous periods in the day occurs at the transition time when the weary dieter arrives home from work.

All too often, the already hungry worker breezes in the door closer to the driveway and enters the kitchen with an attitude that says, "I'm free at last ... and it's happy hour!" What often follows this declaration, of course, is a high-risk eating binge that I have termed "grazing." The process begins with a couple of Michelobs ... during which the beer-quaffer feels an irresistible urge to chomp on an entire bag of potato chips or snack crackers or some other salty and amylose-loaded snacking treat.

In most cases, mind you, the problem isn't really the alcohol ... it's those Ritz Cheddar Crackers or Sour Cream N' Chives Utz Chips that are being gobbled by the handful. Such appetizers are clearly in violation of the Double-0 Secret Weight Loss Code, and as such, they must be resisted! (Try substituting a protein-based appetizer such as shrimp and cocktail sauce.) A better trick is to go into your house through the front door, not the one that goes into the kitchen, then change your clothes, stretch your workday aching back, massage your workday feet and get ready to enjoy family life after this simple, but no-calorie transition. Maybe this is the time to do one or two of those 5 minute jobs you have been postponing for months (besides, when you finally put up that towel rack, the rest of the evening is likely to be much more enjoyable), or put in a few minutes on the exercise bike.

The problem with most of the appetizers on the shelf at the local convenience store is that they contain amylose. To beat the snap-crackle-and-crunch purveyors at their own game, prepare a plate full of snacking goodies and hide it in your refrigerator well in advance of the grazing hour.

If you think about it, you'll quickly realize that there's nothing easier than slicing fruits of various kinds into a handy Tupperware container. Or how about a snack tray that includes cheese,

pickles, artichoke hearts, olives and maybe a bit of bologna and a few smoked oysters?

You can accomplish the same dietary objective at your Friendly Neighborhood Italian Restaurant, by the way, simply by digging into the "antipasto" tray … while making sure your hand doesn't stray toward the bread (of course they give you all you want) basket.

THE EVENING MEAL: A LOST ART?

Like the meal which precedes it, the traditional American supper has been taking a fierce pounding in recent years, as the fastfood restaurants and the shameless manufacturers of the "Frozen Chinese TV Dinner" have joined forces to all but wipe out what was once an endlessly rewarding and soul-nourishing custom. Let's not forget the societal pressures that imply that young Johnny must have several after school activities, each one seemingly finishing at 6:30.

It's a grim prospect, you must admit. How many three-course dinners were you (or your partner) able to cook for *your* super-busy family last week? But the good news about my revolutionary new approach to dieting can be found in the fact that I urge my patients to enjoy every aspect of food as much as possible … and that includes preparation as much as it does consumption. I say, bring back the "dinner hour" (and I mean a full hour!).

To get your evening meal off on the right foot, remember that on my diet, supper is much larger than lunch or breakfast. And no, it doesn't mean that you will store more calories as fat because you ate more calories later at night. Insulin is on-call 24 hours a day. And that's why I usually suggest that you serve a six-to-eight-ounce helping of meat (cooked weight) … along with two different servings of above-ground vegetables and fruit for dessert. (If you serve more than eight ounces of protein, that's okay—but remember that the extra calories will count ... even if they won't be stored as efficiently as high-glycemic calories.)

Take your time in preparing this important meal, while luxuriating in the knowledge that your vegetable choices are unlimited. If you don't believe choosing and preparing this form of nature's bounty can be a rewarding exercise, just take a leisurely stroll through the produce section of any large supermarket. Or try scanning the pages of a good French cookbook to find out what wonders can be achieved with these delectable products of Mother Nature's garden.

You'll probably enjoy that lime-sprinkled butternut squash or those artichoke hearts with pickled mushrooms even more, once you realize that these delightful foods are jam-packed with all the vitamins and minerals your body needs for healthy functioning. Even better, spend a little more time serving food artfully. How much time does it take to add a bright garnish (pimentoes, bell peppers in various colors, mandarin oranges or some thawed and drained raspberries, for example) to a plate of sauteed chicken breasts? The benefits of eating good tasting food, served pleasingly go beyond how long the meal took to cook.

(By the way, I should also point out that you won't be spending your hard-earned dollars on vitamin supplements on this diet, either—because the foods I'm recommending contain more of the As and Ds and Es and other key alphabet letters than you'll ever need.)

Next question: "What about desserts, Dr. Shoemaker? Are you telling us that the only sugar we'll ever taste again will be found in the endless apples, pears and oranges that you're going to make us eat?"

Not to worry, my friends. Among the most pleasing substitutes for fresh fruit on the Shoemaker Dinner Menu are the following:

○ Ice cream, within moderation (no, you may *not* devour the entire carton!).

O Sugar-free dessert ices, available at any supermarket.

O Flavored gelatins (again, look for the "sugarless" variety).

O Any nuts that grow on trees (as opposed, let's say, to pea-nuts … which are an absolute no-no here, for several rea-sons).

O Although you *will* be missing out on the traditional cakes, pies and apple fritters of the American Way of Dessert, the good news is this: if you've eaten all the foods I recom-mended in the quantities I recommended earlier, the odds are high that you won't be hungry at the end (I just couldn't eat another bite) of the meal … and you won't really miss that slice of Aunt Sara's Fudge-Dribbled Pecan Pie all that much!

GETTING BEHIND THE "OLESTRA" CRAZE

If you've been keeping dietarily up to speed in recent years, then you've surely heard all the talk about one food craze or another. Take the current "poster child" of the snack food industry, Oles-tra, for example.

Like Ponce de Leon's magical Fountain of Youth in an earlier era, this no-fat substitute for fat has recently enjoyed star billing as a wondrous elixir guaranteed to solve a chronic health problem —in this case, obesity. Theoretically, a low-fat oil substitute sounds like a great idea.

Too bad the elixir doesn't really work. To understand why, let's meditate for a moment on a thoroughly odd-sounding oxy-moron: "The Low-Fat Potato Chip."

Cook the chip in a non-fat substance such as Olestra, the theory goes, and you'll have done the impossible: You'll have cre-ated a delicious fried snack that doesn't make chip-gorgers swell up like cartoon rhinoceroses!

Sorry, folks. The only flaw in this line of reasoning is the *reasoning* ... which fails to take account of one decisive fact: The real culprit in that tasty treat from the deep-fry boilers of Mama Utz isn't so much the oil (but fat counts!) that the chip was cooked in—but the potato, itself. (Ask yourself: *Where do potatoes grow?*) Because they're crawling with amylose, potatoes simply don't belong in any self-respecting diet—and they will never find a home on mine!

All right, then. If you can't have potato chips for your post-dinner snack, what treat can you rely on to ease the transition to bedtime? How about a basket of fresh hot popcorn? Sounds good! Go ahead and pop it any way you want ... and help yourself to some melted butter, if you wish. (But no "caramel coating" on those clusters of corn, for obvious reasons.)

Another option for the pre-bedtime snacker is baked corn chips. Add a little cheese and/or salsa, and the dish becomes more interesting. Remember, also, that your post-supper beverages should be free of sugar. You're free to drink all the caffeine you wish, however—whether in the form of coffee, iced tea or diet soft drinks throughout the day. If you are like many people, however, a good night's sleep is a treasure, and caffeine can disrupt normal sleep patterns.

TO AVOID CRAVINGS, PLAN "DIET HOLIDAYS"

If you've learned to dread the first few days of any new diet, you're going to be pleasantly surprised to discover that you *don't* feel starved and exhausted after a week or so of "No-Amylose Living." To the contrary, most of the thousands of patients who've followed my 00-2-3 regimen over the years tell me they feel more energy and vitality than they've felt in years. As time passes, they also discover that the environmental cues—sights, smells, advertisements—that so frequently stimulate people to overeat are now being "turned off." Suddenly, those gooey chocolate doughnuts

97

beside the office coffee pot just don't look appetizing, and it's much easier to walk right on past them.

Still, occasional cravings for "taboo" foods are going to erupt now and then. One way to keep them to the minimum is to schedule "diet holidays" under the following ground rules:

IF ... the dieter has scrupulously observed the program during the nine previous days, and without any slippage:

THEN ... said dieter shall be permitted to eat whatever he or she wishes on the tenth day. (The psychological payoff for this simple strategy is actually quite large—since knowing they can look forward to a "day off" now and then gives most of my patients a powerful sense of relief and satisfaction.) This permitted holiday actually brings the best pay-off when the dieter who has been visualizing that baking dish full of lasagna for a week finds out after a few forksful of pasta that the fantasy food was just that —a fantasy. When I hear a patient tell me about their diet holiday, saying "You know, I found out that I really didn't want the plateful after all," I know they are well on the way to successful weight loss.

Another problem that many dieters face is the sheer cost of some no-amylose or low-sugar foods in today's market. Let's face it, such items as honeydew melons ($2 per fruit, at last check) and strawberries (also $2 a pound) can quickly break a careful food shopper's budget. Is it any wonder that obesity continues to attack low-income families in this country ... once you realize that such foods as rice, potatoes and pasta products rank among the least expensive you can buy?

The bottom line is obvious. If you're feeding a family of six, it's much cheaper to give them spaghetti or rice than cantaloupe.

There's no doubt that the 00-2-3 approach to eating is more expensive than eating traditional starchy fare. On the other hand, the dollars-and-cents cost of such obesity-related health problems as hypertension, diabetes, elevated cholesterol and low self-esteem is far higher in the long run than paying for fresh pears, tangerines or Bing cherries at the market.

BUT WHAT IF YOU'RE EATING OUT?

Here are a few tips for that next visit to McDonald's, or maybe Luigi's Spaghetti House down on the corner on Saturday night:

- If you're dining at a fastfood establishment this evening, try ordering the in-house salad and a hamburger. Then eat only the meat and the salad.

- Avoid commercial sauces whenever possible, even when they're marked "low fat" or "healthy choice." (Otherwise, the chances are good that you'll simply be pouring corn syrup onto your Romaine lettuce!)

- At all costs, steer clear of the "bread lady" at your favorite sit-down restaurant. Restaurants know about amylose turning on hunger, when they give you 25 cents worth of coconut muffin, they are selling you a $5 dessert. Sure ... you can go ahead and enjoy the onion soup before your meal ... but do *not* dunk that slab of fresh-cut French bread into it!

- In similar fashion, avoid "breaded" meats, veal cutlets or seafood for example at any restaurant, along with fried foods in general.

- To help keep your sugar consumption to a minimum during a restaurant meal, ask for a "dry" white wine as opposed to "sweet," though your more cynical friends will give you a hard time about this point.

- Whenever possible, order a fruit plate, a salad or some freshly prepared vegetables. Remember that, all too often, the waitress who rattles off the daily "specials" usually also asks you: "And what vegetable would you like with your baked chicken? Do you want baked potato, French fries, macaroni and cheese, or the overcooked, dead string beans from the can?"

99

I always wondered about the vegetables that grow on the macaroni bush. Does it only grow in tropical wetlands?

O   If you must eat dessert in a restaurant, make it fruit. Better yet, go without ... while telling yourself: "I'm on a diet, and this is a good chance to prove to myself that I'm serious about it," not to mention that desserts are big profit items in restaurants.

VACATIONS AND HOLIDAYS: REMAIN VIGILANT

During more than 20 years of experience with dieters, I've learned that "special occasions"—such as vacations and holidays—are frequently responsible for wrecking diets. To avoid this trap, keep reminding yourself: "Whether I'm on vacation in Paris or riding the commuter train to work in Hoboken, the diet comes first!"

The same strategy applies to holidays. From Halloween through New Year's Day, the pressure on most of us is relentless: Eat, eat, eat! But your mission (should you choose to accept it!) will be to chow down as much Thanksgiving turkey and broccoli and salad as you wish ... while passing the bowl of mashed potatoes on to the next diner.

One of the problems with holidays, of course, is that they're usually swarming with friends and family, with ardent well-wishers who quickly become what I call "diet saboteurs." If you want to see what I mean, just try telling that mother-in-law of yours that you don't want to sample her special turkey-with-dumplings ... and you're liable to end up with a casserole dish in your lap or be on the receiving end of a hurtful look.

(Solution: Just tell the saboteur: "Thanks so much. I'd love to eat that great-looking dumpling, but not *this* year. I'm under a dietitian's care. See you next Thanksgiving ... when I'll have three of 'em to make up for what I'm missing here tonight!")

Another problem with holiday eating is the food you end up

eating while travelling to eat too much of the wrong thing. Just hop on a quick flight from Philadelphia for "Christmas in the Rockies" with 140 other crammed-in-passengers. Did you enjoy listening to the child with the ear infection in Row 12 scream bloody murder at take-off? Hey, the food service is a welcome respite. Look, here is the pasta with the tomato-chicken sauce (that means that while the sauce might have been blessed with the passing over of the chicken, there certainly isn't any chicken *in* the sauce), served with a puffy roll, ersatz butter, garden salad (it looks like lettuce and carrots) with lots of Ranch dressing (buttermilk, safflower, and maltodextrins), and the apple pastry for dessert. If you thought that the tomato sauce was safe, taste it. It is laced with sugar.

OK, if the long flights are a problem, how about a jaunt to Orlando, Florida? No kidding, this was my meal not long ago: whole wheat bagel with low fat cream cheese, banana and mega-corn syrup yogurt. And that was followed up with peanuts and sugary breath mints. I was spared the mini pretzels on this flight, but the airline was passing them out on the shuttle on the way home. These are the accepted American fare on a plane!

This year we had to get to New Jersey on short notice. Pack the cooler with grapes, chicken salad and diet drinks or leave the cooler home to make room for the dog? We made it a fast food day with chicken nuggets (no, no sauces and no, no French fries), burgers and high-cost drive-through sodas. Fortunately, the dog didn't throw up in the back of the car.

No wonder travellers gain weight.

THE JOYS OF REGAINING YOUR SELF-ESTEEM

So far I've talked a great deal in this book about the many benefits that will begin to flow your way, once you start to LOSE THE WEIGHT YOU HATE!

Take it from me: You're going to feel better, look better and start enjoying a healthier, more active life.

Instead of feeling isolated and gloomy—*The refrigerator is my only friend!*—you're going to begin gaining a new feeling of value and self-worth.

Instead of wearing your lonely heart on your Size-14 sleeve, you're going to begin telling the world: "I don't have to overeat, in order to feel loved ... and I respect myself because I'm learning how to control my need for instant gratification, via sugar and starch!"

I've said it a thousand times before, and I'll say it again as this chapter ends:

The Double-0-2-3 Program for weight loss and maintenance isn't a diet ... it's a dynamic, high-energy lifestyle that you can go on enjoying for the rest of your days!

REAL PEOPLE, REAL STORIES

CASE STUDY NO. 2: SHELLEY SPRATT

Once upon a time, there was an attractive young woman named Shelley who fell in love with a handsome young mechanical engineer named Jack Spratt.

Equally smitten, the passionate Spratt soon asked Shelley to be his bride.

But they didn't live happily ever after.

Instead, Shelley began to put on weight. It happened slowly at first ... and neither of them noticed it, because they were too busy going out to restaurants to enjoy delicious dinners every other night.

If the truth be told, these two love-birds simply did not enjoy the fine art of cookery—although they did take enormous pleasure in the gourmet fare to be found in the very best of eateries. Secretly, Shelley felt that Jack should cook because she did all the laundry, food shopping and clean-up. Jack felt that Shelley should be like his Mom who did it all for years without complaining.

Nor did Shelley pay much attention to the fact that her tall, slender, 150-pound prince loved to feast on bread, rolls, cakes and other doughy delights. Heedlessly, she joined her lover in these bakery binges, without a single thought about what the future might bring.

Sadly, the future brought fat.

Although she'd weighed only 135 pounds on the day of her wedding, Shelley soon began climbing the scales. As she grew heftier, Jack seemed to grow less attentive. Hurt by the obvious falloff in his ardor, she ate even more to compensate.

Within less than a year, Shelley's weight soared past the 200-pound mark.

Jack grew ever cooler, ever more distant. Frantic now, Shelley plunged into a series of draconian and doomed-to-failure diets. First she tried skipping meals. When that didn't work, she took regular chromium supplements without success. Nearly distracted, she launched a regimen based on daily doses of ginseng. No such luck!

Too bad.

When she finally walked into my office and introduced herself, Shelley tipped the scales at better than 220.

I examined her, listened carefully to her story ... and then began to tell her the good news.

She listened carefully while I explained the complicated workings of insulin resistance and the Glycemic Index and fat-triggering amylose.

"Are you telling me," wailed the astonished Shelley, "that all that bread I ate with Jack was a *problem*? I can't believe it, Dr. Shoe. The other doctors all said that bread was okay ... and that the key to losing weight was to eat no *fat*!"

When I explained to this struggling young woman that her obesity wasn't caused by lack of willpower but by genetic programming over which she had no control, Shelley began to weep. Then she admitted the obvious: She was terrified that her weight problem would destroy her marriage ... and that no one could love a woman who was buried under "a 85-pound layer of blubber!"

We went to work immediately.

Shelley took the plunge, signed on for my Double-0-2-3 No-Amylose Diet ... and soon began to shed the pounds that had been causing her so much torment. But hers was definitely not an "overnight success story." Indeed, it took Shelley a full year to recover her thinner, more attractive self.

As she got leaner, her self-esteem—along with her self-confidence—began to return ... along with the amorous interest of her husband.

Soon she felt so happy to be alive and so hopeful about the future that she—surprise! surprise!—became pregnant.

Of course, she's still got a long way to go before she can claim total victory in the Battle Against The Bulge.

Clearly, the final chapter of Shelley Spratt's story hasn't been written yet.

Still ... the fact that she learned how to control her obesity by controlling the kinds of foods she ate speaks *volumes* about my Glycemic Index–based strategy for healthier living!

She still does most of the cooking, but now Jack is happy to help the woman of his dreams around the house.

7

THE PSYCHOLOGY OF WEIGHT LOSS AND MAINTENANCE

Q. *How many psychiatrists does it take to change a light bulb?*

A. *Only one ... provided, of course, that the light bulb truly* wants *to change!*

After more than 20 years of helping patients lose weight, I'm convinced that the single most important word in the dieting dictionary is the word "attitude."

Like the light bulb in the famous joke about psychiatrists, any aspiring dieter who hopes for success must recognize the crucial significance of motivation, before setting out on this supremely challenging enterprise.

Sounds pretty simple, right?

But it isn't. And that's because—all too often—patients who struggle with obesity are also grappling with the problem of low self-esteem. Like that legendary seafarer, Odysseus, many of these unfortunates find themselves trapped between "Scylla and Charybdis"—between the terrible "monster of the rocks" that is overeating, and the devouring whirlpool that is lack of self-regard.

In this nightmarish scenario, low self-esteem sends the unhappy patient lurching into an eating binge, as the sufferer attempts to soothe painful emotions by ingesting what often ends up being a mountain of food. All too predictably, however, the ensuing weight-gain soon provokes feelings of guilt and self-disgust ... intensely negative feelings that further deplete the patient's dwindling fund of self-respect. The result is usually anger, frustration, increasing social isolation ("I can't attend that class reunion—I look like the Sta-Puff Marshmallow Man!") ... followed, in far too many cases, by the misery of clinical depression.

At first glance, the vicious cycle of overeating-followed-by-loss-of-self-esteem appears far too powerful—and too deeply ingrained—to overcome. How can the obese patient hope to survive the twin assaults of Scylla and Charbydis, after having lived for decades as a victim of both?

It's a foreboding prospect, you must admit. And the problem only gets worse for men and women who are subject to cyclical changes in mood. Women can often blame the second half of their menstrual cycle—the luteal phase—for their chocolate cravings and their amylose binging. But men are also affected by a cycle of hormone-linked feelings. Although subtler in its emotional effects, the male cycle also tends to promote binge behavior.

Eating recklessly, and without regard for adverse personal consequences, sounds like a "substance abuse" problem, doesn't it? And it is ... except that in this case, the substance is amylose. For that reason, those patients who are chemically (genetically?) predisposed toward dysfunctional eating *must* avoid amylose.

Believe it or not, however, there's a bright side to this terrifying problem—and its name, once again, is "attitude."

If you remember the "Odyssey," you no doubt recall that the cagey Odysseus survived his encounter with the Monster Twins by *using his cunning wits*!

In exactly the same way, my Double-0-2-3 No-Amylose Diet allows patients to circumvent the twin terrors of overeating and low self-esteem by first thinking about the problem—and then adjusting their attitude toward the food they eat.

Under my system, the patient's "attitude adjustment" starts during the very first office visit ... at the moment when I begin explaining how obesity is usually the result of genetic programming, and *not* the result of "lack of willpower" on the part of the patient.

I can't tell you how many times I've watched dieters weep with relief, or light up like Yankee Stadium during a night game, as they realized that their "weight problem" (all too often, it's actually their "substance abuse" problem) wasn't caused by moral turpitude or willful self-indulgence, but by genetically triggered insulin resistance, followed by rapid conversion of blood sugar into fatty acids.

Suddenly, a mountain of despair and self-hatred has been lifted from the shoulders of these long-suffering patients.

That's gratifying to watch. And then, while they're still exulting in the discovery that they aren't to blame for their obesity, I give them some *more* good news.

"You're not going to believe this," I tell them happily, "but the fact is that you're actually going to *enjoy* being on this diet!"

(This is the point where they start staring at me like I just got off the 3:40 Express from Planet Jupiter.)

"Dr. Shoemaker ... did I hear you correctly? Did you just say that I'm gonna enjoy being on a *diet*?"

"That's correct," I tell them with a bright smile. "First, I'm going to show you that it's not how *much* food you eat that matters —but what *kind* of food. Then I'm going to give you a list of hundreds of different foods that are perfectly safe under the rules of my diet.

"I'm going to encourage you to eat all of these foods you want [within reason, of course: no 'gorging' allowed!] ... and I'm even going to outfit you with a book of recipes. Get ready for some gourmet-cooking that will make mealtime a blast!"

(They're gaping at me now: *What galaxy hatched this madman, anyway?*)

But it's all true. And once I break it down for them ... by ex-plaining how such starchy foods as bread and pasta work to ele-vate blood sugar—thus triggering an inevitable Fat Attack—the light begins to dawn in the East, and the patient begins to feel some of the joy that goes with knowing: Dieting success is actually possible!

At some time or another, most dieters will challenge my ideas by their *actions*. Perhaps deep down, they don't really believe me. So one fine evening, they proceed to enjoy two jumbo-slices of pizza, with the crust. And guess what happens next? Their weight loss stops, that's what. They start retaining fluid and re-gaining the pounds they worked so hard to lose.

Then they wail at me: "I didn't do very well, doctor—I cheated."

"That's okay," I tell them. "Because what you've *actually* done is to prove to yourself that what I've been telling you is true. You can't afford the amylose. You can eat the pizza sauce and cheese —and you've done that safely in the past. But when it comes to amylose, you are genetically programmed—and you cannot eat the crust because you will store it as fat!

"Now, ask yourself: Who went with you to enjoy that pizza? Did *they* gain weight? No, they didn't. Look, I know that the bio-chemistry of insulin resistance isn't fair—but it's *real*, and you're stuck with it.

"What matters here isn't how *fast* you accept the reality, but that you do it eventually and then change your lifestyle for keeps. When that happens, you will get your weight under control once and for all!"

110

As I've said several times in this book, the good news for my LOSE THE WEIGHT YOU HATE! dieters is that instead of endlessly counting calories or weighing fat grams (or measuring food-portions), they're going to be free to embrace an entire *lifestyle*: a way of living that will bring them more energy and vitality than they've experienced in many years.

TEACHING THE "PSYCHOLOGY OF DIETING"

Spend a few days in my office in small-town Maryland, and you'll be struck by the upbeat—even joyful—atmosphere, as patients and medical staff alike celebrate the fact that losing weight can be an extremely uplifting experience.

Example: I'll never forget the moment that took place a few years ago, when one of the young medical interns who was doing a primary care "preceptorship" in my office spent a few hours in the waiting room (a great teaching technique, by the way), then told me with an astonished laugh: "Dr. Shoemaker ... I never expected to see this, but most of the patients in your weight-loss program are actually *happy*."

I still treasure that remark, because of the way it seemed to underline my primary goal as a healer: To help my patients find more joy and creative energy in their lives, by making them healthier!

As far as I'm concerned, the first step on the road to LOSING THE WEIGHT YOU HATE! is to understand the "psychological dynamics" that lie behind the behavioral aspects of obesity.

To achieve that goal, I break my weight-loss treatment program down into a series of bite-sized discussions—I call them "psychology modules"—in which the doctor and the patient talk about "underlying attitudes" toward food in the patient's life, and their crucial importance as factors contributing to obesity.

Here's a quick breakdown of how the process works, during the first five sessions with a new patient.

Session No. 1: In this session, the goal is to impart some basic knowledge about biochemistry as it relates to weight loss and maintenance. Among the topics I cover (in a light-hearted and easy to follow way) are the following:

O   Fat synthesis;

O   Insulin and how it works;

O   The Glycemic Index;

O   The relationship between protein-sparing and weight loss;

O   The key to successful maintenance;

O   The essentials of the Double-0-2-3 Diet;

O   Medical-legal issues (including informed consent).

Session No. 2: My second session with a weight-loss patient usually takes place two weeks after the first. During this exchange, the following tasks are accomplished:

O   Together, we review the patient's "biochemical profile," based on an earlier, intensive blood analysis.

O   Next, we examine and discuss the patient's "diet diary," which usually opens a window on his or her eating habits. During this session, the details of the 00-2-3 diet are custom-tailored to the patient's own particular biochemistry and psychological profile. For example: Most patients with normal or low insulin need only address their dysfunctional eating behaviors, in order to begin losing weight. On the other hand, those with elevated insulin levels will have to completely re-think their eating patterns and their assumptions about which foods are "okay" to eat. These patients need a new "Eating Lifestyle."

O   During this critically important session, patients will frequently respond to the hard facts about "high insulin" with resistance, denial or some other psychological defense mechanism. Conversely, others will express enormous relief,

112

while typically pointing out: "I knew something was wrong —even if I couldn't pinpoint it before!" (This insight will often empower patients to begin making the lifestyle changes necessary for weight-reduction. Let's face it: Nothing beats the truth!)

Session No. 3: About three weeks after their second meeting, patient and doctor sit down again to measure their progress. Among the usual highlights:

○ By this point, most patients have lost ten to twelve pounds of fat, and the first obvious changes in facial features are beginning to be noticed. Patients often tell me during this session: "I don't know how it happened ... but people keep telling me I look ten years younger!"

What's happening here, in most cases, is that the dieter on the 00-2-3 Program is now regaining lean body mass, after years of eating dysfunctionally. Remember: Effective weight loss isn't really measured in pounds, and the scales don't provide the key yardstick. The real indicator of success here is a change in the percentage of body fat, along with an increase in lean body mass and a reduction of hip and waist circumference. Measure the things that *matter*— and don't be fooled by the scales!

○ In order to reinforce their sense of accomplishment, I usually recommend that my patients have their pictures taken after this session.

○ Because many patients will express enthusiasm and hope during this session, I hammer hard at the idea of self-esteem. I make a point of congratulating the dieter ... and especially in cases where he or she is using a dieting aid such as Medifast™ or an appetite suppressant. In those situations, it's very important that dieters get the credit for doing the hard work involved in losing weight—instead of the dietary supplement!

○ This session also includes "special issues" ... such as the problems caused by potentially diet-wrecking friends and family, along with strategies for remaining on your diet while eating in a restaurant or participating in a family dinner during holidays.

Session No. 4: This session usually takes place during the eighth week of the weight-loss program. At this point, most patients have lost anywhere from 15 to 20 pounds, and their friends and fellow-workers have begun to look at them quite differently. They also find themselves out shopping a lot, as they buy new clothes that will better fit their shrinking frames. Among the subjects covered at this session are:

○ Dealing with the emotional turbulence brought on by sudden, dramatic weight-loss, as friends and family begin to interact with the dieter differently;

○ Preparing for the maintenance section of the program, as the 12-week weight-loss segment winds to a close;

○ Reviewing the reasons for the successful weight-loss, and emphasizing the need for continued vigilance and careful observation of all dietary rules.

Session No. 5: The fifth and final session takes place during the 12th week of the diet. In most cases, this last session seems anticlimactic, since the patient has already learned how to live the Double-0-2-3 Diet, and has fully accepted the idea that he or she must eat differently because of insulin resistance. Among the key steps during this session:

○ Doctor and patient briefly review the patient's daily eating habits and how they will continue indefinitely under the maintenance regimen;

○ The doctor schedules future appointments for those few patients who still require them, although most are now ready to launch the maintenance lifestyle without close supervision;

114

○ If the patient has been using appetite suppressants, the doctor will explain that they must now be terminated for at least three weeks (in order to allow the body to cleanse itself of them), before they can be used again. (In most cases, however, patients discover that if they will follow the 00-2-3 lifestyle closely, they will never need the appetite suppressants again.)

If the patient has been using Avandia *(see Chapter 13)* in a revolutionary new and genetically engineered approach to weight loss, additional blood work will be ordered, in order to make certain that no harm has been done to the liver and that all of the cholesterol parameters are improving.

○ The last session ends with a discussion of future plans, and a reminder that the doctor will always be available, should dysfunctional eating habits ever return. Hopefully, that won't happen, however—since the newly empowered patient now recognizes his or her responsibility to make sure maintenance goals are met!

So much for the session-by-session breakdown of Dr. Shoe's Melt-Your-Flab-Away Program. But one key question still remains: Once a patient has managed to shed the desired amount of weight, how difficult is it to prevent re-gain?

The answer, in a nutshell: Successful maintenance depends in large part on how quickly the dieter masters the principles that underlie the 00-2-3 det. And let's face it: after years of unsuccessful weight-loss attempts (with each failure causing additional damage to self-esteem and ego), many patients simply aren't psychologically prepared to face the real world with their new, slimmed-down shapes.

Not to worry, however: Experience shows that a high percentage of patients who regain five or more pounds within a month of ending their program with me will return for additional consultation, and usually within only two months.

When that happens, I try to use the first follow-up session to focus the re-gainer's attention and energy on re-establishing a restrictive diet.

Interestingly enough, I often find that these relapsed patients belong to the group that was reluctant to have blood work done or to keep a careful "diet diary," per my recommendations. In many cases, the re-gainers turn out to be folks who are also grappling with significant social stressors, and especially with personal conflicts in the home.

Unfortunately, even the most ambitious weight-loss program cannot address interpersonal problems of this kind. But my patients can and *do* learn how to confront life's stresses without resorting to dysfunctional eating—a victory that often leads to enhanced self-confidence and self-esteem.

Another goal of these follow-up sessions is to make sure the patient has not slipped back into believing the old myths that say "eat less, exercise more" is the key to weight loss.

To keep their eyes squarely on the target, I often remind such patients that their recent weight-gain took place because they started forgetting the key principles on which this diet is based. While remaining supportive and non-judgmental, I'll ask them directly: "Why do you think you gained that five pounds back? Haven't you learned yet that you can't get away with eating all that *lasagna*? Perhaps it's time to recognize the fact that your biochemistry isn't going to change. Nor will your special physiological gift for storing starch calories as fat!"

Like cigarette smokers—most of whom fail repeatedly before finally kicking the habit—a high percentage of weight-loss patients find that they need several "tune up" sessions before they finally get it right. And that's fine with me. As I'm fond of telling them: "I don't care *when* you make up your mind to keep this weight off; I just want to make sure that when you're truly ready, you *succeed* in the attempt."

It's also true, of course, that a few patients will not succeed in maintaining weight loss, period. In many cases, these unfortunates are people whose egos have been damaged by a loved one, usually as the result of a painful conflict. This state of affairs is regrettable ... but even in these lamentable cases, I refuse to give up hope. Miracles do happen now and then, and I've also learned over the years that even the most injured patients can be helped significantly—if the doctor is careful to provide support without becoming critical or disapproving.

It's an unhappy fact of life: Not every patient will be able to maintain weight loss. Yet I'm always thrilled to remember that in my own practice, more than 70 percent of those who follow the 00-2-3 program really do succeed in eliminating their obesity and then going on to lead healthier, more energetic lives!

REAL PEOPLE, REAL STORIES

CASE STUDY NO. 3: MISS MARTHA'S HYPOTHALAMUS

Her name was "Miss Martha"—and she stormed into my office like one of those howling "northeasters" for which our Chesapeake Bay region is so famous.

"Dr. Shoemaker," she roared at me, "I can't *stand* it anymore. I want the weight off—and I want it off *now!*"

It took me two or three minutes, but I finally managed to calm her down. Then I settled back to listen. Miss Martha had an amazing story to tell ... the story of a 45-year-old woman who had been struggling to control her eating patterns for more than a decade and a half.

As it turned out, Miss Martha was a classic "Yo-Yo Dieter." Perpetually overweight, she would periodically starve herself until she had lost 25 pounds. That painful strategy would take her down to 139, which she regarded as the "ideal weight" for her size and frame.

Within a few days of her achieving her goal, however, the unfortunate Miss Martha would get walloped once again by the Yo-Yo.

For reasons that she couldn't understand, she would take off on eating sprees that ran completely out of control. All too often, these sprees would be set off by eating a single slice of bread ... and they wouldn't let up until she'd gained most of the 25 pounds back.

119

In medical terms, Miss Martha's problem was the result of hyper-activity in her hypothalamus—a tiny gland, located deep inside the brain, which performs many tasks related to metabolism. Specifically, her obesity was linked to over-activity of the ventral lateral nucleus (VLN) ... an area of the hypothalamus which serves as the "hunger center" and thus controls appetite.

Like many other metabolic processes, the activities of the VLN are keyed to changes in the level of blood sugar. Any sudden drop in blood glucose will "turn on" the VLN, which then powerfully stimulates the appetite and often leads to over-eating. (And that's precisely why my "00-2-3 Diet" is designed to *prevent* such rapid falls of blood sugar!)

Once Martha turned on her hypothalamus by eating food containing amylose (a bagel, for instance, or a ripe banana), she became ravenous. Why? It happened because, as her blood sugar soared, her insulin level rose quickly, and then her blood sugar level began to *fall* rapidly—an event which soon clicked on her hunger center.

In Martha's case, the actual culprit was the rapid rise in blood sugar following a meal containing amylose. That rise triggered the insulin surge, and the resulting dropoff in her blood sugar soon led to the release of several key hormones (known as the "counter-regulatory" hormones), such as glucagon and epinephrine. These organic agents boosted the glucose in her blood, countering the insulin effect—but that quick boost was accompanied by predictable symptoms that the counter-regulatory hormones cause, symptoms that were instantly, but mistakenly diagnosed as "hypoglycemia" by the doctors who were trying to help her.

Of course, these counter-regulatory hormones produce some marked biochemical effects of their own that cause the "hypoglycemia" symptoms. For example: Patients scheduled for a colonoscopy examination of their intestinal tract are often given an injection of glucagon in order to "dry up" potentially disruptive secretions in the bowel. Quite often, these patients will then complain of feeling "queasy" and slightly nauseated, even as their skin begins to feel "clammy." In the same way, patients who receive shots of epinephrine often break into a "cold sweat," while also complaining of feeling "light-headed." (These complaints are alarming, by the way, and in a few unfortunate victims, cause the physician to react by ordering misguided tests like a "5 hour glucose tolerance (GTT) test." Fortunately, an important position paper that appeared in the New England Journal of Medicine put an end to most of the egregious GTT orders.

It took only a few minutes and a few simple lab tests to determine that Miss Martha's obesity was the result of sharp fluctuations in her blood glucose levels—and that those surges had been turning on her hypothalamic eating centers, and thus triggering the eating binges. Happily, my 00-2-3 diet helped her to shut down the elevator and thus to turn off the biochemical cascade that leads to fatty acid–manufacture and eventually to fat storage

Although she didn't meet the medical criteria for the eating disorder known as "bulimia" (she never purged, for example), her eating sprees were awesome to watch. As she told me during our first meeting: "I can buzz through four or five doughnuts before I even taste the first one!"

It didn't take me long to convince Miss Martha that the key to avoiding the binges was to "turn off" the "insulin response"— and thus to shut down the hunger-provoking enzymatic activity of her hypothalamus.

To achieve that goal, I quickly put her on the 00-2-3 diet, which reduces glucose-intake and eliminates amylose from the diet entirely.

The results were impressive, to say the least. As she began to shed her flab, Martha's frequent episodes of "feeling bad" became less frequent. And the palpitations, cold sweats, nausea and dizziness which had accompanied those episodes gradually disappeared.

All too often, Miss Martha's "attacks" (they usually followed an amylose- or glucose-loaded meal) had been repeatedly called hypoglycemia by her multiple prior physicians, even though her lowest glucose never dropped below 75—well within the normal range—during these years of "Yo-Yoing."

Now 50 years old, Miss Martha has dropped below her 139-pound "ideal weight." She controls her hunger by eating several small meals each day, and by avoiding amylose. And she no longer rides the Dieting Yo-Yo several times each year.

Ask her to describe the effect of the Shoemaker Diet on her life, and this hard-charging university secretary won't miss a beat. "I've never felt better in my life," says Miss Martha. "I'm the living proof that the Yo-Yo doesn't have to defeat you.

"The key to success is to make sure you know exactly what you're eating—and then to avoid the stuff that sets off the surge in blood sugar."

8

ACHIEVING MAINTENANCE OR ... "THIS ISN'T A DIET— IT'S A LIFESTYLE!"

Question for Successful Dieters: Is there any joy on earth like the joy of slipping into a 20-year-old bathing suit ... without hearing the sound of groaning, protesting fabric?

Second Question for Successful Dieters: Now that you've achieved the weight-loss goals you established for yourself 12 weeks ago, how are you going to keep that unsightly flab from returning?

For weight-watchers everywhere, the good-news answer to Query #2 is that you *can* design and maintain a lifestyle guaranteed to keep you looking slim and also vibrating with newfound energy. How? In this chapter, we're going to take a close look at the Essentials of Maintenance—the key strategies that lie at the heart of my program for joyful, creative and flab-free living.

YOU RANG, DR. PAVLOV?

In order to understand the psychology of successful weight-maintenance, let's take a step back for a moment and think about a very interesting household pet—a loyal and thoroughly predictable canine known as "Pavlov's Dog."

As you probably recall, Dr. Ivan Petrovitch Pavlov was a Russian scientist who won the 1904 Nobel Prize in Medicine for his groundbreaking research on how living beings often respond to "environmental cues" without even knowing it.

In order to study "unconscious responses" to external stimuli, the clever Dr. Pavlov created an experiment in which a dozen hungry dogs were allowed to chow down only after a loud bell was rung.

It took the dogs about 45 seconds to figure out the drill: *When I hear the ding-dong, it's Alpo-time!*

After his dogs had been fully "conditioned" in this manner, the good Dr. Pavlov made a startling observation: Whenever the bell rang, the barking mutts would begin to salivate ... even when their expected food never arrived.

In scientific terms, the dogs had come to "associate" the ringing of the bell with being fed, and their bodies responded accordingly: When the bell chimed, they drooled!

Thank you, Dr. Pavlov, for providing millions of dieters with a crucial lesson:

○ If you're going to keep the weight you've lost from returning, you must become conscious of the "environmental eating cues" that trigger your own tendency to load up on fat-building glucose and amylose.

WHEN IN DOUBT, SLAP A STICKER ON IT!

According to scientific researchers, one of the most important eating cues is location—any physical space (whether at home or at work) in which you have grown accustomed to wolfing potato chips and cheese doodles, while downing endless Nehi belly washers and burping contentedly.

Think about it for a moment. Do you have a favorite "snacking hideaway?" What about that plump-pillowed easy chair in the Rec Room ... the one located exactly ten feet from the jumbo-sized Color Zenith?

Or are you a Secret Auto Snacker ... one of those shadowy, elusive figures who spends at least an hour each day zipping up anonymously to fastfood drive-in windows, then cruising the streets with an open 20-piece box of Chicken Nuggets on the passenger seat and a bubbly Choco-Shake clutched in your steering wheel-hand as you zoom along?

If you think about your snacking binges, you'll soon discover that they usually take place in few predictable locations.

So how can we become more conscious of our eating patterns, each time we respond to an "environmental cue" from the surrounding landscape?

One helpful approach can be found in my smoking cessation program, during which I routinely ask patients to slap a fluorescent orange sticker on areas where they frequently smoke cigarettes. Within a few days, the stickers blossom near telephones, on auto dashboards, beside the coffee pot and in many other locales where the urge to puff on the weed often breaks out. The stickers carry the patient's initials, along with the phrase: "I WON'T SMOKE HERE!"

If you plant a big, dayglo-hued sticker on that easy chair, you'll instantly create a "Snack-Binge No-Fly Zone" ... making it much more difficult to sit there with an open package of Ranch-Flavored Chipsy-Doodles in your hand. (After all, you gave your word that you wouldn't eat in the Orange Sticker Neighborhood!)

GETTING PAST "TRANSITION TIME"

Another environmental cue for starch-snacking takes place during key moments of the day ... moments in which we are emotionally vulnerable to these cues because of fatigue, anxiety or other emotional states linked to shifts in our daily activities.

One of the most challenging of these "transition times" is the arrival home from work each day. With dinnertime still an hour away and snack-foods crooning like golden-haired sirens from counter tops and cabinet shelves, is it any wonder that so many of us wind up neck-deep in Goldfish crackers and foaming root beer ... or that this snacking behavior actually makes us eat *more* at the meal that follows?

During two decades of counseling weight-loss patients, I've learned that a high percentage of diet-failures occur during the interval between dinner and bedtime. "I do fine during the day," many patients have told me, "but at night, I just can't stop eating!"

Whenever I hear that line, I ask them: "Okay, but what was in that dinner you ate? Did it contain bread or pasta or rice or potatoes—or even worse, *several* of those high-amylose foods at once? If so, is it any wonder that your insulin/counter-regulatory hormone responses drove you to snack relentlessly before you finally hit the sheets?" That snack-generating evening meal costs even more if you had a sandwich for lunch or a few cookies at the mid-afternoon break (call it the second meal effect when you talk to the bariatricians about it).

Another especially threatening transition for the dieter is the shift from family time to bedtime. How can we really hope to get a decent night's sleep, without first downing a massive slab of Aunt Nellie's Crumbly Peach Pie and a glass of ice-cold milk?

The bottom line is simple. Because most of us are especially vulnerable to these "transition attacks" and "environmental cues," we must learn to recognize and anticipate both. One helpful strategy is to prepare a healthy (and tasty) snack-food in advance of any situation where you fear that your hand may stray toward that box of Cheddar Nips or that cellophane bag of *guacamole* chips. Another is to make sure that you have something interesting to do waiting for you at home (check the African violets, feed the tropical fish, talk to your family about what they learned in school this week), and if nothing appeals to you, maybe this is the time to go for a walk with your spouse and say hello to your neighbors.

Just remember: If you eat Transition Foods, select them carefully (translation: no glucose or amylose!), so you should be able to eat them without worrying that you're back on the road to Fat Oblivion.

The next step in the Shoemaker Strategy is designed to blunt the kind of response that good old Dr. Pavlov observed in his dogs ... by teaching yourself to respond to the environmental or transitional cue by *reaching for the prepared snack, instead of the crackers or chips.*

One very good approach to this problem, obviously, is to avoid buying the chips, crackers and other amylose-loaded goodies in the first place—by learning how to "shop the perimeter" of your local supermarket, rather than falling prey to all those mouth-watering displays of delectable snack-foods at the center of the shopping-action! Most grocery stores will place their produce, meat and dairy goods—along with frozen foods—along the outside walls of the store. The inner aisles, meanwhile, are jammed with hidden land mines—with dietary danger-zones full of bread, pasta, processed foods, syrup-laden fruit and sugar-added cans of soup, among many other fat-making foods. If your grocery store manager has figured out your shopping strategy and plants the fresh bread displays in your carefully selected path, just laugh and keep on walking.

GETTING OUT OF THE FAST LANE

Another key step on the road to weight-loss is learning how to practice better "time management," so that you can stop running from stoplight to school to playing field to music lessons and back to stoplight long enough to feed yourself the foods that will best protect your health.

When it comes to the art of preparing healthy meals, we can take another lesson from that ancient Chinese philosopher, Lao-Tze, who summarized his philosophy for successful living in a pithy apothegm: "Make haste *slowly!*"

For millions of Americans today, life in the "fast lane" simply means life in the "stress lane," as we race from one frenetic, nerve-jangling deadline to the next. Ask yourself: Is it any wonder that half the nation now takes tranquilizers of one kind or another (along with acid-blockers designed to ease the agony of peptic ulcer disease) every hour *on* the hour?

And what shall we make of the weirdly paradoxical fact that we keep getting fatter and fatter ... even as the speed at which we live increases day by day?

I say it's time to write ourselves a National Speeding Ticket, and then to begin scrutinizing our behavior—especially in the kitchen, where such culinary horrors as the "Frozen Diet Mexican *Jalapeno* Chili And Fried Ice Cream TV Dinner" long ago became standard fare for millions of nutritionally deformed Americans.

My solution: Why not spend a few of the hours we normally reserve for the Boob Tube in the *kitchen*, learning about good nutrition? Or maybe you could take the kids on a jaunt through a supermarket—while pretending that you're on a school field trip to a science lab? (Remember: the key to better nutrition is gaining accurate knowledge about the food you're putting in your mouth!)

Don't make the mistake of preaching this sermon to the typical single mother, however, or she'll quickly inform you that working two jobs and raising two demanding kids by herself leaves precious little time for the Tube—or anything else! Instead of preaching, look for every possible way to help her ... perhaps with medications, and perhaps also with lifestyle modifications.

After more than 20 years of counseling overweight moms and pops, I'm convinced that most of us can find the relatively few minutes required to make healthier eating choices. And those choices will be easier still, if we can keep track of our daily food intake by maintaining a "diet diary" from one week to the next.

What about those women who must struggle with such issues as weight-gain during and after pregnancy?

When it comes to the special nutritional problems of these brave souls, we must be careful to remember that pregnancy often triggers a massive surge in placental hormones that act exactly like insulin in the bloodstream. The problem of weight gain in pregnancy can be compounded by development of diabetes in some women (resistin again?)

Such high-powered hormones as chorionic gonadatrophin and placental lactogen help regulate the growth of the fetus—while also boosting cellular uptake of glucose. (That's why expectant mothers often report that they feel "starved" ... and why they tend to snack relentlessly while carrying their infants to term.)

The greatest challenge faced by these mothers-to-be can be found in the fact that their surging hormones often cause blood sugar-levels to drop precipitously. These patients must eat, eat, eat.

In too many cases, however, the exaggerated feeding behavior caused by the hormonal activity will culminate in subsequent weight-gain for the new mother. That happens primarily because mom's cells, freed from the task of pulling in extra glucose to feed the developing child, quickly begin making fat instead. Is it any accident that a high percentage of my new weight-loss patients come from the ranks of new mothers? When I hear "I gained all my weight in my last pregnancy and I can't take it off," it is time to get out the day-glo stickers again to help deal with the learned eating habits forced on Mom by the hormones of pregnancy must be re-learned.

Although many women are concerned about timing of pregnancy and they are prescribed "hormone therapy," research shows that hormones such as unopposed progesterone treatments to prevent conception often cause unnecessary weight-gain. Just ask the women who spent over $1,000 each for implantable contraceptives about this problem—and many will tell you how they gained 25 pounds or more.

OBESITY: AN EQUAL-OPPORTUNITY ILLNESS

Sure, many pregnant women do wind up gaining extra weight, but the twin problems of over-eating and resulting obesity are by no means limited to these moms-to-be. For many men aged 35–45 (and especially those who were active in sports), growing fat in middle age seems to be an inescapable fate ... and especially in a culture where males so frequently play an under-active role in purchasing and preparing food.

For the beer-quaffing and snack foods-by-the-handful-devouring menfolk who watch NFL football every Sunday afternoon, the challenge of slimming down becomes doubly difficult—once they begin to realize that it will probably involve learning how to cook, and even learning how to shop for nutritional foods at the supermarket!

Yet the news is also good, even for these culinary unfortunates ... many of whom tell me that they experience a wonderful feeling of liberation when I tell them: "My friend, it's high time you learned how to *cook*!"

Along with these struggling menfolk, several other groups of "nutritionally challenged" citizens frequently find that they face a formidable challenge, once they decide to get their eating habits under control. For those struggling with diabetes, elevated cholesterol, high blood pressure or pain from degenerative arthritis in weight-bearing joints, the task of avoiding fat-building foods often seems especially difficult.

Among these long suffering patients, no group faces more harrowing obstacles than the adult-onset (Type II) diabetics, whose disorder—lack of proper insulin effect required to move blood sugar in and out of cells—rarely improves from day to day. As I've told a thousand diabetic patients in recent years: "You have to remember that diabetes doesn't care if you're sitting at a fancy restaurant or attending a gala cocktail party with a corporate president. Regardless of the social setting, if you make a dietary mistake, you're going to *pay!*"

THE WORKPLACE: A "HAZARDOUS EATING" ZONE?

Although many dieters don't realize it at first, one of the most hazardous environments on earth (when it comes to weight-gain) is the ordinary American workplace.

If you want to understand what I mean, just pause for a moment to draw up a mental picture of daily life in your office. If you're like most Americans in today's Flying Fastfood Circus, your mental picture probably includes the following:

O A bright pink cardboard box, crusted with powdered sugar and marked: *Dunkin' Donuts;*

O A softball-sized pasteboard container that bears the immortal American legend: *Big Mac*;

O A cellophane bag the size of a bedroom pillow, overflowing with orange-hued fried corn twists known as *Chee-zee Delites*;

O Enough Candy Kisses, Reese's Pieces and Tootsie Rolls to completely outfit a Halloween trick-or-treater.

O Where are we going to order our lunch today? Are we going after the pizza from the bowling alley ... or the bread and turkey sub from the mega-roll lunch provider?

What is it about "work," anyway, that makes people so eager to vacuum up every easily worn carbohydrate in the neighborhood? Whenever I ask myself this question, I remember how the owner of a local beauty shop sent me six of her employees a few years ago. Happily, all six met their weight-loss goals. But they were soon back in my office, seeking additional help ... because the boss had failed to halt her long-standing practice of hauling doughnuts, sandwiches, cookies and potato chips into the shop so that "her girls" would have something to "nibble on" during the long workday.

That problem was fairly easy to fix (the beauticians were soon munching on apples slices and dried apricots, instead of chips). But what do you tell a harried employee—a marketing executive, let's say—who must attend sales dinners and receptions and "cocktail hours" day in and day out? For these calorie-challenged individuals, eating too much glucose and amylose represents nothing less than a "workplace hazard."

In order to reduce their exposure to these fat-triggering substances, I urge patients who work in such over-fed settings to follow a few tips.

Example No. 1: Instead of eating the amylose-loaded sandwich that you felt compelled to order while hosting an important client at lunch, just eat the filling! You won't lose the sale if you're "allergic to bread." Who knows, you might launch a fascinating discussion of gluten and amylose, and thus show off your encyclopedic knowledge of fat manufacture!

Example No. 2: If you're being pressured to dig into the baked lasagna (from Sysco, no doubt) at the Company Office Party, explain to one and all that you're saddled with "a different biochemistry than other people ... and darn it, it just isn't fair!" In most cases, you'll find that your fellow-revelers immediately begin to sympathize—even as they start easing up on the culinary pressure.

Example No. 3: Start actively throwing up, the moment the boss' wife demands that you eat a slice of her raspberry jam walnut tort with whipped cream. No, on second thought ... maybe you better eat that dessert (it probably came from Sysco as well), and add three more days to the length of your diet. On the other hand, if you have a job already lined up somewhere else ... well, I better leave that decision up to you!

OVEREATING: TOO OFTEN, IT'S A "FAMILY AFFAIR"

Another major threat to the nutritional safety of weight-loss patients often lurks in an unlikely-sounding and yet common setting: the family gathering.

Ask yourself: Is there any social pressure on earth quite as fierce as the pressure that radiates from beaming Aunt Clara, at the moment when she pleads with you to sample her "Prizewinning Mississippi Mud Caramelized Pecan Pie?" The solution: Tell her that you know she'll understand—sensitive lady that she is!—the fact that your dietitian has laid down the law, and that eating her Pie could seriously jeopardize your health. (It's the *truth*, after all!)

Then stand firm. Remember that you are not obligated to eat foods you don't want in order to satisfy someone else's emotional needs. Learn from Shakespeare's Polonius, who offers the dedicated dieter some very useful advice in *Hamlet*: "To thine own [nutritional] self be true!"

Remember, also, that family gatherings are usually diet-killers. "Did you get enough to eat?" is a standard after-dinner question. Just look at how the media glamorize and hype the act of overeating. Have you seen the one where everyone is eating too much at the Olive Garden Restaurant ... everybody from the blushing bride to the beaming grandfather? And what about those "All You Can Eat!" pitches from the Red Lobster (Fried Everything —And Don't Forget the Unlimited Hush Puppies!)?

What else would you expect, really, from a country that celebrates a *national holiday* in honor of binge-eating? (It's called Thanksgiving.)

"Oh, why not? You only live once!" Maybe so, but does "living once" have to mean dieting the rest of the year?

This family diet-sabotage often involves simple jealousy, even if no one will admit it. "I was always thin, and she was always fat! And now she thinks she can one-up me, does she? Madeline, have another croissant! I'm sure it won't upset this strange new diet of yours!"

There's no doubt that families in this culture express love with food. And who can turn down expressions of love from loved ones?

In most families, telling "too much truth" is not only politically incorrect—it can get you banished from the next holiday celebration! But the truth is best. "Aunt Maude, you know I'm on a diet that doesn't let me eat amylose—and here you are, insisting that I eat this herb bread that you baked just for me!"

Sometimes, of course, you might have to eat a little herb bread to keep peace in the family. Just remember, on those occasions, that this capitulation will cost you some extra time on your diet.

AMYLOSE: HOW MUCH IS TOO MUCH?

The first thing to understand—when thinking about daily amylose-intake during the maintenance phase of my program—is that safe amounts will vary from person to person, depending on insulin levels. Here are some other considerations that you should keep in mind, while figuring out the correct amylose-limit for your particular situation:

○ The fasting insulin level, measured by a blood test, is controlled genetically, and while it cannot be reduced below its genetically programmed level by diet, weight loss or wishful thinking, it can be raised artificially by overeating or eating dysfunctionally. Remember to divide the number 70 by your fasting insulin level. The quotient you get will tell you number of servings of amylose you're allowed, per week.

○ If your insulin level exceeds 30, you are permitted only two servings of amylose. (Remember that a "serving" includes only a single sandwich or muffin or potato—not an entire plate full of starches!)

○ Patients with insulin levels in excess of 20 should allow themselves no more than three servings of amylose per week.

○ If your level is 15 or under, you can safely permit yourself one serving of plant starch every other day.

○ Those patients with insulin levels of 10 or less can enjoy up to one amylose-serving per day. For those with levels lower than 10, experience shows that being overweight is usually the result of "sloppy" eating habits. In this one case, "more exercises and fewer calories" is, indeed, the correct prescription for weight loss.

But these 10-and-unders are a decided minority; my clinical research shows that 95 percent of my weight-loss patients became fat because they ate too much amylose, period.

The good news for obese patients everywhere is that they can learn to "count amylose" quite easily during my 12-week program. Most patients are also thrilled to discover that they feel much better—more energetic and alive—after only a few weeks of avoiding fat-triggering foods. In many cases, I've also learned, sticking "before and after" pictures of the dieter near the bread-and cracker-jammed pantry can be quite helpful in fending off sudden amylose attacks!

Most important of all, perhaps, is the encouragement that a successful weight-loss patient often receives from family, friends, and also his or her beaming physician.

I can't tell you how many times I've enjoyed the sight of watching a weight-loss patient smile as big as the full moon, after hearing me tell her the simple truth: "Say ... you look *terrific!*"

MAINTENANCE FOOD CHOICES

The maintenance diet is different from the weight-loss diet. Depending on the patient's insulin level, amylose can be added. The number of weekly amylose-servings that can be "safely" eaten without significant regain of weight is your fasting insulin divided into 70.

The following "diet diary" reflects the food choices made by an individual with an insulin level of 10. This person was able to eat one serving of amylose a day without regain.

The food choices in the diary are featured in the recipe section, but I want to emphasize here that each of these meals was inspired by my "living-life-fully" principle of healthy eating. Food should be plentiful, prepared well, spiced properly and served attractively—so that it provides a pleasing backdrop for conversation.

Please take a close look at the amylose selections in the diary … and don't forget that these meals can also be enjoying during the weight-loss phase of my program—provided that all of the amylose is eliminated.

MAINTENANCE MENU—ONE AMYLOSE DAILY

Sunday
Breakfast

> Sliced strawberries, pineapple, kiwi
> Freshly squeezed orange juice

Lunch

> Clam chowder with scallions
> Spinach salad with red peppers, blue cheese,
> Spanish onions, mushrooms
> Rounds of thick crusted Greek bread

Snack

> Tortilla chips with melted cheese

Supper

> Slow-baked turkey breast
> Smoked oysters, chick peas, onion,
> mandarin orange stuffing
> Steamed asparagus with hollandaise sauce
> Romaine lettuce salad, parmesan cheese; oil and vinegar
> Cantaloupe and blueberries
> White wine

Monday
Breakfast

> Mushrooms, red pepper (from salad night before)
> and cheddar cheese omelet

Lunch

Sliced turkey, letovers go "in the lunch box"
Apple slices

Snack

Tray of pickles, smoked oysters, artichoke hearts, cheese

Supper

Hamburger cooked on the grill
Garlic bread
Broccoli
Spinach salad with feta, black olives
and sliced cherry tomatoes
Iced tea with lemon

Tuesday

Breakfast

Sausage and hominy

Lunch

Chef salad, oil and vinegar

Supper

Sweet-and-sour chicken with fried rice
Egg rolls

Dessert

Frozen raspberries

Wednesday

Breakfast

Grapefruit
Cantaloupe slices

Lunch

Sliced turkey, still tastes great
Romaine lettuce salad with Parmesan, oil and vinegar

Snack

Popcorn

Supper

Eye of round
Oven-baked potato wedges
Cole slaw

Dessert

Kiwi, honeydew, seedless red grapes

Thursday

Breakfast

Raisins, dried apricots, shelled sunflower seeds,
cashews and plain, low corn syrup yogurt

Lunch

Grilled chicken breast
Spinach salad with pineapple chunks, mushrooms
and papaya slices

Supper

> Steamed clams, sesame shrimp
> Corn on the cob

Dessert

> Blueberry pie (hot recipe pie crust)

Friday

Breakfast

> Huevos rancheros
> Tomato juice
> Cantaloupe slices

Lunch

> Chick peas, olives, turkey chunks, artichoke hearts,
> green peppers

Snack

> Tortilla chips with salsa

Supper

> Zucchini, cheese, sweet Italian sausage casserole
> Homemade French bread

Saturday

Breakfast

> Princess Anne goop, with the special stomach
> settler, santolina

Lunch

Apple, cheese, pickle

Supper

Oysters Rockefeller
Smoked roast beef
Vegetable salad with cauliflower, yellow peppers,
pimentos and green olives

Dessert

Raspberry sorbet

CASE STUDY: FATTY LIVER

Sarah Roses didn't drink alcohol, didn't smoke either. She liked cereal for breakfast, a sandwich for lunch and potatoes with her supper. Her HMO physician had sent her to a gastroenterologist to have additional work up done on her liver because her blood tests showed abnormally high liver enzyme levels. No obvious cause was found.

The gastroenterologist performed a colonoscopy and a stomach scoping, with lots more blood work, but still no cause was found. Ms. Roses needed a liver biopsy to find out what was wrong. Fortunately, the biopsy only showed fat deposits in her liver. Unfortunately, the fatty liver can be serious, possibly causing cirrhosis.

Ms. Roses weighed 210 pounds. She was 5' 2" tall with a waist of 39" and hips of 42". She had classic truncal obesity, usually seen in men. I knew from looking at her that her liver problem was simply due to hyperinsulinemia. Sure enough, her insulin was 23 and her GGTP, a pertinent liver test, was 255, six times normal.

Sarah lost 45 pounds in 18 weeks, using thiazolidinedione medications (the new ones are safe for livers) and the No–Amylose diet. She looked great and felt great. She learned to live without amylose and didn't miss it.

She came to her last office visit looking like Gary Cooper in "High Noon." "Well, did my liver improve?" Yes, it had. Her GGTP was 23 and her other liver function tests were normal. What a relief! The diet saved her liver.

143

I see these stories every day, only one of 10,000 in the Fat City. When insulin levels are over 20, fat frequently is stored in the liver. The No-Amylose diet mobilizes fat from liver fast. Reduce the insulin storage effect and watch the healing begin.

Sarah's mother, Pansy heard about this magical cure. Pansy had Type I diabetes. She needed insulin shots to stay alive. Even worse, Pansy was losing a tremendous amount of protein in her urine. She had markedly abnormal liver tests, worse than Sarah's. The same gastroenterologist had done a liver biopsy, confirming a diagnosis of "nonalcoholic steatohepatitis, with nephrotic syndrome." She didn't feel well at all and certainly couldn't say her diagnosis twice quickly. Fatty liver is easier to say.

Pansy tried the No-Amylose diet, with extra protein added to balance the amount lost in the urine. This is another success story. Pansy watched her insulin doses carefully, discarded her ADA diet, and with very close careful medical supervision, was rewarded by an unbelievable improvement in liver and kidney function.

Coincidence perhaps? In an experiment in nature, Pansy went back to her old diet. You guessed it, her previous world class elevation of GGTP began to return. Stop the bread, the pasta and the rice! Her liver tests went back to normal again. No, this isn't coincidence. The deposition of fat in livers of non-alcoholics responds beautifully to the 00-2-3, No-Amylose, protein-sparing diet.

9

APPETITE SUPPRESSANTS: PROCEED WITH CAUTION!

The house lights dim, and the audience quickly falls silent.

It's showtime!

Good evening, ladies and gentlemen, and welcome to the mysterious, flickering world of Dr. Presto, the spell-binding magician of the instantaneous weight-loss!

Tonight, before your very eyes, Dr. Presto will cast his spell over an obese patient, then ask him to swallow a magical potion that will result— ka-POOOOF!—in a sudden weight-loss of more than 30 pounds!

o   o   o

Wouldn't it be wonderful if medical doctors could actually prescribe "magical potions" that would cause patients to lose weight overnight ... and then to *keep* it off?

145

Wouldn't it be terrific if those of us who struggle year in and year out with the threat of obesity could swallow a pill, or boil a herb, or maybe even synthesize a new gene in order to make losing weight easy?

(And while we're dreaming a little bit … how about a scenario in which the genetically based illness known as "obesity" spontaneously cures itself and vanishes from the long list of human diseases?)

Sorry, friends, but the answer to all three of those questions is: "No such luck." Magical thinking of this kind has no place in a science-based weight-loss program!

After 20 years of leading patients through successful dieting and maintenance programs, I can tell you with complete certainty that achieving sustained weight-loss always requires them to change both their eating behaviors and the kinds of foods they daily consume … based on their genetically programmed ability to store starch calories as fat.

There's nothing magical or mysterious about the key ingredient necessary for dieting success—the willingness to stop eating those foods which trigger fat storage in the human body. As many sadder-but-wiser health care consumers have learned in recent years, merely swallowing a pill daily can never substitute for the careful, thoughtful process of changing lifestyles and eating habits in order to become slimmer and healthier.

Thankfully, losing weight and keeping it off doesn't require any hocus-pocus from *Dr. Presto*!

But does this mean that there's no place at all for the many powerful diet-drugs that have been developed by the pharmaceutical industry in recent years?

Of course not.

As you're about to discover in this chapter, "appetite suppressants" (the most common type of dieting medication, by far) can be quite helpful to dieters who wish to lose weight faster than would be possible by controlling food intake, alone. That's because many patients who have struggled and failed to lose weight on their own simply need a "jump start" in order to shake off that extra poundage.

In other words, these valuable dieting tools—when *properly* prescribed in a carefully monitored clinical setting—can speed up a weight-loss program considerably. As with any medication, however, there's a price to be paid for this biochemical assistance, and its name is: "side effects."

In order to understand how the appetite suppressants work and the risks involved in using them, we need to step back for a moment and take a look at a few of the well-known dieting drugs that have dominated the U.S. weight-loss industry in recent years.

FENFLURAMINE AND PHENTERMINE: LESSONS FROM THE CONTROVERSY

If you're like most Americans today, you probably remember the alarming news stories about a "miracle" combination of dieting drugs, "fen-phen," that had proved amazingly successful at helping its users to lose weight ... until a shocking 1997 report by researchers at the Mayo Clinic suggested that the "fen" (and its cousin, dexfenfluramine, Redux) might have caused abnormalities in the heart valve structure of many patients, along with being implicated in at least one death.

Soon after that disclosure, America's plaintiff lawyers moved in for the kill. Before they finished their work, the pharmaceutical companies had reportedly agreed to a $5 billion national settlement ... an agreement that took place after they apparently convinced the court that American Home Corporation had knowingly withheld information about the safety of taking Redux and fenfluramine, according to later published reports.

Were the health claims regarding fen-phen substantiated by

clinical experience? No. But you wouldn't have known that from the media hype that has surrounded this issue—a firestorm that left many Americans with the exaggerated impression that the fen-phen combo of weight-loss drugs were a single deadly substance!

In fact, the fen-phen regimen that was used by millions of Americans during the early 1990s actually consisted of two different drugs: fenfluramine (sold as Pondimin™, and later pulled from the market) and FDA-approved phentermine (still on the market). These two chemical substances worked effectively to suppress hunger-impulses in the hypothalamus of the human brain.

As it turns out, both drugs had been prescribed routinely by U.S. weight-loss physicians for many 20 years.

But that scenario changed fast during the late 1990s, as the U.S. Food and Drug Administration (FDA) made headlines all around the country by yanking both Pondimin (fenfluramine) and dexfenfluramine (Redux™) from the American market—after concluding that they posed significant health dangers for the millions of dieters who had been using them. (Phentermine remains FDA-approved to this day.)

Although some health researchers initially classified both fenfluramine and phentermine among their more powerful cousins, the amphetamines, later studies showed that fen-phen actually works on a different principle than the infamous "speed" pills of earlier dieting eras. Extremely potent, amphetamines continue to be used today to treat severe behavioral disturbances, chronic fatigue syndrome and attention deficit. These substances, which "turn on" the brain's satiety center and thus reduce appetite, are also subject to abuse by drug-takers in search of the high-energy "rush" that they provide—before causing the abusers to "crash," sometimes into severe depression and even psychosis.

Fortunately, however, both fenfluramine and phentermine possess far less addictive firepower than amphetamines and thus lack the potential for illicit use.

Available under several brand names, phentermine and several related medications have been sold generically for 40 years. This drug works to suppress the hunger center in the hypothalamus, part of the central nervous system. Millions of women who had babies during the 1960s and 1970s will probably recall how their obstetricians routinely recommended phentermine to prevent weight gain after delivery, and also as a pharmaceutical magic agent that would stop the "postpartum blues" in their tracks. Fortunately, however, such cavalier and no-questions-asked prescribing of phentermine no longer meets the standards of medical practice, and has become a thing of the past in most doctors' offices.

Pondimin has a different story, however, in that fenfluramine appears to calm—rather than excite—the central nervous system. Widely praised during the mid-1970s as the first "anorectic" (appetite-suppressing) drug that could be prescribed at high doses without narcotic effects that would lead to abuse, Pondimin actually works as a sedative for many patients who take doses larger than one 20mg dose per day. The FDA considered Pondimin so safe that it would allow patients to take as many as six 20mg tablets per day.

In my own practice, however, I never needed to use more than one 20mg tablet per day for weight-loss benefit. And this approach seemed especially prudent, later on—because the complications involving an additional problem allegedly related to use of fenfluramine, pulmonary hypertension, and the heart valve abnormalities, all occurred at the higher doses.

Although Pondimin also produces peripheral effects (including, frequently, a temporary boost in glucose uptake), the drug's key impact occurs in the hypothalamus where it has proved effective at stimulating the satiety center, thereby shutting down appetite.

WHY DIET PILLS, ALONE, AREN'T ENOUGH

Coincidentally enough, my own early career as a family practice physician was greatly influenced by a research program on hypertension, obesity and appetite suppressants that I joined while serving out my residency at Williamsport Hospital in Pennsylvania, back in the 1970s. That program had been assembled by Albert Stunkard, M.D., who would go on to become recognized as a leading U.S. weight-loss researcher and theoretician at the University of Pennsylvania.

The research team at Williamsport also included psychologist Kelly Brownell, who today publishes widely from his research post at Yale University.

Dr. Stunkard's breakthrough research called for experiments in which he and his staff combined behavior modification techniques with regular doses of fenfluramine. The program included input from psychologists, nutritionists and resident physicians, all of whom combined their expertise in an ambitious schedule of therapies ranging from individual and group discussion sessions to classes on behavior modification. By using the drug in concert with aggressive counseling from our in-house psychologists, we were able to correlate weight-reduction with declines in blood pressure—a finding that should have had a significant impact on the entire weight-loss industry, but didn't.

One of the most useful outcomes of our work occurred when we were able to help patients suffering from obesity and high blood pressure with *both* problems, by designing a weight-loss program for them that relied heavily on drugs. In the end, several of the Stunkard-authored studies showed that appetite suppressants—when combined with behavior modification programs—could be used effectively in weight-reduction programs, and many patients visited our hypertension-and-obesity clinic each day to obtain prescriptions for the medication. These patients did well ... remembering, of course, that those with high-blood-pressure were required to provide additional informed consent before they

150

could receive the prescriptions.

Under the Stunkard regimen, the weight-loss patients did well at first, and it was gratifying to see how their blood pressure fell as they shed their excess poundage. But our success was short-lived; all too soon, these same patients began re-gaining the weight they'd lost. Their blood pressure also began to rise again. What had we missed? Increasingly puzzled, we analyzed every aspect of the program, but came up with nothing that would explain these relapses into obesity. (What we failed to challenge, however, was the assumption that the low-fat-and-reduced-calorie diet required for our program actually made nutritional sense! In fact, it did not.)

Looking back on that early experience, I remain amazed that the same kinds of nutritional fallacies espoused as "the whole truth" back then continue to enjoy almost universal acceptance today.

It took several more years of research at my Chronic Fatigue Center in Pocomoke, Md., before the truth finally emerged in the form of two crucially important words: "protein burning."

As it turned out, all of the money spent on psychology and "eating tips" had been wasted—because most of these patients failed to eat adequate amounts of protein, even as they went right on consuming amylose.

In short, the obesity experts of that day failed to understand what most of their colleagues still refuse to acknowledge in 2001: Amylose restriction is truly the key to successful weight-loss!

During the years of research that followed my stint at Williamsport, I came upon a key insight: the realization that both fenfluramine and phentermine exacerbate the human body's tendency to burn protein (rather than fat stores). And yet the basic strategy for successful weight maintenance—as I've pointed out elsewhere in this book—depends heavily on protein sparing, rather than protein burning. Indeed, the entire *point* of the maintenance, Low-Glycemic Index diet is precisely that dieters must teach themselves how to burn fat, while sparing protein.

151

Unfortunately, however, both of these appetite suppressants are notorious for increasing protein loss (catabolism) in dieters.

After reviewing the results of Dr. Stunkard's Williamsport project 20 years later (along with several other fen-phen programs), I came to the conclusion that dieters who rely on pills alone—without carefully following a protein sparing diet—will inevitably re-gain every pound they lose. I also realized in retrospect that Dr. Stunkard's approach had been based almost entirely on the strategy of "Eat less fat and exercise more," which amounts to nothing less than the same prescription for failure of maintenance that we see today as we saw back then.

Both Dr. Stunkard and Dr. Brownell have remained influential figures in the world of weight-loss to this day ... even though they seem to have overlooked the crucial fact that *maintenance* is the real test of a diet-program's effectiveness. Yet their well-intentioned but mis-directed thinking about obesity, which has since been embraced by the Medical Establishment, continues to dominate the government health bureaucracies and the news media to this day. Example: Only a few months ago, I received an urgent phone call from a medical reporter at the Philadelphia Inquirer (Marian Uhlman). She explained that the mayor of her city was leading a citywide weight-loss campaign, and that she wanted to report on this issue. Startled by my rather unique theories about body mass, protein sparing and amylose, Ms. Ulhman responded to our lengthy interview by asking me point-blank: "Why are you saying something so totally different from what all the *experts* say?"

My response to that question was a simple one: "Please go ask the 'experts' to tell you their maintenance-rates! Then you might want to ask them why they are considered to be 'the' experts. Perhaps you can help them catch up by passing on some of the nutritional information I just gave you!"

This important lesson has not yet reached most of the U.S. weight-loss industry, however. As a matter of fact, the pharmaceutical companies seem to be working harder than ever these days to create powerful dieting drugs that can be sold as an "easy fix" for the problem of obesity. "Take our pill," says the breathless manufacturer, "and watch that ugly fat melt away!" What the glossy brochures usually fail to point out, however, is that dieters must also find the patience and determination to stay with a protein-sparing diet, if they expect to keep their lost pounds from returning within a few months.

Looking back from today's perspective, it's easy to see how the over-reliance on "chemical fixes" was reflected in the FDA's short-lived decision to certify the weight loss drug, Redux. This medication also targeted the satiety centers of the brain—but its side effects included the threat of memory loss. Expensive, and also plagued by some other safety concerns, Redux fell by the wayside when the FDA did an about-face and yanked it from the market in the late 1990s.

During its brief lifetime, Redux was heavily promoted as a "magic bullet" for obesity ... perhaps because its high cost ($3 a day) ensured large profits for manufacturers. Although Redux advocates argued that it could be taken long-term without health risks, I was not convinced. In my view, the long-term risks clearly outweighed the benefits, and I decided not to prescribe it for any of my patients.

FEN-PHEN: ONLY A SHORT-TERM SOLUTION?

The *Saga of Fen-Phen* began with the publication of a series of papers, starting back in 1991, detailing the landmark research studies conducted at the University of Rochester by Dr. Michael Weintraub and a team of investigators. In those highly publicized experiments, patients had been given a combination of phentermine and fenfluramine (that combined medication soon became known as "fen-phen") over the course of a long-term experiment.

The Rochester study showed that the weight-loss patients were able to maintain their lower weights, provided that they continued to take the appetite suppressants under careful medical supervision. Because the side effects were minimal, this study made huge waves throughout the U.S. weight-loss industry.

Suddenly, weight-loss physicians from Portland, Maine, to Portland, Oregon, were besieged by patients who insisted on being given prescriptions for fen-phen.

But the fen-phen bonanza soon became a health disaster—and in order to use appetite suppressants effectively and safely, we need to understand *why*.

The most important thing to know about the biochemistry of appetite suppression is that these substances act as "releasing agents." Translated, this simply means that when a nerve is stimulated with these appetite suppressing medications (and other appetite modulating drugs work differently), it will release extra quantities of "neurotransmitter"—the chemical compound that carries messages from one brain cell (neuron) to the next.

Simply stated, the neurotransmitter transports the brain's electrical messages across the spaces ("synapses") between neurons.

Many appetite suppressants work on the principle that says: "Add more of a specific neurotransmitter to a specific brain circuit, and the message will grow stronger accordingly."

In essence, the phentermine suppressant worked by using a neurotransmitter known as "norepinephrine" to boost the power of messages to the brain's hunger center. Those messages said: "Be quiet!" ... but in a voice that was much louder, after the neurotransmitter-enhancer had done its work.

On the other hand, the fenfluramine suppressant worked to boost signals to the brain's satiety center (thereby suppressing appetite), by drenching the pathways to it with "serotonin," another powerful neurotransmitter.

What a combination! All at once it seemed obvious that stimulating the satiety center and suppressing the hunger center with the two drugs that made up fen-phen would rapidly reduce obesity in most patients. (And they were right: to this day, many patients will tell you that this combination produced the most effective weight-loss drug they ever took.)

There was a serious drawback, however.

Although most researchers didn't realize it at the time, the end-less bombardment of the neurons in order to increase secretion of neurotransmitters soon caused a kind of "chemical fatigue" to set in. After about 12 weeks of low-use dosage (and in a shorter time of high dose usage), in fact, the neurons are no longer able to se-crete extra amounts of the key neurotransmitters, serotonin and norepinephrine. The chemical cupboard is bare.

At this point, most weight-loss patients hit a "plateau"—a pe-riod of time in which further weight-reduction from medication becomes impossible. Frustrated, the patient and the doctor agree on what turns out to be a dangerous strategy—increasing the dosage of the suppressants, in the hope that taking more of the drug will allow the patient to overpower the plateau. The cup-board is still bare. Increasing the doses and the duration of treat-ment simply exposes patients to additional and more serious side effects.

Instead of taking this reckless step, doctors and patients should allow for a three-week "washout" period in which the patient takes no weight-loss medications at all. Such a pause allows the over-taxed nerve to restore its own supply of neurotransmitter chemicals. Merely "upping the dosage" is like whipping a mule who's already on his last legs: It simply didn't work.

This important insight emerged during lengthy research in which I monitored results among more than 700 patients whom I'd followed since 1993.

In the end, I concluded that the regulatory agencies had been correct to provide guidelines or suggestions advising that fen-phen be used only in the short-term. In too many cases, I eventually discovered, patients who relied exclusively on the drug for long-term maintenance were not successful. At the same time, by burning protein as the preferred fuel because amylose was permitted in the diet, they were creating substantial health risks for themselves. Protein-burning simply isn't good for your health, and the appetite suppressants burn protein.

The bottom line was easy to read: Diet pills should never be used as a substitute for behavior modification and proper dietary management. (And "proper management" does *not* mean "Eat less and exercise more!") Quite simply, suppressants work much better when used in combination with the No-Amylose diet. This strategy virtually guarantees that patients who succeed in meeting their weight-reduction goals will be able to prevent the shed poundage from returning. There is no need for appetite suppressants as maintenance aids, not when the Low-Glycemic Index diet does so well.

Such reservations aside, however, there's no doubt that the "miracle" diet drug-combo helped millions of patients in their battle against obesity between 1992 and 1997, as more than 6 million Americans (mostly women) joined the fen-phen bandwagon, usually with gratifying results. So lucrative was the practice of dispensing the stuff that some doctors ended up devoting their entire practices to buying the drugs wholesale, then dispensing them right in the office. Others launched "fen-phen practices" —aka known as "mills"—where the only medical criterion required for a prescription was the presence of a checkbook.

I could understand the attraction, however. My own weight-loss program generated a loss of up to one pound of fat per week. With fen-phen, the weight loss (but not necessarily the *fat* loss) doubled to *two* pounds per week.

Fen-phen was an extraordinarily effective weapon in the battle against fat. But when a few greedy doctors prescribed it irresponsibly and indiscriminately at high doses for long periods of time, with some frightening results, they took that powerful tool away from the rest of us. Indeed, the fen-phen gold rush was so ferocious that Dr. Weintraub, himself, soon became appalled by it, telling reporters: "In truth, I never thought there would be fen-phen mills. And I never thought of it as a magic pill. Every time I hear that word, I sort of cringe."

What Dr. Weintraub and the other researchers who studied fen-phen had never realized was that it can cause significant damage to serotonin-sensitive tissues in both the heart and the lungs, if high dosages are maintained for too long without careful medical supervision.

In July of 1997, that chilling fact was starkly underlined—when researchers at the world-renowned Mayo Clinic in Minnesota discovered that 24 women who had been taking the combination-drug were suffering from a potentially lethal heart valve abnormality.

Within a few months, several hundred other longtime fen-phen users were found to have damaged heart valves as well.

Having racked up more than 18 million prescriptions in 1996 alone, the fen-phen boom generated more than $4 billion in gross revenues for the pharmaceutical companies before it came to a screeching halt in the summer of 1997.

By then, of course, many obesity patients had been told they were suffering from the heart valve disorders triggered by the "miracle drug." Although there is still considerable debate today about the scope of the damage caused by fen-phen (several major studies are ongoing that don't show any health effects), one fact is not in doubt: The FDA and the academic research centers must do a better job of discovering the known effects of new drugs (and new drug combinations) in the future.

At the same time, America's 650,000 physicians must be more cautious about prescribing inadequately tested "miracle drugs," merely in order to satisfy surging public demand for them.

But it's also true that the "heart-valve epidemic" hasn't happened yet ... leading some jaded observers to suggest that the undisputed benefits of fen-phen—for so many potential patients —were wiped out by some greedy doctors, pharmaceutical companies and lawyers (but not necessarily in that order).

o   o   o

THE FIRST RULE OF MEDICINE: "DO NO HARM"

Soon after the first reports of potential injury from fen-phen began to surface in 1997, I carefully reviewed the charts those patients in my practice who had taken the combination of fenfluramine and phentermine.

I was both relieved and pleased to learn that there was no evidence of either heart valve problems or primary pulmonary hypertension among my patients. As always, they had been monitored carefully. I had insisted on regular cardiograms, for one thing, while also requiring that patients using fen-phen take physical exams on a monthly basis.

As a matter of longstanding policy, my usage of diet pills was restricted to those who really needed them—and for periods that never exceeded 12 weeks, with dosages carefully limited to one of each pill per day.

All too often, at the height of the "craze," it seemed that doctors were dispensing fen-phen like vitamin C, without appropriate controls on duration of therapy, quantity of daily medication or regularly scheduled monitoring of patients. In some cases, physicians were even prescribing the drug on the Internet, where effective medical supervision of the substance was nil.

The fen-phen debacle called worldwide attention to the ongoing search for an effective weight-loss medication—a substance that could give chronically overweight patients a boost in the struggle against fat, but without triggering hazardous side effects. And indeed, that so-far-futile quest today forms one of the most discouraging and frustrating chapters in the annals of modern medicine. Today there are more than 60 weight-loss drugs under development by the pharmaceutical companies, all of whom are doing their best to come up with the one compound that will hit the jackpot.

THE SEARCH FOR A SAFE, EFFECTIVE DIET DRUG

Even as medical experts around the world were warning against the dangers of fen-phen, which appeared to cause heart disorders in some patients because of the way it continually bathed tissues in powerful neurotransmitters, the search continued for an appetite suppressant that would be completely safe.

For a while, it looked as if the researchers had found just such a drug, after they synthesized a new compound, sibutramine, that worked on an entirely different principle than fenfluramine or phentermine, yet provided users with the same result.

Instead of stimulating the brain to churn out large quantities of the two "anti-hunger" message transmitters (norepinephrine and serotonin), sibutramine was designed (as a "reuptake-inhibitor") to prevent the brain from breaking down these naturally occurring appetite suppressants.

Simply described, sibutramine worked to inhibit the process by which serotonin and norepinephrine are removed from the critical nerve regions that controls weight-loss: the synapses of nerves in the hypothalamus. In effect, sibutramine merely enhanced the ability of already present neurotransmitters to do their job—thus providing a major boost for those who were struggling to control their daily food intake, and without undesirable side effects.

The best way to show how this principle actually worked is to look at a case study involving my good friend and former weight-loss patient, Beth Anderson.

159

Beth is a dedicated public school administrator. She makes a good living and has had a major impact on the lives of kids. Cheerful and energetic most of the time, Beth seems to enjoy life to the fullest. She works very hard, of course. She also lives in an elegant Victorian house—complete with gables and an eye-catching portico—that she restored herself. She plays a mean game of tennis doubles at the local country club, when she isn't playing Bach or Schubert on her Yamaha baby grand piano.

At first glance, most people would never suspect that Beth Anderson was also grappling day in and day out with the serious illness known as "obesity." But she was. The simple fact is that this dedicated teacher has a genetic weight problem; she was born with high insulin and will have it forever.

At 5-10 and 178 pounds when I first met her, Beth Anderson had already qualified for the "obese" designation. She was 32 percent fat.

But she was a gutsy, determined fighter—a fact that became clear as soon as I started interviewing her.

"You're not going to believe this, Ritchie, but only four months ago, I was 28 pounds lighter!"

"Of course I believe you, Beth. Regaining all that weight must have been pretty frustrating. What happened?"

She shook her head, then sent up a rueful laugh. "Fen-phen is what happened, Ritch! I lost about 30 pounds with that stuff, starting back in 1996. But then last year when the news about the heart problems broke … well, I stopped taking it right away, just like everybody else.

"I figured, what the heck, I'd proved that I could lose all that weight! I mean, keeping it off would be *easy*, right? I kept getting lots of exercise, and I tried to watch everything I ate.

"But you know what?" She groaned mournfully. "Without fen-phen, I started gaining pounds every week. I couldn't believe my eyes, each time I stepped on the bathroom scale.

"So here I am, right back at Square One. I need your help, because I definitely don't want to carry all this weight! Lose it, gain it, I feel like a Yo-Yo."

She sighed, then closed her eyes for a moment. It was the same look of defeat that I'd seen many, many times during my two decades of treating obese patients. "Beth, it sounds to me like you've got a great deal of self-discipline and determination."

She was nodding earnestly now. "It's nice to know that someone actually understands."

"Of *course* I understand, Beth. Why wouldn't I? I live with the Yo-Yo Problem, myself! If I'm not careful, my weight will balloon out of control within a matter of weeks.

"I've treated hundreds of patients in your situation over the years, and nearly every one of them had to battle the Yo-Yo in order to stay thin. After tracking these folks for a few years, I've determined that about 70 percent of my patients are able to keep their lost weight from returning. But the remaining 30 percent quickly re-gain most of the weight they've managed to lose.

"I invented a new a medical category for those struggling patients: I call them 'The Y-Y 30 Percent!' And I take great satisfaction from that low figure of 30 percent ... because every other diet program I've heard about would require a 'Y-Y 99 Percent' category!"

She was laughing again. "Y-Y for 'Yo-Yo'?"

"You got it. Over the years, I've determined that the Y-Y 30s need special help, if they're going to avoid riding that well travelled path back to obesity.

"Many of them are professional people like you, Beth. They face special stresses on the job that frequently involve food. For example: How often does your work require you to attend professional luncheons. I'll bet you do two or three of them a week. Am I right?"

"You sure are. I spend half my life at study seminars or community meetings, with every one of them organized around lunch.

Club sandwiches with three slices of bread are just the prelude to huge slices of cake or pie for dessert. I must've eaten a thousand of them over the years!"

I nodded. "This is a pretty familiar story, Beth. You'd be surprised how many patients come through that door with stories about how their jobs require them to get fat!"

We had a good laugh, and then I went on to give Beth the good news.

As a certified member of the "Y-Y 30 Percent," she belonged to the category of weight-loss patients who succeed very nicely at "losing the weight they hate" … but who for one reason or another simply cannot achieve continuing "maintenance" and quickly climb the scales back to obesity.

For these folks, I explained, a dietary "boost" is not only in order, but medically *required*. These patients are suffering from a chronic illness, after all. They're grappling with a health-threatening disorder basically no different in chronicity than asthma or diabetes. Obesity isn't a "winter problem" or a "post-partem problem" for most of us. In fact, it amounts to nothing less than a lifelong struggle between our genetics and our lifestyles. Ask yourself: Would anyone wish to tell a struggling asthma patient that taking a medication for the condition is inappropriate?

Beth listened carefully while I went on to impart the best news of all. After several years of prescribing a new, carefully tested weight-loss medication for scores of patients, I was convinced that sibutramine (brand name: Meridia) could safely provide the "boost" necessary to help the 30-Percenters successfully achieve maintenance.

After appropriate cardiac-testing and a complete physical exam, I put Beth on 15 milligrams of sibutramine daily. She liked the fact that she could take the dosage in a single pill, and that there were no potentially harmful side effects to worry about. She was getting the benefits of fen-phen without the health risks!

Intent on living up to her low-amylose maintenance program, and while continuing her own personal lifestyle of frequent walking and tennis, she went on to lose 33 pounds during the next six months.

As I listened to the exuberant Beth Anderson brag about her "new, slimmed-down lifestyle," I couldn't help wondering: Had I finally discovered the magic-bullet solution to the problem of weight-loss maintenance?

Unfortunately, it didn't turn out that way.

What I didn't realize at the time has since come clear: the disturbing fact that even this "wonder drug" contained a serious flaw —its tendency also to encourage "protein burning" (sounds familiar, doesn't it?) in patients. Because so much of her weight loss had been based on the robbing of vital protein-stores rather than fat, Beth's weight gradually returned, once she stopped taking the wonder drug. (In her case, the re-gain was only hastened by her aversion to eating meat, which kept her protein-intake to the minimum and exacerbated the imbalance in her metabolism.)

It was at this point that I finally began to understand that successful weight-loss maintenance could *never* be based on drugs— no matter how effective they might prove to be in the short run.

The secret to maintenance isn't in the chemistry—but in changing the dieter's lifestyle!

APPETITE SUPPRESSANTS *CAN SPEED RESULTS, HOWEVER*

Although they never were intended to be used for permanent weight-control, there's no denying that appetite suppressants such as fen-phen gave weight-loss patients a tremendous psychological boost. Let's face it: Watching 25 pounds evaporate within 12 weeks can do wonders for your self-esteem ... especially as pant-sizes and shirt-sizes begin to shrink, and long-retired bathing suits are retrieved from the attic!

After this initial surge of euphoria, patients often gain an enhanced sense of confidence in their ability to maintain their weight loss with the low-Glycemic Index diet. As a result, they don't regain their weight. Some cycle the No-Amylose diet for a few weeks into their maintenance program and continue to lose weight. Over the years, I've found that I can often help patients tap into this positive energy by capitalizing on the new self-esteem they gained as a result of the initial weight loss. "You proved you can do it," I will often tell them, "and you can keep *on* doing it, if you really decide that successful maintenance is important to you!"

Is there any doubt that our society insists on "instant gratification" in most areas of life? Americans want to see goals reached *fast* ... and if you doubt that, just spend a few minutes watching their behavior at drive-through restaurant windows. As long as the food keeps arriving at breakneck speed, things go smoothly. But slow the process down for even a minute—*Where's my fried chicken?*—and the rage is apparent on almost every face.

You can be sure that most dieters in this country are equally impatient. That's why they sign up in droves for the Very Low-Calorie Diet (VLCD) weight-loss programs, which now offer the fastest weight-loss results (up to 3 pounds a week) in the U.S. According to recent surveys, using phentermine with a diet (up to 2 pounds a week) ranks second in popularity among dieters —with the No-Amylose diet (about a pound a week) currently holding down third place. (While evaluating several other weight-loss programs in recent years, I found no convincing evidence that they provide reliable maintenance.)

Although some dieters benefited greatly from suppressants such as fen-phen, we must always remember that the drugs aren't candy —and that like all medications, they harbor many potential side effects. Still, these possible negative outcomes are often overstated by cautious physicians, in my experience. During more than two decades of using them regularly and safely with thousands of weight-loss patients, I encountered only five situations where dieters were forced to stop taking the medications due to harmful reactions.

My results with appetite suppressants were actually quite favorable, when compared to the well-documented national dropout rate of six percent for use of placebos in drug trials. During my survey of 700 patients, for example, I expected at least 42 dropouts (about six percent), instead of the five patients who were forced to suspend their use of the medication.

On the other hand, my patients may have been better-motivated than those who participate in national drug trials. For this reason, I'm quick to suggest that proper patient selection and careful follow-up of those prescribed appetite suppressants is the key to avoiding potentially dangerous side effects. Hopefully, the "dieting mill" approach to weight loss ("How ya doing; here's your B-12 shot; here are your pills; pay the lady $60 cash; credit cards accepted; see you in two weeks!") is now a thing of the past!

To achieve their full potential, then, appetite suppressants must be integrated into responsible, carefully managed weight-loss programs operated by caring, ethical practitioners.

USING SUPPRESSANTS EFFECTIVELY: THE STEPS

Once a patient has decided to make appetite suppressants part of his or her weight-loss program, we sit down for a lengthy review aimed at discovering whether or not there are any contraindicating factors that might make such usage hazardous for that specific patient. (The list of such contraindicating factors is contained in the standard Physicians Desk Reference, or PDR.)

After this review, the patient undergoes a cardiogram in order to make certain that his or her heart function is normal. (The presence of any heartbeat abnormality instantly disqualifies a patient from using appetite suppressants, under my dieting guidelines.)

My dieting program also excludes patients with manic-depressive illness that requires lithium. The same rule applies to my pregnant patients, who should not take diet drugs until after childbirth and after they have finished nursing their infants. In addition, I insist that patients suffering from glaucoma obtain permission from their attending physicians before beginning to take these medications.

Although the medical standard of care—as reflected in the language of the PDR—at one time allowed patients with controlled hypertension to use appetite suppressants, my dieting program does not permit such usage by those who have elevated blood pressure or those who take medication for that condition. My rule is a simple one: Patients may not take these substances until their blood pressure returns to normal.

I think it's unfortunate that some patients treat appetite suppressants with cavalier disregard for the health risks involved ... while also assuming that because they're taking a diet medication, they don't have to be careful about the foods they eat. Is it really surprising to learn that such patients invariably regain their lost weight?

Recent research shows clearly that appetite suppressants cause the human body to burn protein. For that reason, you can be sure that if you eat the standard American diet, any weight-loss you achieve through pills will eventually be erased, as protein is consumed and fat is spared. Thus we see the importance of the No-Amylose diet. If dieters can learn how to prevent the rapid surge of insulin by avoiding glucose and amylose starches, their bodies will be able to mobilize fatty acids from fat stores—a process which will consume fat.

The situation is very different, however, for patients who are losing weight only by virtue of burning protein. In most cases, these bedraggled souls feel tired, perpetually exhausted. Yet they don't sleep well at night. Their skin grows pasty, and their hair loses its luster. Facial muscles sag, and snappish irritability quickly sets in. Soon these unfortunates are wrestling with excess stomach acid, constipation, and even bowel spasms.

Such is the life, unhappily, of the "yo-yoing" and protein-burning weight-loss patient.

TAKING RESPONSIBILITY FOR WHAT YOU EAT

Patients who decide to use any appetite suppressant as a supportive medication in my dieting program should always obtain their prescriptions for it only from physicians who will combine the drugs with a comprehensive approach to nutrition and an emphasis on maintenance of weight-loss. Don't let the P. T. Barnums of the diet pill industry make a sucker out of you!

During the first few days of taking this medication, you can expect to feel somewhat "jittery" and shaky. But this side effect usually lasts for only two days or less. And I'm happy to report that I've never had to stop a patient from using appetite suppressants because of this early, short-lived response.

After the first few days have passed, the effects are so mild that many patients begin to doubt that they're receiving any real benefit from the medication. All too often, they end up telling me: "I need something stronger, doctor. I don't have that 'hyped-up' feeling that the pills gave me at first."

In this situation, I quickly tell them that the "hyped-up" reaction was a mere side effect ... and that it had nothing whatsoever to do with their weight-loss.

To summarize, then: On average, appetite suppressants will help the typical weight-loss patient to lose an extra pound a week, compared to the weight-reduction produced by my no-amylose diet, alone. If you do the math, you'll see that a 12-week program—using both tools—should allow you to lose about 25 pounds. Those patients who need to lose 100 pounds or more can do so by engaging in repeated "cycles" of pill-taking, spaced around three-week "washout" periods in which they take no diet medication at all.

Using this strategy, a patient can ratchet his or her weight down steadily, without much risk of long-term complications. In most cases, however, my patients find that they don't really need the pills after the initial 12 weeks. As a doctor, I find it immensely satisfying, each time one of them tells me that the "Double-0-2-3 Diet" alone is enough to continue losing weight steadily!

The key point to remember is that appetite suppressants provide dieters with a quick fix—and with the instant gratification that so many desire. I can't tell you how many times I've heard an obese patient say: "If you'll just give me some success early, I'll be willing to live on a diet later."

The appetite suppressants serve an important supportive role —both emotionally and physiologically—in successful weight-loss. Their great drawback, however, is that they tend to lift responsibility for weight maintenance from the patient ... who frequently begins to believe that losing weight involves nothing more than "better living through chemistry."

Wrong! To avoid sliding into this misconception (which will quickly lead to patients regaining all of their lost weight), we need to keep emphasizing the basic premise of this diet—the idea that effective weight-loss and maintenance requires significant changes in lifestyle and eating behaviors ... along with careful avoidance of sugar and amylose.

Accomplishing those things is simple enough, once you understand the basics of the Shoemaker approach to dieting. But the first step is always the recognition of one basic fact:

To win the battle against fat, we must take responsibility *for what we eat*—instead of mistakenly relying on chemical compounds and other gimmicks to do it for us.

CASE STUDY: JIM BOB'S CHOLESTEROL

Jim Bob's father died suddenly of a heart attack at age 46. His unlit cigarette was found next to the bottle of insulin he was supposed to have used that morning. After his 40th birthday, Jim Bob wondered what he should do so he could celebrate his 50th birthday.

Jim Bob's wife knew he probably had diabetes, just like his father. The sweets, candy and sodas didn't help. Indeed, with a blood sugar of 330, weight 235, BP of 180/110, cholesterol 295, triglycerides 340, HDL 35, LDL 175, apo A1 of 110, apo B of 204, and Lp (a) of 25, Jim Bob was a metabolic time bomb. His lipid phenotype was type II A.

My 00-2-3 diet can correct his blood sugar. No insulin will be needed for Jim Bob. His cholesterol, as you will read, cannot be fixed by diet alone. He needs medication. Whether the most important determinants of cholesterol, apo A1 and apo B, can be corrected, will determine how many candles are on Jim Bob's last birthday cake.

This is a success story, with statin drugs successfully lowering his cholesterol to 230, HDL 34, triglycerides 280, and LDL 141. The apo A1 and apo B didn't change. Then, with the same medication and the 00-2-3 diet, the cholesterol was 192, HDL 46, triglycerides 110, LDL 124, apo A1 128, apo B 125, Lp (a) 18, blood glucose 117. The diabetes medication prescription was never refilled.

169

I didn't expect the apo A1, and apo B to improve so dramatically with the 00-2-3 diet. I will not guarantee similar results for you. As you read this cholesterol chapter, remember that there are significant errors of logic made by physicians first, by telling people to eat low fat diets, and second, by just concentrating on HDL and LDL as our most important parameters for evaluating cholesterol health.

All members of the statin class of cholesterol lowering drugs work by blocking the enzyme, HMG CoA Reductase, that makes cholesterol. The most important stimulator of this enzyme is insulin. By following my No-Amylose, 00-2-3 diet, Jim Bob essentially reduced the insulin effect on his cholesterol. This is why you can eat protein, eggs and butter (in moderation) and watch your cholesterol fall as you simultaneously lose weight.

Now, if I could just convince Jim Bob to quit smoking cigarettes ...

10

CHOLESTEROL: THE STORY BEHIND A GREAT AMERICAN MYTH

Listen my children, and you shall hear ... a Grim Fairy Tale!

Once upon a time, in a kingdom far away, there lived a terrifying Ogre who held the entire populace in his merciless grip.

The monster's name was long and ugly, and once you heard it, you never forgot it again:

CHOLESTEROL!

And wherever he went, sobbing women fainted and grown men blanched with sudden fear.

From one end of the great kingdom to the other, all lived as slaves of the Ogre, while trembling at the sound of his taunting cry:

"Go ahead ... eat some egg yolk ... and DIE!"

Roaring with laughter, the Ogre would then open his gnarled, horny hands to reveal ... half a dozen soft-boiled eggs running with creamy yellow ... while the populace shuddered in fear.

This is the story of how Ogre Cholesterol ruled his kingdom for 20 years.

(But it's also the story of how he was finally overthrown!)

CHOLESTEROL: GETTING BEHIND THE MYTHS

Ask the typical American citizen to define the word "cholesterol," and the odds are high that you'll soon find yourself listening to a catalogue of health horrors that would rival those spawned during the darkest hours of the Black Plague.

"It's a white, waxy substance—like Crisco—and it piles up in arteries and causes people to have heart attacks in the middle of dinner!"

"It's liquid fat, bright yellow, and it seeps into your lungs and clogs them until you're gasping for air!"

"It's twice as dangerous as cigarettes, and if you don't believe me, go eat a couple of eggs. Next thing you know, they'll be strapping you into an ambulance. ..."

After more than 20 years of non-stop bombardment from the U.S. Medical Establishment, is it any wonder that John Q. Citizen has learned to live in fear of cholesterol ... a perfectly benign and very useful substance that helps strengthen cell membranes in the human body, while also performing several other essential tasks?

If you're like most people, you probably don't realize that the human body, *itself*, is the largest single source of daily cholesterol ... and that it manufactures, on average, about 1,200 mg of this important substance each and every single day regardless of what you eat.

Many readers will also be surprised to learn that the vast majority of Americans who are now eating low-fat diets—while also avoiding eggs and following the American Heart Association dietary recommendations for lowering their risk of heart disease —are actually fooling themselves.

Ask yourself: How many times have you listened to the endlessly repeated advice from "medical experts" supposedly in touch with the latest health research: "The key to preventing a heart attack is to lose weight, eat low-fat, and exercise?"

And when the low-fat diets predictably don't work, how long does it take the doctor to begin writing prescriptions for expensive cholesterol-lowering medications?

As shocking as it may sound, that strategy of low-fat-diet-followed-by-cholesterol-drugs is the *wrong* strategy for preventing heart disease in most people!

Before the U.S. Medical Establishment starts aiming its heavy artillery in this direction, however, let me hasten to point out that, yes, there are some patients (about 20 percent of the populace) with a genetically controlled abnormality that results in overproduction of cholesterol. These "Type II" patients (and you'll be reading more about the special challenges faced by these "Frederickson Lipoprotein Phenotypes" later in the chapter) really *must* take medications in order to lower their cholesterol.

But what the *rest* of us need in order to avoid heart disease isn't a drug. Instead, we need to learn the workings of cholesterol (both dietary *and* internally manufactured) inside and out. Most of all, we need to know how this important substance is made, so that we can arm ourselves with the most powerful weapon we have in the battle against heart disease: accurate knowledge!

The bottom line here is simple and easy to understand. It consists of five crystal-clear principles that explain why limiting cholesterol intake is a wrong-headed approach to the problems of cholesterol-buildup and heart disease.

Principle No. 1: There are actually two sources of cholesterol. One type (endogenous) is manufactured in the human liver; the second

173

type (exogenous) comes in through the food we eat. In most cases, dietary cholesterol is far less important as a risk-factor for heart disease than cholesterol manufactured internally.

Principle No. 2: The cholesterol we make internally far exceeds the amount we take in—and the human body will discard most excess dietary cholesterol, based on how much of it is being produced in the liver at any particular time.

Principle No. 3: The trigger that controls this critically important endogenous manufacture of cholesterol and prevents disposal is actually insulin ... which means that eating sugar and amylose not only makes you fat—it also will result, over time, in elevated (and health-threatening) levels of cholesterol!

Principle No. 4: The manufacture of endogenous cholesterol is activated by an enzyme, HMG-CoA Reductase. The speed and efficiency of this "organic trigger" is most powerfully controlled by insulin, which regulates the performance of the enzyme at every moment.

Principle No. 5: When it comes to heart disease, there are two basic types of patients: those at risk for a premature heart attack (before age 65), and those who have outlived this health risk, but who remain vulnerable to heart disease caused by age-related deterioration of coronary arteries and other blood vessels. (There's some very good research evidence, by the way, to show that those who experience premature [reminder: premature means before age 65] heart attacks must henceforth keep cholesterol as low as possible to avoid a repeat attack.) Also: Keep in mind the differences between a person aged 65 who has high cholesterol—but who has never had a heart attack—and a person aged 65 who *has*. Obviously, the same medical recommendation cannot fit both patients!

If you're like most American readers, you're probably gasping with shock right now, as you tell yourself: *Wait a minute. If Dr.*

Cholesterol: The Story behind a Great American Myth

Shoemaker's right, then we've been blaming the wrong culprit for cholesterol-related diseases during the past 20 years. The culprit isn't dietary cholesterol —it's dietary glucose/amylose!

It's the sad truth, ladies and gentlemen.

Medical Research Bulletin from Dr. Shoemaker: Only 20 percent of the U.S. population is affected by the genetically programmed condition known as "high blood cholesterol." For this relatively small group of citizens—and this group only—controlling cholesterol with medications is important, in order to prevent long-term damage to blood vessels (atherosclerosis) and related heart attacks. These patients—the Lipoprotein Phenotype II's—make up the population that is most susceptible to premature heart attacks. Type II patients need to do everything they can, including cutting back on saturated fat and dietary cholesterol, to prevent heart disease. But mostly they need to take medication. The rest of the people at risk for heart attack related to cholesterol need to recognize how to control their weight and their cholesterol by understanding how insulin and amylose control levels of cholesterol and triglycerides. Those non-Type II cholesterol patients who won't follow a low-amylose diet or whose physicians/dieticians don't prescribe a physiologic diet in the end will have to take medications to control their cholesterol since a low-cholesterol, low-fat diet won't.

Although recent research shows that these folks with genetically elevated cholesterol are at significantly higher risk for cholesterol-related heart disease, the good news is that they can control their cholesterol blood-levels rather easily by taking one of the "statin" medications designed to prevent enzyme reactions essential to producing the substance. Don't forget that all of the HMG-CoA-Reductase inhibitors (the statins turn off HMG almost as fast as insulin turns it on) have potential risks that have been identified since 1988. Rarely, statins damage muscle fibers which can overload the kidneys with the muscle protein, myoglobin. Statins in these few cases can become killers. Fortunately, that side effect is detectable well ahead of time by monitoring tests of muscle

175

enzymes. Statins more commonly damage liver cells, so when you are stuck with a statin prescription, make sure you have liver and muscle blood tests done repeatedly.

For the remaining 80 percent of patients—and this fact will probably come as a shock to many—*the vast preponderance of the scientific evidence shows very little relationship between dietary cholesterol and heart disease!*

That's right. You read that correctly. But just so there's no mistake, let me say it another way: *For four-fifths of the population, monitoring and limiting dietary intake of cholesterol will not significantly reduce the buildup of cholesterol deposits on arteries, or help stave off atherosclerosis.*

Not only have we been hoodwinked by the Medical Establishment into mis-identifying the cause of most heart disease—we've also been gulled into spending hundreds of millions of dollars each year on "cholesterol-lowering" drugs that we wouldn't need, if we actually were given the chance to understand the process by which cholesterol is made! Our lives, our bodies, our choice.

Having uttered this heresy, let me pause for a moment to make sure that my message is crystal-clear. Am I denying that heart disease remains the number-one killer of Americans, here in the first few years of our new century? No, I am not. Am I denying that high cholesterol is associated with heart disease? Absolutely not. What I *am* saying, however, is that for most people, the amount of cholesterol contained in food we eat has very little impact on the risk of developing a heart ailment. And for most patients with mild cholesterol problems (problems *not* related to being a Type II, mind you), eating low-fat and low-cholesterol foods is a prescription for angioplasty and a new stent added to a coronary artery.

For too many years, now, millions of Americans have been falling victim to the famous *modus ponens* logical fallacy, when it comes to the subject of cholesterol. This notorious mistake in reasoning occurs whenever an observer garbles the logical relationship between two propositions—a misstep that usually produces absurd conclusions.

In most cases, the *modus* fallacy takes place when an observer leaps from the assertion "If *a,* we may then conclude *b,*" to "from *b,* we can then derive *a.*"

A good example of the fallacy at work would be: "Turtles have four legs, and a turtle is an animal. Therefore, if I know an animal has four legs, then it must be a turtle!"

The same false logic of the *modus ponens,* when applied to the relationship between cholesterol and heart disease, might read as follows: "High levels of bloodstream cholesterol are associated with an increased risk of heart disease." But if we leap from that assertion to: "Lowering heart disease risk means lowering high cholesterol," we have once again made the mistake of deriving *a* from *b*—and we have once again become snarled in a logical fallacy.

In this case, the *ponens* (Latin for the "bridge"—the *pons*—that connects both propositions) shatters to smithereens ... the moment we realize that heart disease is actually linked to many "confounding variables" (such as aging, smoking, high blood pressure, a family history of diabetes and maybe a chronic infection from an organism such as chlamydia, which can cause inflammation in blood vessels in heart and brain), in addition to Ogre Cholesterol.

Let's face it: when it comes to the subject of cholesterol, logic usually winds up standing on its head—while common sense goes flying out the window!

CHOLESTEROL: WHAT IS THIS STUFF, ANYWAY?

As you might imagine, the biochemistry involved in the metabolism of cholesterol is staggeringly complex. But so what?

Welcome, readers one and all, to the first diet book in the history of publishing that does *not* patronize you by assuming that

177

you cannot grasp some basic science!

Here are a few basic facts—as opposed to myths—about one of the most unfairly vilified chemical compounds on Planet Earth:

- O Cholesterol is actually an essential building block for human beings, and the body relies on it to repair damaged cell walls.

- O Cholesterol also plays a key role in the manufacture of such important "sex hormones" as estrogen and testosterone.

- O Cholesterol serves as a biochemical factor in the digestion of fat and performs several other valuable tasks in maintaining cell function in brain and nerve tissues.

- O Most of the cholesterol for these functions is produced in the liver. But humans also take in dietary cholesterol each day—the vast majority of it from meat, eggs and other dairy products, such as cheese.

- O A whitish, greasy substance, cholesterol looks like smeared chalk when observed in arteries or bodily tissues. This highly specialized form of fat travels through the bloodstream on complex vehicles comprised of "recognition molecules" called apoproteins, combined with bits of specialized triglycerides and additional "structural" proteins known as "lipoproteins." Built by the liver, these unique entities ferry the cholesterol through the blood with great efficiency.

CHOLESTEROL-LEVELS: A MATTER OF "PHENOTYPE," NOT INTAKE

If you recall my earlier chapter on the genetic basis for insulin resistance—the key factor in obesity—it will come as no surprise to discover that our genes *also* determine how our bodies manage cholesterol. When diseases like obesity, diabetes and high cholesterol are discussed by "experts," just listen to how quickly the idea of diet is brought up before genetic considerations are reviewed, as if diet took priority over genetics. And just for fun, when you pick up an article on treatment of high cholesterol, substitute "blue eyes and blonde hair" for high cholesterol. The comments about low-fat and exercise sound comical regarding eye and hair color, just as they are comical when we think about dietary treatment of genetically high cholesterol.

Some years ago, one of the nation's leading researchers on the physiology of metabolism—Dr. D. S. Frederickson—was the first to suggest that cholesterol phenotypes (the observed expression of the genetic code of an individual) could be identified by a lab procedure known as "electrophoresis." This new tool would soon have a major impact on our understanding of how genes actually dictate cholesterol levels for most people.

Within a few years, Dr. Frederickson's innovative measuring device would help science to establish the presence of five basic cholesterol types, I-V, each of which is based on a genetic difference in the lipoproteins and apoproteins involved in transport of cholesterol from bloodstream to liver to human tissues and back again to the liver.

Because they involve uncommon genetic abnormalities affecting specific enzymes (you will meet lipoprotein lipase, LPL, shortly), Types I and V are relatively rare. Type III is more common, and involves a variety of insulin response flaws. But Types II and IV are extremely common and are extremely important to our understanding of cholesterol transport. Type II, for example (whether IIA or IIB), works with remarkable efficiency to increase LDL production in the liver, seemingly without the control applied by the body to the other phenotypes, and thus contributes to high LDL cholesterol (the "bad stuff") that ends up in the arteries of the 20 percent of the population in whom this gene is expressed.

Because of this super-efficiency, the "Type II's" clearly face the greatest risk of hardening of the arteries, heart disease and heart attack. For that reason, these patients need to be treated aggressively with medications on a continuing basis—regardless

179

of their LDL or total cholesterol-level on any given day. You need to know if you are a Type II!

Type IV, on the other hand, is by far the most common of the phenotypes. Although IV lacks the extraordinary artery clogging efficiency of Type II, numerous studies show that it also carries an increased risk of heart disease from elevated cholesterol. These studies also demonstrate that high triglycerides are markers for the process by which insulin shuts down the benefit of the "LPL Effect." Wait just a bit for the LPL discussion, and take time to remember that high triglycerides are not a disease but are the result of disruption of normal handling of triglycerides by insulin. (Question for everyone: Does it come as any surprise to find high insulin levels in adult onset, insulin resistant diabetes are highly associated with both Type IV lipids and high triglycerides? No, of course not!)

The use of the Frederickson phenotypes fell by the wayside when we entered the statin era. Who cared what the phenotype was when the health problems posed by high cholesterol levels disappeared when the statins were prescribed. These drugs were so good at what they did that many physicians no longer had to think about the ultimate sources of the cholesterol levels, the genetic make-up of the patients. To this day, I still get annoyed when "statin era" lab tech sees my request for a lipoprotein electrophoresis, and because she doesn't do those tests often (if at all), runs a protein electrophoresis test instead. The patient has to have their blood test redrawn. As asimple example of the effect of the statins on lab testing is that a standard "lipid profile" no longer includes a phenotype.

Regardless of the diet-changes urged a few years ago by the American Heart Association (AHA), the reality is that Type II high cholesterol patients cannot be helped by eating less fat and less cholesterol—and the AHA diet only helps Type IVs (the vast majority) minimally. What most of the Type IVs *really* need is to lose the flab hanging over their belts because the mechanism they use to lose the belly is the same mechanism they use to drop their cholesterol: the no-amylose diet. In short, they need to reduce the "insulin response" they get from eating all those starches—*because that response is the actual culprit behind their high cholesterol, by virtue of setting off the activation of HMG CoA Reductase, that makes the liver produce large amounts of it internally!*

Complicated? Not really. Now that you understand a few of the basic steps involved in "cholesterol physiology," you'll be delighted to learn that my Double-0-2-3 Diet works beautifully to help you lose weight *and* keep your cholesterol down. Only three steps are required for guaranteed success, and here they are:

Step One: Ask your family doctor for a lipoprotein electrophoresis blood test to determine your cholesterol phenotype. Be specific and assertive. In the next section, I'll tell you why to insist that assays for Apo A1, Apo B and Lp(a) also be done.

Step Two: If you should turn out to be a Type II (one chance in five, remember), ask the physician to put you on the appropriate cholesterol-lowering medication immediately and take it faithfully. But don't take the prescription without the electrophoresis test proving that you must take medication. Make sure the routine blood monitoring tests get done (your physician will thank you for helping with the reminder).

Step Three: If you end up in the Type IV pool (the most likely scenario), forget about low-cholesterol diet advice altogether and simply follow the steps in Dr. Shoemaker's No-Amylose Diet. You'll lose weight, and your cholesterol level will also come down ... and you won't have to spend your precious free time counting fat grams *or* calories—or waste your precious paycheck on cholesterol medications that you don't need.

As a side-note, a particularly eager "drug rep" visited me recently. He wanted to sing the praises of his new wonder-drug, a cholesterol-lowering compound so powerful that we might call it a "gorilla-statin" without fear of exaggeration.

"Tell me, doctor," he asked excitedly, "whom do you treat with statins?"

Answer: "Only my Type II-A and II-B patients who have not had a heart attack, along with *all* patients—regardless of phenotype—who have."

The drug rep blinked at me, then confessed that he hadn't heard *this* kind of comment in his travels before. "That makes so much sense, how come I don't get that answer to my question from everyone?"

"Here's a suggestion," I told him. "Why don't you ask your prescribing physicians if they use 'phenotype' as a basis for determining treatment, and see how many are even aware of this key diagnostic tool?"

When the rep returned a few weeks later, he shook his head sadly ... then reported that only two doctors (both were cardiologists) out of the hundreds practicing medicine in his sales territory were profiling patients patient-risks by phenotype!

So I asked him: "Well, Mr. Representative, what do you want to know about your *own* cholesterol-associated risk, now that you're an expert on your medication?"

He answered: "Doctor, that's easy. I sure do want my phenotype done, along with my apoproteins and my Lp[a] that we talked about last time. We've got good information available, these days, and I want to use very bit of it in order to make up my own mind about fat and a diet that is healthy for my heart and my arteries. I've got young kids, you know, I want to see them graduate from college!"

FAT AND CHOLESTEROL: A FANTASTIC JOURNEY

In order to understand the biochemistry behind *Shoemaker's Cholesterol Heresy*, we're about to take a "Fantastic Cholesterol Journey" through the human digestive tract and bloodstream ... where we will witness the thrills and spills that take place when this re-markable substance is "packaged" and then "unpackaged" for its endless voyages throughout the human body.

Our Fantastic Journey begins when a slice of breakfast bacon plummets through the esophagus into the stomach, setting off an astonishing series of enzymatic reactions that are known in their entirety as "digestion."

As we ride our magic-carpet bacon slice through the stomach and intestines, we will be meeting some of the major players involved in fat manufacture and storage—including "HDL" and "LDL," along with some characters that are actually far more im-portant to cholesterol-linked heart disease than either of them—including apoprotein A, aproprotein B, and Lp(a). And you just have to get to know your best fat friend, lipoprotein lipase (LPL). Don't get confused by LPL and LDL, they aren't the same.

Before we climb aboard our carpet, however, let's arm ourselves with a few definitions. For starters, let's remember that there are several different types of cholesterol ... but that two of them in particular have become quite familiar to most of us in recent years:

O   High-density lipoprotein (HDL) cholesterol is known as the "good cholesterol" because it is associated with a low risk of heart disease. HDL cholesterol contains a higher per-centage of lipoprotein than the other cholesterol carriers, and thus has some added chemical basis that helps it to "chip away" deposits of cholesterol (known as "plaque") from artery walls. HDL also works effectively to transport cholesterol to the liver, where it can be converted for other uses or eliminated via excretion in bile. Don't forget, either, that there are at least *five* different types of HDL, and that each one has a different effect on health—a fact which is still handily overlooked by most physicians and the media, who long ago became accustomed to endlessly chanting the same over-simplified mantra: "We want your HDL to go up, in order to protect against heart disease!"

183

O Low-density lipoprotein cholesterol, on the other hand, is known as the "bad cholesterol"—because research shows that it poses an elevated risk for subsequent development of heart disease. The health problem occurs when this form of cholesterol is added to deposits of plaque on the walls of arteries, but only after the LDL has been oxidized inside human cells. When these deposits "harden," they reduce the flexibility of the vessels and narrow them as well.

The result can be atherosclerosis, which reportedly causes more than half a million heart attack-deaths each year in the U.S. alone. Before blaming cholesterol for causing all of this havoc, however, we should remember that such "small molecules" as those found in apoproteins A and B1, along with Lp(a), are actually larger factors in the development of heart disease than total cholesterol or HDL or LDL.

Regardless of their importance, however, most dieters have never even *heard* of these key molecular players ... most of whom you'll be meeting on your approaching Journey Through The Human Gut.

(And don't forget that researchers continue to identify new sub-types of A and B apoproteins each year—which means that the Cast of Cholesterol Characters will only grow larger in the days ahead.)

Although detailed knowledge of the biochemical dynamics involved isn't necessary for most dieters, they should know that apoprotein A (apo A) provides the main "docking station" that allows HDL to "lock onto" the molecular vehicles that transport it throughout the bloodstream. Apoprotein B (apo B), meanwhile, acts in similar "lock and key" fashion to permit LDL to dock securely with the molecules of its cardiovascular transporter.

Question: Why do these apoproteins play such an important role in the manufacture, transport and utilization of cholesterol?

Answer: The apoproteins are controlled genetically and not altered by diet; only rarely are they altered by medications (including statins). For these reasons, these vital forms of protein—and especially apo A—actually determine the efficiency with which cholesterol is used by the body. Like blood-patrolling "cholesterol traffic cops," they have a huge say in how this substance is packaged and transported throughout the body. Example: if you turn out to be one of those dieters with low production of apo A and high production of apo B, you will probably need to lower your blood-cholesterol any way you can ... *regardless* of your genetic phenotype. You are a walking LDL time bomb, even if you aren't Type II, though most Type II patients have too much Apo B as well.

Of course, the often overlooked Lp(a) also has a major impact on the process by which cholesterol-building triggers heart disease in many patients.

According to the latest research, Lp(a) works to accomplish two key tasks in the development of heart disease. First, it locks onto molecules of oxidized "bad" LDL in the developing plaque in a blood vessel wall. Second, it then links these harmful molecules together with blood platelets, where they immediately begin the heart-threatening process of blocking arteries. This process eventually results in a mature plaque, one that can cause reduction of supply of vital oxygen and nutrients to heart, brain, and peripheral arteries.

For the record, here's a brief rundown on how these small protein molecules affect heart disease rates:

O Individuals blessed with high apo A's are rarely attacked by cardiovascular diseases, and usually enjoy lengthy life spans regardless of total cholesterol and LDL levels;

O Those unfortunates who display elevated levels of apo B (and especially when accompanied by a reduced ratio of A to B) will face a heightened risk of heart attack. (This biochemical fact helps explain the curious anomaly that takes place when patients with cholesterol in the 180–190 range, independent of their phenotype, nonetheless develop hardening of the arteries and "premature" heart attack.)

O Lp(a) exacerbates the health condition in which plaque-hardened arteries gradually constrict blood flow by promoting the clotting of platelets. Such "traffic jams" can put unhealthy stress on hearts already struggling to move blood through compromised vessels.

So what's the bottom line, when it comes to understanding the actual biochemistry involved in cholesterol-related heart disease?

Simple. In this arena of disease (and disease prevention), we must never forget Shoemaker's Controlling Principle, which tells us: *Ultimately, the events that matter most in the development of cholesterol-linked heart disease are those which occur at the molecular level. And because they're controlled genetically, most of these events remain impervious to diet-based therapies.*

Instead of alerting the public to this very real health hazard—especially insulin as a major factor in triggering over-production of endogenous cholesterol—the Gurus of the Conventional Medical Wisdom continue to mystify us with the Mythology of the Cholesterol Ogre, by endlessly perpetuating several long-discredited myths, including these:

O Getting 30 minutes of strenuous exercise each day will significantly reduce your unhealthy LDL!

O The key to lowering the amount of cholesterol circulating through your bloodstream is to eat less fat—and especially saturated fat—which can best be accomplished by eating low-fat foods!

O The best way to fend off the merciless assaults of Ogre Cholesterol is to entirely avoid those foods (such as egg yolks and animal organs) that are highest in this dangerous substance!

FAT AND CHOLESTEROL:
ALL ABOARD FOR THE FANTASTIC JOURNEY!

Now let's get back to our piece of bacon.

If you could look at that pork under a microscope, you'd quickly see that it consists of both muscle fibers and surrounding fat. When you swallow the bacon, stomach enzymes quickly go to work separating these two elements. A few minutes later, when the fat and the protein reach your small intestine, special enzymes manufactured in the pancreas (the "lipases") go to work breaking the fat down into long chains of fatty acids ... which are then absorbed by special cells located farther down the intestine.

These intestinal cells are highly efficient packagers of fat. By quickly linking three fatty acids to a glycerol, they perform the necessary repackaging of the individual components of fat molecules to make a transportable substance, a triglyceride. These particles are then wrapped together in several layers of lipids, along with special apoproteins and free cholesterol to form the basic vehicle that will move the fatty acids building blocks throughout the body: the chylomicron.

Next step: once the chylomicron has been assembled, several other intestinal enzymes can work on it. Their job is add cholesterol to the package, where required (a control feature that affects and is affected by cholesterol production by the liver, except in Type II cholesterol patients), and also to convert that same cholesterol into an inactive—and harmless form—known as the "cholesterol ester." Once this step has been accomplished, cholesterol can be shipped all through the body in an easy-to-manage form that presents no threat to blood vessels. Maintaining a healthy balance of cholesterol-to-cholesterol-ester ratios in the chylomicron is the key to good cholesterol management—and all of my recommendations to patients are based on that observation.

So much for the "packaging." But what happens when it's time to take cholesterol out of the package and free it for its many tasks —including cell membrane-repair and manufacture of hormones,

187

among other jobs?

At this point, another key enzyme, lipoprotein lipase (not LDL), steps in to provide the chemical catalyst necessary to "free up" the bound cholesterol, so that it can go to work. This important enzyme, attached to the inside lining of blood vessels, acts like the mouth-parts of a mosquito—in effect by penetrating the round globe of the chylomicron, then withdrawing fats and breaking them down into harmless compounds.

Although the public statements about most cholesterol research and what primary care physicians read in current literature usually don't reflect an awareness of this crucially important fact, LPL's activity is remarkably reduced by insulin ... which turns out to be a decisive factor in the regulation of blood cholesterol. Once again, the message is clear: If you "spike" your insulin-level by consuming glucose and especially amylose, you're sending a biochemical signal to your body to manufacture and then transport large amounts of cholesterol.

Even worse, without LPL removing cholesterol from the chylomicron and then loading it onto the nascent form of HDL (HDL-3)—which soon becomes the carrier form for cholesterol *removal* (HDL-2A) ... guess what happens to HDL? Answer: The levels fall like a stone.

And if the LPL remains inactive, what happens to the triglycerides in the chylomicrons? Answer: they stay inside the chylomicrons, which continue to circulate through the blood.

In other words, when a patient is described as having "a high triglyceride-level, with low HDL and moderately high total cholesterol" you can just about be sure that his or her lipoprotein lipase isn't working correctly because insulin has shut it down. Recognize the phenotype of this individual? It is a Type IV. Translation: If you're a Type IV phenotype (the usual situation, remember) with high triglycerides, the winning diet-strategy is to activate your lipoprotein lipase by shutting down your insulin.

(All together now: How do we shut down the insulin? DON'T EAT AMYLOSE!)

Once again, the message is clear: If you "spike" your insulin-level by consuming glucose and especially amylose, you're sending a biochemical signal to halt the process of breaking down cholesterol and triglycerides. In short, the spike permits Lp(a) to do its insidious job on your excess oxidized LDL building blocks—thus giving the green light to plaque-buildup in your arteries.

When thinking about the movement of cholesterol through the human body, it really is important to remember that the process is *also* regulated via a second level of control—a biochemical mechanism that allows the digestive system to adjust for changes in dietary intake of this key substance.

This "second circuit" is always monitoring cholesterol. But it kicks into high gear whenever too much cholesterol gets loose into the bloodstream. When that happens, enzymes in the intestinal wall immediately begin to sense the over-abundance of the fatty substance. If I knew how, I would surely tell you here.

The key point here is that these intestinal enzymes exactly mirror those found in the liver. By reversing the process by which the liver packages and distributes cholesterol, the second circuit protects against imbalances in the production and distribution of this form of fat throughout the body.

Although science does not yet understand how this monitoring occurs, it's clear that the link between liver and intestinal enzyme function plays an important part in the monitoring process. And when the cholesterol-monitors sound the alarm, the body responds by activating in yet *another* enzyme (LCAT) inside the lining cells of the small intestine to once again convert the cholesterol into its harmless form, the ester.

(At this point, however, we must be careful to remember that a second form of LPL—found in the liver—continually monitors and balances the enzyme-regulated activities of the bloodstream LPL. Of course, this enzymatic variant also remains firmly under the control of insulin, as well.)

Although this biochemical balancing act sounds complicated, the underlying logic couldn't be simpler. What's happening here is that, based on your genetically controlled cholesterol level, *the more cholesterol you take in with your food, the more actively the body "compensates" for it by "binding" it harmlessly, via the ester. And conversely: If you eat very little cholesterol over a period of days, the body will compensate by "telling" the liver to make more of the endogenous cholesterol.*

Pictured another way, you might simply describe the body's cholesterol-management system as a delivery service—FedEx comes to mind—in which "boxes" containing fats, cholesterol and protein (the technical name for the boxes is "lipoproteins") are endlessly being assembled, delivered and then taken apart in the bloodstream, in order to provide the cells with cholesterol.

This depiction of the process helps us to understand the key role played by "packaging" in cholesterol-management. In fact, the *amount* of cholesterol we take in matters far less than the type of vehicle (or lipoprotein) which delivers it. And that's because the human body uses some types of packaging far more efficiently than others, and thus delivers much greater amounts of "free cholesterol" to waiting cells in situations where the vehicle features this extra efficiency.

Once again, we are faced with the parallel to the thermodynamics issue. "Cholesterol in equals cholesterol out." No, "cholesterol in" is just the first step of a remarkable journey of this necessary substance, a journey full of packaging, enzymes, lipoprotein carriers, recognition molecules and renegade Lp(a), through the human body. Provided we avoid the dangerous packages made by insulin responses and our own genetic make-up, we have nothing to fear from the **Cholesterol Ogre.**

11

W*HY DO WE KEEP FEEDING THE CHOLESTEROL OGRE?*

Question for Ogre-Fighters Everywhere: If only 20 percent of the population needs to worry about high cholesterol, how did the nation become convinced that this harmless, fatty stuff is more lethal than arsenic?

Answer for Ogre-Fighters Everywhere: The myths about cholesterol and heart disease actually got their start way back in 1987, when the National Institutes of Health (NIH) released the results of five widely publicized studies on the subject. These studies targeted white males aged 40–65, and two of them were restricted to Scandinavians. Nonetheless, their findings became the statistical foundation for the National Cholesterol Education Program (NCEP)—a massive project aimed at "waking America up to the dangers of cholesterol."

Although the demographics were limited, the five studies did establish that among middle-aged white men, at least, cholesterol levels over 240 are associated with an increased risk of heart disease (and especially in the presence of other risk factors such as diabetes, smoking or high blood pressure).

Remarkably enough, however, the NCEP somehow managed to leap from this narrow finding to the conclusion that *anyone* with a cholesterol level of more than *200* milligrams per deciliter of blood should immediately launch a low-cholesterol diet, along with a high-powered exercise program. What? Reminder: when you hear consensus opinions of panels of experts, look out! Find out who is paying the experts for their time.

Within a matter of months, it seemed, these mere opinions of the NCEP became the Conventional Wisdom on cholesterol. All too soon the entire nation was talking about the "dangers of LDL"—and refusing to even *look* at egg yolks, cheddar cheese, T-bone steaks and all the rest of the high-cholesterol foods. And it wasn't long before every lab slip in America listed the normal value of cholesterol to be under 200.

Although I don't want to slide into cynicism on this issue, I can't help asking: What was the motivation behind saying that "200 is better than 240," in the absence of scientific proof? Maybe that NIH panel of experts truly believed that if lowering your cholesterol a little bit (down below 240) was good for your health ... then lowering it a *whole lot* (way down below 200) would be even better. Still, I can't help wondering: Is there anybody out there besides me who suspects that the "200 decision" might have been influenced in some way by external forces that were in favor of establishing an unreachable goal for serum cholesterol levels?

As remarkable as it seems, Americans soon proved willing to make draconian changes in their eating habits, based on these NCEP declarations ... *even though all of the studies involved told us virtually nothing about women, African-Americans, Hispanics or young people!*

Make no mistake: the trend-setting recommendations about lowering cholesterol and fat intake came directly from this first panel and its unsubstantiated *opinions*. Just try to find a clinical lab now, however, that doesn't put an asterisk on the 200 value for the upper limits of normal for cholesterol, even though there is no proof that 200 is the magic number.

A second NCEP panel (1993) discovered that focusing on low-fat, low-cholesterol diets—while also demanding a reduction in total cholesterol—didn't really have a measurable impact on cardiac health, as had been opined by the first NCEP study-group. But the scientists on the second panel weren't discouraged by these disappointing findings; they moved quickly to recommend that the citizens reduce their unsaturated fat intake (while also "increasing their HDL") as the next logical step in the War on Ogre Cholesterol. No one talked much about the genetics of HDL. The number might fall if the patient smoked and went up some if the patient drank an alcoholic beverage, especially red wine, moderately. Ignore for a moment the fact that the rise in HDL in the red wine drinkers occurred in a metabolically inert form of HDL (the jury is still out on this point). Who really believed that we could raise our HDL? Many people were convinced, after all the NIH was the NIH, right?

It wasn't long, however, before the target shifted again, as you knew it had to. The diet has no chance of working; I have showed you why low cholesterol intake activates compensatory metabolic reactions that increase internal production of cholesterol and why HDL is never going to be raised by diet. By 2001, the latest (NCEP III) in this never-ending series of NCEP panels was focusing squarely on the arch-villain of the entire melodrama: LDL cholesterol. The bottom-line recommendation: Drug treatment should be prescribed vigorously for *all* those with high cholesterol. Get ready for the rise in statin-associated morbidity!

A travesty of scientific research? You bet. What's needed, of course, is a panel with the courage to step forward and point out the obvious—that the only people who really need cholesterol-lowering medications on a daily basis are the Type II patients with chronically high cholesterol ... and that the rest of us who have never had a heart attack require nothing more elaborate than losing some weight and reducing our daily intake of dietary amylose!

In many cases, the clinical decision-making that followed on the heels of these unsupported recommendations bordered on the absurd. Example: In one notorious case study, a 22-year-old female athlete was found by her clinician to have a cholesterol level of 220. In spite of the fact that her body fat represented only 15 percent of her body mass and that she was in superb physical condition, the doctor felt required to tell her: "You have a cholesterol problem!"

The medical brouhaha over the NCEP opinions began immediately, and it has not yet subsided. And with good reason … because there are two basic trends that blew the lid right off the NCEP's eat-less-fat-and-exercise-more approach to preventing heart disease:

First, the studies showed clearly that the "Type II" high-cholesterol patients could not be helped by dietary changes, since their daily cholesterol outputs were the result of genetic programming.

Second, the same studies made it clear that cutting down on dietary cholesterol among the remaining 80 percent of the public had no effect whatsoever on reducing heart disease rates!

Even worse, a related series of highly disturbing studies showed that patients who followed low-fat diets in an attempt to lower cholesterol eventually experienced an average weight-*gain* of slightly more than eight pounds per year. Ironically enough, their weight increases, which came primarily from low-fat (read, "high-corn syrup") foods and "wholesome diets containing six-to-11 servings per day of complex carbohydrates" (read, "amylose"), actually *drove up* their cholesterol!

Interestingly however, the CDC's continuing discussion of the "trend toward obesity" in the United States completely failed to mention the powerful role played by low-fat diets.

Step right up, ladies and gentlemen, and meet the Cholesterol Ogre!

GETTING BEHIND MYTHICAL "200 CHOLESTEROL"

What *is* it about cholesterol that makes otherwise intelligent people become so strangely compulsive and irrational?

Let me tell you for a moment about one of my medical colleagues —an outstanding practitioner, beloved by her patients—who seems to be afflicted with a terrifying aversion to the ordinary egg yolk.

Example: I've heard her describe more than once how she opens eggs and then carefully pours the whites into a container for her breakfast. (The yolks go straight into the trash.) This good woman has apparently decided—in spite of the medical evidence and in spite of my urging—that biting into an egg yolk will bring on an instant aneurysm ... or perhaps lead to a fatal blood clot deep inside a coronary artery.

Do you think she listens to me when I describe the life-history of another friend—a commercial fisherman in Maryland who ate 30 eggs, fresh from the hen house, daily for 50 years, before finally dying of an ailment completely unrelated to cholesterol at age 86? (Question: What were his apo A and Lp[a] numbers?)

Regardless of the evidence, however, people like my doctor-friend continue to insist that eating too much of the wrong kind of cholesterol (translation: fear about LDL cholesterol, but LDL isn't in our food, it is a lipoprotein carrier!) will rapidly destroy your arteries and bring on a heart attack or a stroke or both.

Much of the blame for this absurd mythology rests with the news media, which has been bombarding us with LDL "scare stories" for more than a decade now. Flip on a news program or pick up the afternoon paper, these days, and you're likely to receive a dramatic health warning: "The oxidation of LDL must be prevented at all costs."

Of course, the same voices often urge us to "include more vitamin E and C, along with extra beta carotene," in order to make certain that the dreaded LDL-oxidation does not take place. But these melodramatic warnings inevitably fail to include a very valuable piece of information—the undisputed fact that oxidation of LDL always takes place inside the cell.

As any undergraduate biology major will quickly tell you, antioxidants such as vitamins E and C only rarely penetrate human cells ... and certainly have little effect on the sequestered, membrane surrounded, LDL-receptor complex inside the cell. In other words: there isn't a shred of scientific evidence to support the notion that consuming these vitamins has the slightest impact on heart disease rates.

Even more disturbing than this deception, however, has been the continuing stream of misinformation about the adverse health role that cholesterol plays among the elderly. According to a recent and highly influential report by the NIH (NCEP, Adult Treatment Panel II, 1993), there are significant heart-health benefits to be gained by prescribing cholesterol-lowering medications for patients over 65 whose blood-cholesterol exceeds 200. As the report notes on page IV-4: *Drug therapy may have a role in some high-risk elderly patients, particularly those who are in good health.*

This remarkable observation—one of several in which the Panel gives tacit approval for widespread use of cholesterol-lowering drugs among people over 65—was offered to a believing public ... even though there are no primary prevention studies whatsoever to demonstrate that over-200 cholesterol has any impact at all on heart disease in the elderly!

Interestingly enough, the NIH panel readily admits—in Part IV, Section A1 of its own report—that there is no hard evidence for concluding that elevated cholesterol in the elderly is associated with heart disease. As the Panel points out:

"Primary and secondary prevention clinical trials have included relatively few elderly patients, and the question can be raised whether results

carried out in middle-aged patients can be extrapolated to the elderly. Since the basic pathophysiologic processes underlying coronary atherosclerosis and CHD probably are similar in middle age and later life, extrapolation across the life span in principle seems reasonable. Moreover limited trials of drug and dietary treatment of elevated cholesterol levels among elderly subjects indicate that they are at least as responsive as younger persons. Thus this document regards it as reasonable to predict that cholesterol-lowering regimens will have similar effects on the pathogenesis and prevention of CHD in middle-aged and elderly people."

I can't agree that the heart-health characteristics of a 39 year old guy with his second heart attack are related in any way to the 79 year old man who has lived long enough to also have calcifications in his heels, his shoulders, and his cartilages as well as his arteries.

After admitting that there are no hard data to support the "extrapolation," this extraordinary document goes on to cite only one controversial—and deeply flawed—study that appears to provide evidence (but only "by analogy") of a link between CHD and cholesterol in the elderly, as follows:

This conclusion seems bolstered by analogy from the positive outcomes of trials of CHD prevention in the elderly, notably, the recently completed Systolic Hypertension in the Elderly Program (SHEP). In this trial, which included a significant proportion of subjects in their seventies and eighties, reduction in isolated systolic hypertension among otherwise healthy older persons substantially reduced cardiovascular complications, both CHD and stroke. A similar result can be anticipated in therapy for CHD prevention through cholesterol lowering in older persons. The extent to which this potential benefit can be translated into reality in practice, however, has not been fully determined.

Convincing?

Hardly. Here's my question for the cholesterol gurus at the NIH: How can a single study—itself allegedly flawed—that is based entirely on high blood pressure data serve as the basis for conclusions about CHD and cholesterol in the elderly?

Let the readers of this book answer that key question for them-selves!

Regardless of the deep flaws in this NIH assessment of the is-sue, however, the net result was that several million older Ameri-cans—many of them on fixed incomes—soon wound up with prescriptions for expensive cholesterol medications that they sim-ply didn't need. With the generalizations of NCEP III in 2001, the dollars spent on cholesterol medications will sky-rocket. Add a national program to pay for prescription drugs and Pandora's payment box is wide open. An appalling failure of leadership? You bet. But a great deal of the responsibility for creating the "Ogre" also lies with the U.S. Medical Establishment, which has spent many years needlessly frightening the public about the dangers of cholesterol—even as the pharmaceutical companies (who fund most of the Establishment's "scientific research," after all) have been making millions peddling their cholesterol-low-ering medications. The drugs are safe and work well, no ques-tion about that. But who are the at-risk patients who truly need them?

Does this sound harsh, even cynical?

Is Big Science really for sale in this country—and are most of the highly regarded "academic scientists" at the major universi-ties and government "think tanks" unwittingly participating in a conspiracy to sell people health products that don't improve their health?

Before you decide that Dr. Shoemaker has "gone around the bend" on this topic, read what one of the prestigious medical journals in the U.S. (the New England Journal of Medicine) published as an editorial on the conflict of interest at work in situations where scientists conduct research paid for by drug com-panies.

According to a May 18, 2000 editorial, "IS ACADEMIC MEDICINE FOR SALE," the continuing conflict of interest amounts to nothing less than a national scandal:

The ties between clinical researchers and industry include not only grant support, but also a host of other financial arrangements. Researchers serve as consultants to companies whose products they are studying, join advisory boards and speakers' bureaus, enter into patent and royalty arrangements, agree to be the listed author of articles ghostwritten by interested companies, promote drugs and devices at company sponsored symposiums, and allow themselves to be plied with expensive gifts and trips to luxurious settings. ...

Academic medical institutions are themselves growing increasingly beholden to industry. How can they justify rigorous conflict of interest policies for individual researchers when their own ties are so extensive? Some academic institutions have entered into partnerships with drug companies to set up research centers and teaching programs in which students and faculty members essentially carry out industry research.

What is the justification for this large-scale breaching of the boundaries between academic medicine and for-profit industry? ... When the boundaries between industry and academic medicine become as blurred as they now are, the business goals of industry influence the mission of the medical schools in multiple ways. As the critics of medicine so often charge, young physicians learn that for every problem there is a pill (and a drug company representative to explain it).

Ask yourself: Does the above argument by the august editors of the NEJM sound convincing, or what? As the judge always says in the courtroom, while banging his wooden gavel: "Next case!"

I want to be clear in my message: I also have received research support from pharmaceutical companies that also make cholesterol lowering medications. I have no quarrel with drug companies funding basic science and research, but every consensus panel and every expert must come clean with anything that might be a conflict of interest. While I am not saying that any scientist's opinion is for sale when a study is done, and mine certainly isn't, the public needs to know who did a study, who paid for the study and who edited the results of the study for the payor's benefit.

SOME GOOD NEWS FOR NO-AMYLOSE DIETERS

After more than 20 years of watching people struggle to lose weight—while also studying the biochemistry involved in the process—I'm convinced beyond a reasonable doubt that counting milligrams of dietary cholesterol is mostly a waste of time ... especially if you happen to be one of the 20 percent of Americans who are cursed with genetically programmed high-cholesterol. In that case, you must take medication to counteract your physiology. Just be sure you know that all medications can hurt us.

If you're a Type IV, on the other hand, you need to forget about counting cholesterol—and start counting amylose!

Regardless of the continuing debate over cholesterol and heart disease, the good news for millions of people today is that keeping your weight down by limiting your intake of glucose and amylose will *also* work to keep your cholesterol at rock-bottom. (For more detailed facts about the biochemistry involved, see the upcoming chapter on rosiglitazone and PPAR-gamma: Chapter 13.)

Why? It's actually quite simple. To review the steps in the argument one last time:

○ First, the problem with ingesting large amounts of glucose and amylose is that they cause the body to release large amounts of insulin.

○ Second, along with transporting sugar molecules across cell membranes, this powerful substance is assigned the task of "turning on" the key enzyme involved in the production of cholesterol.

○ Third, as soon as this reaction-galvanizing enzyme gets a "green light" from the insulin surge, it goes to work boosting cholesterol production in the liver.

○ Fourth, if you eat those three slices of bread with dinner—or that heaping bowl of *spaghettini*—you're not only telling your body to make fat ... you're also telling it to manufacture lots more cholesterol.

As I've told thousands of dieters over the years: "If you can shut down the scenario in which your body converts starch calories to fat, you will be lowering your cholesterol in the bargain!"

That's all the typical dieter really needs to know about food intake and cholesterol. But it would also be helpful for most weight-loss candidates to sit down with their family physician and learn something about the particles that actually count most, when it comes to hardening of the arteries—the apoproteins, along with Lp(a), which determine the dynamics of cholesterol-management in the bloodstream.

Regardless of the complex movements of these particles, however, the bottom line is always the same: the controlling factor for all of them is insulin response!

THE COST OF FEEDING THE OGRE—IN DOLLARS AND CENTS

If you don't think there are Big Dollars to be made out of the "cholesterol scare," consider the following scenario, which gets played out in America millions of times each day. Imagine a recently retired individual, 65 years old, who's living on a fixed income. One fine morning, he or she drops by the doctor's office for a regular checkup.

"Uh-oh," says the doc, while scanning a report from the laboratory. "Your cholesterol is too high … why, it's still over 240!"

"Sounds bad, doc! I sure don't want heart disease. I've been exercising like you said. And as much as I hate those fake eggs and awful tasting low-fat foods, I've been sticking to the diet. Tell me what I need to do."

Within a matter of minutes, the physician is writing this older patient a prescription for a "cholesterol-lowering medication" … a pill, I might add, that these days costs anywhere from $3 to $4 each. (In many cases, of course, the doc winds up prescribing *two* of the pills to the unsuspecting patient, in situations when one tablet daily does not meet the "200 goal.") Yet the patient has already outlived a premature heart attack.

The results are painful to think about. Imagine a retiree living on $750 a month from Social Security ... and spending, let's say, $200 a month for the cholesterol medication that he doesn't actually need!

Don't let this happen to you, reader.

And don't make the equally tragic mistake of destroying your quality of life by spending time worrying needlessly about cholesterol and fat grams. Sure, you need to be thoughtful about the foods you eat. If you're a Type II phenotype, you need the daily medication ... and if you've had a heart attack in the past, you should *get that LDL-level down under 100*. The medical literature, independent of studies sponsored by drug companies, is quite clear on this point.

Enough said. Once all appropriate precautions have been taken, it's time to stop worrying about cholesterol and enjoy your dinner!

Each time I give a patient this advice (as often as possible!), I'm reminded of the 1992 Olympics in Barcelona ... and in particular of a feature newspaper story written by a U.S. reporter about life in that beautiful city.

Obviously disgusted, the reporter went on at length about how appalled he was by the Spaniards' lifestyle. Why ... the taverns in Barcelona were simply *jammed* with folks guzzling red wine, eating chin-high servings of greasy food, and puffing on fat cigars. But when the reporter asked one Spaniard "how in the world you people manage to live so long, with this kind of lifestyle," the amused wine-bibber snapped back:

"The problem with you Americans is that you're afraid to live. You print warnings on your cigarettes and your bottles of beer, and you're terrified to eat an egg.

"Here in Spain, we don't die any sooner than you—but our lives are full of *life*!"

Why Do We Keep Feeding the Cholesterol Ogre?

I think we can all take a good lesson from that merry Spaniard ... by worrying less about the fat and the cholesterol in our lives. Instead of fretting needlessly, let's start putting that energy into *enjoying* the food we eat!

12

THE FACTS ABOUT EXERCISE AND WEIGHT-LOSS

ONCE CONSIDERED A "MAGIC BULLET" FOR OBESITY, GETTING MORE EXERCISE TURNS OUT TO BE A BLANK

Key question for hopeful dieters: How much do you know about the actual role of exercise (as opposed to the public myths) in losing weight and keeping it off?

To test your factual knowledge of how working out actually affects weight-loss, just mark the following statements "True" or "False."

O If you exercise every day—while also avoiding fatty foods —you can lose several pounds a week, guaranteed.

O High-energy aerobic exercises burn calories at a rapid rate —which means that you could "burn off" a hot fudge sundae, let's say, merely by running around the block for 10 minutes.

205

O When you exercise, your body relies exclusively on cholesterol for fuel—which means that working out is a surefire way to reduce your cholesterol-level.

O Exercise prevents heart attacks, because breathing hard for extended periods prevents harmful plaque deposits from building up on the walls of arteries.

O The human body was designed for exercise, so people who launch strenuous exercise programs such as running or weight-lifting don't have to worry about injury, regardless of their age.

O   O   O

If you answered "False" to all five of these questions, you deserve a round of applause—for having the common sense required to fend off some of the most pervasive myths in all of American life.

These absurd myths, endlessly promulgated in the news media and in the doctor's office alike, tell us that the "secret to losing weight is getting more exercise and eating less fat!"

Wrong, wrong, wrong.

After more than 20 years of practicing sports medicine as an important part of my outpatient practice, I never fail to be amazed by the inflated list of "health benefits" that supposedly flow from even the lightest exercise, as America's surreal obsession with "working out" grows more frantic by the day.

How did we wind up, as a nation, in the extraordinarily paradoxical situation of "worshipping exercise" ... even as the U.S. Centers for Disease Control and Prevention (CDC) warns that more *than one-third of all Americans* are now officially classified as "obese," and that the cause of our obesity is mostly our sedentary life style?

Exercise is routinely listed by experts as beneficial for a weight loss program. And it is, if the patient exercises to a high level for at least *12 hours per week*. Exercise is also listed as a recommended method for raising HDL as part of a cholesterol risk reduction program. That is also true, but only if the patient avoids the foods that cause insulin to shut down lipoprotein lipase, the enzyme that loads cholesterol onto HDL-3, making HDL-2. Without the activity of the enzyme, HDL levels of all classes fall, as does total HDL.

For the rest of us non-Olympians—ordinary folk who struggle to find even 20 minutes to take a walk each day—gaining "accurate knowledge" about obesity, insulin resistance and exercise is an absolutely essential step on the road to good health.

When it comes to understanding weight-loss and maintenance, the real enemy is misinformation—false knowledge based on a flawed understanding of how the human body actually responds to exercise at the biochemical level.

Read the health news these days, and the odds are high that you'll end up thinking of exercise as a "magic bullet" cure for just about every ailment that torments the human race ... everything from obesity to diabetes to asthma to alcoholism to clinical depression.

Too bad that most of these glowing assessments of exercise actually amount to little more than breathless hype.

Please don't get me wrong, however: Exercise *can* provide some real health benefits (along with a lot of fun!) for those who know how to get the most out of it. And the first step in that process is resisting the hype—while keeping the actual relationship between dieting and exercise in clear perspective.

To show you what I mean, let's return to our "True or False" quiz and take a quick look at each of the "Exercise Myths" described there.

MYTH: *If you exercise every day—while also avoiding fatty foods—you can lose several pounds a week, guaranteed.*

REALITY: Exercise actually burns calories at a relatively slow rate, so unless you spend many hours each day out on the running track, the ultimate impact on your body's fat-storage metabolism will be minimal. In the same way, eating less fat will have little if any effect on how your body converts glucose and amylose to fatty acids, which is actually the key factor in making most people overweight.

MYTH: *High-energy aerobic exercises burn calories at a rapid rate— which means that you could "burn off" a hot fudge sundae, let's say, merely by running around the block for 10 minutes.*

REALITY: In fact, even most the strenuous physical exercise actually burns calories at a relatively low rate. *(See calorie-tables in Appendix 5.)* To make up for that hot fudge sundae, for example, you'd probably have to run around the block for an hour, not 10 minutes. The bottom line: You can't depend on exercise to melt away the weight you hate!

MYTH: *When you exercise, your body relies exclusively on cholesterol for fuel—which means that working out is a surefire way to reduce your cholesterol-level.*

REALITY: This is nonsense. Although tiny amounts of cholesterol do get used up during physical activity, the basic "fuel" burned by the body is glycogen, a complex carbohydrate storage compound for glucose. Regardless of how much you exercise, you can't change the genetically programmed dynamics that control how your body stores and transports cholesterol.

MYTH: *Exercise prevents heart attacks, because breathing hard for extended periods keeps harmful plaque deposits from building up on the walls of arteries.*

REALITY: The medical condition known as "atherosclerosis" occurs when oxidated cholesterol hardens into plaque on the walls of arteries and other blood vessels. We have a lot to learn about the complex series of events that involve apoproteins, platelets, cells that comprise the blood vessel walls, white blood cells that migrate into blood vessel walls, compounds with unusual names like plasminogen activating inhibitor that appear to enhance clot formation in plaque and prevent dissolution of the clot, substances involved with inflammation (the unusual names abound here), and cholesterol and atherosclerosclerosis. But it is safe to say that breathing hard has nothing to do with hardening of the arteries. Elevated cholesterol is a vastly overblown risk factor for four-fifths of the American population, and is actually far less important in most cases than other factors such as smoking, diabetes and high blood pressure.

MYTH: *The human body was designed for exercise, so people who launch strenuous exercise programs such as running or weight-lifting don't have to worry about injury, regardless of their age.*

REALITY: In fact, such high-impact sports as jogging, basketball and racquetball place enormous stress on hip, knee and ankle joints. Weight-lifting also includes a significant risk factor (especially among those avid participants who enjoy doing "bug-eye" bench presses!) for rotator cuff injuries and shoulder-impingement syndromes. These strenuous activities can also injure muscles and tendons through overuse. For these reasons, middle-aged patients (and especially those over 50) should not launch ambitious exercise programs without consulting a physician (don't settle for lip-service) first. Learn to stretch before you try to run!

EMPTY CLAIMS AND UNREAL BENEFITS

As a former competitive wrestler in high school, I'm a great fan of both organized sports and physical exercise. I'm also convinced that these activities provide some important health benefits for their participants—including improved muscle tone, heightened aerobic performance and refinement of dexterity, coordination and the motor skills required for effective running, throwing and jumping, for example. Another huge payoff for this kind of activity is the personal sense of accomplishment and satisfaction that accompanies the proud statement: "I have *done* something!" Great, I'm glad you made the time to enhance your fitness.

My reservations about the health value of exercise are restricted entirely to the false claims that have been made on its behalf in recent years by a Medical Establishment that seems intent on spreading misinformation about the physiology of working-out.

Perhaps the most egregious example of this "disinformation campaign" can be found in the area of cardiac medicine, where proponents of the "Exercise More and Eat Less Fat School" of preventing heart disease never seem to tire of singing the praises of the exercise machines to be found at your local health club.

In spite of the fact that "cardiac rehab" has become a fast-growing medical industry in recent years, the claims for this approach to preventing heart attacks have remained depressingly hollow.

Let's face it: The Public Relations Machine that feeds the Exercise Myth is fueled by "true believers" (and there are millions of them out there), along with a huge number of truly dedicated physical fitness enthusiasts. Who can blame this latter group for taking so much pride in the Daily Workout? And why *shouldn't* the sizeable U.S. population of "obligate runners" (they crank out at least six miles a day) take satisfaction in their "lean-and-mean" appearance, after spending so many hours huffing and puffing along rural highways and city sidewalks?

Still, there's no doubt that this group of "Just Do It!" workout-fanatics represents a small minority—and that most of us simply don't have the time for such extended jogs across the countryside.

The blunt fact is that you can't "Just Do It"—if all you have is 20 minutes per day (or per *week*) to hit the tennis court or the weight room at your local health club!

Still, the current tendency to regard exercise as a cure-all for every illness is hardly a new one. To this day, I haven't forgotten my first encounter with the issue ... back during my days as a medical student at Duke. It happened one afternoon in 1975, as I watched the head of the Department of Medicine—a leading internist in the mid-Atlantic region—examine a heart attack survivor during a follow-up visit.

Gathered around the patient's beside, we medical students were listening avidly, intent on gleaning any pearls of insight or wisdom that might fall our way.

Along with our professor, we listened carefully while the heart patient in the bed described the wonders of his new "exercise regimen" ... a daily routine that included many sit-ups and push-ups, along with lots of time spent walking and jogging on a treadmill.

More than once, our professor/internist smiled at the patient's newly found faith in the benefits of exercise.

But once we'd said our good-byes and then reassembled out of earshot 20 yards down the hallway, our teacher turned to us and pointed out: "At least this patient will be in good physical condition—when he dies of his next, inevitable heart attack!"

After more than two decades of caring for heart attack victims and patients suffering from other forms of heart disease, I can tell you that the professor's words are as true today as they were in 1975 ... regardless of the "exercise hype" that flows non-stop from such citadels of popular culture as the CBS Evening News, Women's Day, Prevention Magazine and Sports Illustrated.

EXERCISING FOR WEIGHT-LOSS HAS ONLY ONE DRAWBACK—IT DOESN'T WORK!

In order to get a handle on why exercising more and eating less is an ineffective strategy for achieving permanent weight-loss, let's take a quick at the highlights from several recent studies that actually measured the impact of jogging and swimming and all the rest on fat storage in the human body.

For many of us—accustomed as we are to the endless (and "politically correct") prattle about the "benefits of exercise"—these numbers will come as a shock. Why? Because they make it perfectly clear that our current attitudes about "working out" aren't based in scientific fact—but in cultural mythology.

Example: How many times have you heard a friend or neighbor brag loudly: "Oh, I *never* use a cart when I play golf—walking those four miles is such a great workout!" (The reality: If you stretch a four-mile walk out over four hours and 18 holes, the actual impact on your metabolism will be minimal. If the fellow had just said, "I get a terrific benefit from being outside, seeing Nature up close and getting away from the hectic life at the office," I would not argue about the benefit of the golf game.

Or how about the tennis fanatic who tells you: "We just spent an hour playing doubles—a terrific workout!" (The reality: Playing tennis doubles usually amounts to nothing more strenuous than standing in place for long stretches at a time, in between taking an occasional whack at the ball. For most players, the most strenuous part of the game consists of bending over to pick up loose balls—which doesn't make a dent in the calories from the two or three beers, the overstuffed roast beef sandwich and the bowl or two of pretzels they'll enjoy later in the clubhouse!)

BURNING EXCESS CALORIES: THE STOPWATCH DOESN'T LIE

Ever wondered just how many fat calories you can burn off by walking, running, swimming or riding a bicycle? *(See Appendix 6.)*

If you're like most readers, you may be surprised to discover that it takes a great deal of physical effort to make even the smallest inroads on your body's storehouse of fat! Some examples:

○ If you walk at a moderate pace … you'd have to keep it up for more 37 minutes, just to burn the amount of calories contained in the average serving of chocolate ice cream (193).

○ Pedaling your bicycle over hill and dale won't save you from fat—not when it takes 31 minutes of such high-energy exertion just to burn off the calories contained in an ice cream soda (255).

○ So you like to swim laps—hard laps—at the local YMCA pool? Sounds good … but it won't protect you from fat attacks caused by high-calorie foods. Example: You'd have to swim those laps for 48 minutes without stopping, in order to shed the calories contained in the average TV chicken dinner (542).

○ Although running does burn a few more calories than most other forms of exercise (provided that you don't just "shuffle" along), even this strenuous activity won't provide you with a "magic bullet" for fat. To "run off" that same TV chicken dinner, for example, you'd have to keep running around the block for at least 28 minutes.

○ ○ ○

DESIGNING A REALISTIC EXERCISE PROGRAM

Although exercise won't save you from the fat-penalties that accrue from eating too much glucose and amylose, there's nothing wrong (and indeed, there's an awful lot *right*) with exercising as a way to improve cardiovascular fitness—while also toning up muscles that may have lain dormant for too many years.

Before launching an ambitious exercise regimen, however, it's *very* important to remember that most "ballistic exercises"—activities that involve running and jumping—will send major shocks ripping through your heels, ankles, knees, hips and lower back. If the muscles that support these joints haven't been strengthened (or if you fail to stretch them adequately during warm-ups), the result could be joint discomfort or even injury.

Instead of frustrating yourself and winding up on a non-steroidal anti-inflammatory medication, why not design a realistic exercise program that starts very slowly with stretching activities, then graduates bit by bit to more dynamic pastimes such as basketball and distance running?

If you want to gain a real appreciation for the value of stretching, just watch a professional athlete prepare for "game day." Ever noticed how a professional tennis player will spend a full 15–20 minutes stretching legs and arms and lower back—*before* he or she gets down to the serious business of hitting the ball?

Question: How do you know when you haven't been stretching leg, arm and back muscles enough before engaging in strenuous exercise?

As in most things, common sense can be your guide. If you notice soreness or discomfort when you stretch a muscle group—of if you notice restriction in joint extension or flexion—you can be pretty sure that you haven't stretched those aching muscle fibers enough.

For many obese patients, the most obvious effects of exercise-related dysfunction can be found in the "hamstring" muscles (hams), which often become truncated and inflexible from carrying the patient's excess weight. Too see what I mean, just take a look at how the big belly on the character we'll call "Belly Man" pulls his center of gravity forward. In order to keep from falling on his face, Belly Man is forced to arch (extend) his back. But that maneuver leaves him in an unnatural position—leaning far backwards—which puts enormous pressure on his inter-vertebral disks, while also requiring him to bend his knees slightly. (Of course, this postural distortion continued over time also accounts for most of the chronic low back pain and sciatica to be found in those suffering from obesity.)

214

With his stressed body distorted in these various ways, Belly Man typically develops a dysfunctional kind of walking in which his hamstrings remain in constant flexion. All too soon, this unnatural posture begins to alter the bio-mechanics of the knee, so that the inside cartilage (medial meniscus) is subjected to subtle increases in torque and tear. Experience shows that in most cases, the first structure to be damaged in the knees of overweight patients is the severely stressed medial meniscus ... and that this injury syndrome clearly ranks as the most common cause of knee replacement among overweight patients.

Still, there are several other forms of this dysfunction—all of which may require extended stretching in order to restore abused muscles and tendons to normal use. Among the most common of these muscle disorders are the following:

- trapezius muscle spasm, upper back pain, headache
- rotator cuff syndromes, shoulder pain, worse with hands above shoulders
- impingement syndromes, shoulder pain, hands moving up to shoulders
- extensor and flexor epicondylitis, elbow and wrist pain
- carpal tunnel syndrome, wrist pain and hand numbness, overuse
- costochondritis, pectoralis muscles insert on sternum, chest pain
- piriformis muscle spasm, buttock and hip pain, mimics sciatica
- patello-femoral syndrome, knee pain, especially in teen age women athletes
- anterior compartment syndrome, lower leg, worse with excessive pronation seen in runners—look for wear on the shoes
- achilles tendinitis, pain with use of calf muscles

215

O   plantar fasciitis, morning heel pain

This rather grim-sounding list of muscle disorders underlines what's wrong with the "eat less and exercise more" approach to weight-loss—namely, the disturbing fact that asking overweight and under-stretched patients to suddenly become two-hour mall walkers will often cause significant micro-trauma to individual muscle fibrils.

When that happens, local swelling and fluid retention are the inevitable results, with inflammation following not far behind. And what happens next? It's simple: Somewhere between the heating pad (or am I *supposed* to use ice packs—who knows?), the MRI, the cortisone shots, the Synvisc injections (three of them, at $800 a pop), the arthroscopy procedures and the binges of Tylenol, our would-be weight-loser throws in the towel ... and gives up both the weight-loss *and* the exercise programs!

In spite of these hazards, however, the malls and the jogging tracks of America are crowded each day with lost souls who wail: "Just look at me—if I don't start exercising daily, I'm gonna keep on gaining weight!" Unfortunately, these misguided strivers have not been taught that the impact of exercise on calorie-burning is minimal ... and that they're significantly increasing their risk of injury when they suddenly start exercising for all their worth.

But this repeatedly observed scenario doesn't have to happen to you—not when you can rely on the instructions in LOSE THE WEIGHT YOU HATE! to help you shape an exercise regimen that will protect your body from injury, even as you gradually re-build and strengthen de-conditioned muscles.

STAY AWAY FROM THE "EXERCISE MACHINES"— ALONG WITH THE PUSHUPS AND BENCH PRESSES!

Here's a fun suggestion for all of us who've ever been tempted to spend "only $39.99 a month" on a slick-looking exercise machine

... after being promised: "Your best friends won't recognize you at the beach, as you show off the kind of lean, muscle-rippling physique that most people only dream about!"

Turn off the sound!

That's right—just go ahead and hit the "mute" button on the Zenith and watch that next "Exercise Infomercial" without benefit of the verbal sales pitch. By focusing exclusively on the visual come-ons contained in the video, you should be able to separate the reality from the hype. Why, look at all those gorgeously sculpted models, each one outfitted with sleek biceps and wasp-slender waists! Surely *you* can become one of these lean and elegant sirens ... merely by working out three times a week on one of the chrome-plated, Space Age exercise-contraptions these sylph-like creatures seem to enjoy so much!

Better take a closer look, however—before you start stressing your heart *and* your wallet.

Those are actually professional models ... and they undoubtedly get paid to spend four or five hours a day working out furiously, in order to assemble the kind of evanescent and incredibly short-lived physical beauty that leaves us salivating in front of the TV screen.

It's a scam, my friends. It's nothing more than a modern, high-tech variant of Ponce de Leon's Sixteenth-Century quest to locate (and then commercially bottle) the "Fountain of Youth"—a magical elixir guaranteed to postpone the effects of aging, while promising endless physical beauty to all who drink the secret potion.

(Ponce never discovered the Fountain, by the way.)

And you won't, either—no matter how many hours you spend riding the latest version of the "Great Titanium Nordic Colossus" sold by the blonde bombshell celebrity-of-the-month. (Don't worry—the Colossus will end up in the closet, along with the barbells and the "rowing machine" you bought ten years ago and never used.)

217

But wasting your money on needless exercise equipment is only one of the bad things that can happen, if you allow yourself to be seduced by these unscrupulous Infomercials for Stair-Steppers (there go the hamstrings!), ski devices (stand by for a Nordic hyper-extension of the spine!) or rowing machines (welcome to your impingement syndrome!).

All too often, these impressive-looking machines simply end up promoting asymmetric development of the targeted muscle groups. That happens because the infernal devices usually do not provide balance, flexibility or effective range of motion. Instead of stimulating healthy muscle development, they often contribute to various overuse syndromes, along with impingement of the shoulder's range of motion.

Machines aren't the only villains in the drama called *Exercise Your Way To Injury!*, however. Among the other contenders for the False Bill of Goods Championship are the following popular exercise delusions:

PUSHUPS ARE THE KEY to a beautiful upper body! Sorry, folks, but the key just broke off in the lock. Doing endless pushups at home usually guarantees problems with anterior shoulder musculature, hands down.

I CAN BENCH-PRESS MY WAY to a stunning body! Would that it were so. A more likely scenario, however, is that you'll end up wearing ice-packs and gulping anti-inflammatories, soon after you damage your shoulder muscles and under-used rhomboids with ill-advised weight-lifting.

ONLY 20 MINUTES OF AEROBIC EXERCISE a day will erase all those cellulite-bulges and leave me looking thinner than Twiggy! Will somebody please explain to me how "20 minutes" recently became the two biggest buzz words in the world of physical fitness? The last time *I* looked, 20 minutes was still exactly 1,200 seconds ... which is far too short a time on which to base such ludicrous health claims! (Why 20 minutes? Did it happen after some Madison Avenue marketing whiz realized that this is the amount of time that busy people would think they could spend on themselves? 30 minutes, no way. 10 minutes, not enough. 20? Just right.)

TAKING THE STAIRS INSTEAD OF THE ELEVATOR up to the second floor at work will quickly melt away all my flab, so that I'll wind up looking better than Tab Hunter at the height of his storied appeal. (You're *kidding,* I hope? About the health value of walking the stairs *and* Tab Hunter?)

Ladies and gentlemen, can we "get real," as teenagers like to say?

KEEPING YOUR FEET AND HANDS IN CONSTANT MOTION will allow you to burn off calories by the bucketful. Not true. And the danger with this approach is that it could leave you looking both overweight and jittery at the same time!

RISING UP ONTO YOUR TIPTOES FOR THREE MINUTES EVERY HOUR will keep you razor-thin. Although the women's magazines and the "family health" publications continue to crank out an endless stream of daffy articles such as *Ten Ways To Get All The Exercise You Need Without Leaving Your Office!* and *Exercise Your Way To Great Health By Standing On Tiptoe For Three Minutes A Day!*, the blunt fact remains: Most forms of exercise burn calories so slowly that their impact on weight-loss is insignificant.

Instead of building a Taj Mahal of false expectations around pushups, sit-ups and knee-bends, why not develop a modest, regular routine that includes walking, swimming, and biking in a pleasing combination you will actually *enjoy*? Putting together a realistic program of this kind will allow you to improve your muscle tone and your cardiovascular efficiency, and you'll probably feel more alive and energetic as a result.

Please keep the wonderful benefits of exercise right where they belong: in a fitness program—and not a weight-loss program.

EXERCISE AND TRAINED ATHLETES: A VERY DIFFERENT STORY

Although 20 minutes of exercise per day does not affect fat storage and glucose metabolism, there's no doubt that trained and dedicated athletes who spend three *hours* a day or more working out can expect major benefits in cardiovascular fitness and weight loss. They will undoubtedly have a lower percentage body fat, too.

The key physiological advantage for the trained or professional athlete, of course, can be found in the way he or she is able to greatly increase the efficiency of the mechanism that stores glucose-energy in glycogen. In this situation, the loose insulin–liver receptor and the insulin–muscle receptor interaction become more efficient by virtue of an increased *number* of receptors, and perhaps also by an increased *affinity* of the receptors for insulin, itself. But insulin resistant patients will simply regain their weight when they stop exercising if they start eating amylose again.

As we have seen in earlier chapters, the second mechanism for disposal of glucose from elevated blood sugar depends on the attachment of insulin onto the receptor of a fat cell. Paradoxically, however, the affinity of insulin for the fatty acid receptor in the fat cell is reduced with exercise ... even as the *number* of those receptors is similarly reduced. And this reduced affinity of the receptor is what allows the trained athlete to mobilize fat quickly —without having to wait for the end of the eight-hour period during which insulin remains bound to the receptor site. This freedom from time constraints is precisely what permits the release of fatty acids—so that the latter can be used directly as fuel by muscle cells.

Trained athletes have often described what happens when— after exercising at a high level for a long period of time—they finally exhaust their glycogen reserves. At that point, they suddenly "hit the brick wall" ... after which their bodies begin to release free fatty acids for energy burning. This process culminates in the famous "second wind"—that fabled "last blast of energy" that often accounts for the winning touchdown in football, or a buzzer-beating, last-gasp three-pointer in basketball.

According to recent health research, the phenomenon of the "second wind" leaves behind a biochemical residue that can be detected rather easily in blood serum and urine. This residue consists of particles called "ketones," and these can also be found in the exhalations of athletes who are exercising at peak intensity. Is it any wonder, given this fact, that the biochemical "signature" of low-calories diets such as Medifast™ is the presence of these ketones in both breath and urine?

The source of the ketones is easy to pin down—they emerge when the body burns fat directly, which is precisely how Medifast triggers weight-reduction. Still, these substances can slow down an athlete, if they reach significant levels. To avoid that, most dedicated athletes soon learn how to carry along sugar and water replenishments during competition in order to avoid ketosis.

In the past, more than a few diets (now outmoded, of course) tried to take advantage of the ketone phenomenon by encouraging dieters to eat fat exclusively—in the hope that this rather bizarre approach would result in the increased production of ketone bodies. Unfortunately, however, the dieters soon realized that increased ingestion of fats would *not* lead to mobilization of one's *own* fat stores.

After years of watching patients lose weight (and keep it off) with my protein-sparing 00-2-3 diet, I've proved beyond a reasonable doubt that this approach helps the patient reduce fat stores by diminishing the effect of insulin on the fat cell receptor —regardless of whether or not the dieter happens to be a trained athlete. If you are like most of us and would rather spend an extra 10 hours per week with our families and not alone on a bike or on a running course, stay away from amylose. If your family exercises together (and just look at the bikes mounted on top of vacationers' cars), know your insulin before you assume that the extra exercise will prevent health problems of high cholesterol and obesity.

If you have to mow the grass or double-dig the organic garden, get your work done and enjoy how beautiful everything looks in the long rays of a summer sunset. The hard work provides many emotional and physical benefits, but don't kid yourself; the garden work won't pull the extra pounds.

DAILY EXERCISE: GETTING IT RIGHT

Here's a quick breakdown of the steps involved in working out a realistic exercise program that will help you reclaim your physical fitness.

FIRST ... recognize that every exercise workout must begin with a lengthy period of vigorous stretching of all major muscle groups.

SECOND ... sit down and think your way through a *realistic* daily routine that will actually allow you to meet your goals. (Example: Don't schedule a daily 30-minute walk in Chicago in January, if you know that you *hate* fighting your way through snowdrifts!)

THIRD ... you must create a "support system" that will help you stick to your exercise regimen. (Example: Why not find an exercise partner who can give you "pep talks" when you need them, and vice versa?)

FOURTH ... Go get your picture taken while you're in the middle of exercising. (Believe it or not, experience shows that such photos provide a major boost to motivation, by proving that the dieter does, indeed, *need* to shed some poundage via exercise ... and also that our determined exerciser is doing everything he or she *can* do to achieve that worthy goal. For best results, try taking your photos every three weeks. But remember: Don't confuse fitness with weight-loss!)

FIFTH ... set up a system that will allow you to measure simple fitness parameters—such as calf circumference and degrees of extension of hamstrings. You can obtain another helpful yardstick by counting the number of breaths you take per minute, after climbing three flights of stairs.

HOW LONG SHOULD YOU EXERCISE?

As I've told more than one interviewer in the past, there are no magical properties to be found in the "twenty minutes a day" formula.

Instead of locking yourself into a prescriptive cliché, why not use a few simple yardsticks to measure exercise—such as continuing the activity until you feel *tired*? Start modestly, and don't push past the "fatigue point," even if that turns out be 10 minutes at first. (Remember, also, that once you start getting into shape and thus prolonging the exercise-period, you can begin monitoring your pulse rate in order to gain further knowledge about how your body is handling the load.)

Another helpful yardstick for measuring duration in the veteran exerciser is to simply continue the activity until you "break a healthy sweat." Although this suggestion doesn't apply to swimmers, obviously, it will allow those of us who punish ourselves on the treadmill or exercise bicycle to know that when the "sweat has begun to drop off your chin," to measure the time to fatigue. As you become more fit, the time to fatigue will be prolonged, but learn when to stop when fatigue sets in, before cramping begins.

Finally, remember that other helpful formula for measuring the intensity of exercise: the ability to *talk*. If you can recite a longish sentence (such as this one) in one breath while working out, you probably aren't exercising hard enough. Which is why most highly trained athletes agree: When it comes to achieving peak perform-ance, silence is golden!

THE PLATEAU: SMOOTHING OUT THE CURVE

Another clear-cut benefit from exercise occurs when the dieter has reached the well-known "weight-loss plateau."

What happens, typically, is that an obese patient on a protein-sparing diet will lose weight steadily—up to the point where about 15 percent of the poundage has been dropped. At that point, however, the weight loss will level off ... regardless of whether or not the individual tips the scales at 170, 270 or even 470 pounds.

The "metabolic down-regulation" that occurs during every diet will cause the patient's weight-loss to slow down dramatically at the 15-percent point. But it is precisely here that exercise can provide significant assistance. When combined with sweating and free fatty acid mobilization, such exercise will help to smooth out the curve of weekly weight loss—while preventing the jerky "stop and start" pattern that often begins after the plateau is reached. (Remember: If the weight-loss patient is using Avandia, the plateau only kicks in at 25-percent weight-loss.)

Of course, it's also true that any exercise regimen should be based on the physical condition of the patient. Those dieters who are 100 percent or more over their ideal weight must avoid weight-bearing exercise, in order to avoid injury. The exercise bicycle can be an effective tool in this situation—but the swim-ming pool clearly ranks at the top of the list of exercise locales that are ideally suited to patients who need to lose more than 50 pounds. Don't trade in the weight problem for an orthopedic problem.

GETTING THE MOST OUT OF A WORKOUT: SOME SUGGESTIONS

O Remember that each exercise period should start with 30 minutes of stretching that involves all of the joints. While you probably can stretch for a shorter period of time if you weren't sore after your workout a few days before, for many, stretching can bring a profound sense of inner peace that supercedes the benefits of exercise.

O Early on, don't worry about counting pulse rates, unless you're engaged in a cardiac rehabilitation program.

O One especially effective form of stretching is "proprioceptive neuromuscular facilitation," also known as "PNF," in which the goal is to maximize the contraction of opposing muscle groups. As an example, look at the overweight patient using PNF to develop enhanced flexibility and stretching of the hamstrings. He sits on the floor with legs held straight out in front. At regular intervals, he contracts the quadriceps (thigh muscles) as much as possible, in order to straighten his legs. This activity stretches the opposing muscle groups, the hamstrings. When the thigh muscles are contracted "to the max," the patient should try to flex his ankle, bringing his big toe "up to his nose," which requires even more contraction of the quadriceps. What happens here, ideally, is that the knee will actually straighten 3–5 degrees more, while the hamstring muscle gets an even better stretching. You can repeat the PNF stretching for any pair of muscle groups.

O Remember that muscles can only perform two basic functions: They can be stretched by the movement of other muscle groups, or they can contract on their own. Stretching moves individual myofibrils within the muscle cells a bit farther apart. Although the range of motion seems small, when viewed from outside the muscle, its effect at the molecular level is actually quite significant. By stretching these

225

muscle cell units periodically, normal joint-motion will be enhanced. In addition, the process of reducing spasm of muscles that overlie anatomically damaged joints (by stretching) will allow those joints to move more easily.

O Another benefit from PNF exercise occurs when muscles are contracting—a process that produces lactic acid within muscle cells. This phenomenon takes place when glucose is broken down without an adequate supply of oxygen. Such lactic acid buildup can contribute to a number of exercise-related problems, such as cramping. The lactic acid, itself, can then contribute to reduced blood flow, which only adds to the problem of lactic acid retention. Profound stretching releases lactic acid and as a result, blood flow is increased.

The reduced amount of blood flow (a primary cause of oxygen depletion) occurs when muscle fibers squeeze against blood vessels, causing fluid retention within affected muscles. And it is this retention that accounts for the hugely swollen musculature you see in bodybuilders such as movie star Arnold Swartzenegger. Stretch, Arnold!

(Sorry, Swartzenegger fans, but the major factor responsible for Arnold's added "amazing build" is nothing more exotic than H2O!)

This kind of fluid retention can cause sharp consternation among dieters at times. Example: A young woman called me recently to complain bitterly about the fact that although she had been "doing aerobics" for an hour a day, she simply wasn't losing weight fast enough. When I asked her about stretching, she readily admitted that she hadn't done any. Imagine her dismay when I pointed out that a one-hour aerobic workout without adequate stretching can stimulate significant amounts of fluid retention in muscles, with weight gain as a result.

Because a one-hour workout burns relatively few calories, the fluid retention that accompanies a failure to stretch can actually negate—or slightly surpass—the superficial weight-scale measure of burning the calories. This unhappy fact is surely the basis of the common and comical fallacy that "a pound of muscle weighs more than a pound of fat." As any great physicist will tell you: One pound of something must weigh exactly as much as one pound of something *else*!

The point here is that when a muscle develops fluid retention through exercise, it looks bigger and feels harder. The result, usually, is an enhanced self-image for its owner. When the exercise stops, the fluid retention also stops and the muscle quickly loses its size. Stretch to obtain maximum benefit from your exercise.

DO YOU NEED A STRESS TEST?

Those dieters interested in building an effective, exercise-based weight-loss program right now for themselves will be delighted to hear my one-word answer to this question: "No!"

Well, maybe the answer is "not necessarily." In most situations at my office, I'm content to give dieters who want to launch an exercise program a simple, modified version of the old-fashoned, but nonetheless useful Masters 2 Step Test. No, this stepping test isn't as sensitive as a $2000 radionuclide stress test. If the patient's resting EKG is normal and the medical history doesn't include any cardiovascular problems (such as chest pain, unexplained fatigue, skipped heartbeats or shortness of breath), then I simply ask the dieter to step quickly atop a stool with one foot after the other ... and then to return to the floor in the same way. Over the years I've learned that de-conditioned individuals will begin to experience an increased respiratory rate within ten seconds.

The bottom line for me is this simple step test. If the individual is able to continue the stool-stepping for 30 seconds—while also displaying normal blood pressure and pulse response—then I don't insist that he or she spend the money required to undergo a routine stress test performed under standard conditions. There are exceptions to every rule, of course.

The normal blood pressure-response to exercise is a slight rise in the systolic reading, accompanied by a corresponding drop-off in diastolic pressure. Given these facts, a systolic pressure–drop in a de-conditioned patient should be a red flag that requires a stress test. In similar fashion, a rise in diastolic pressure calls for the test. Although these rules aren't set in stone, they do serve as handy guidelines for most situations.

LONG-TERM EXERCISE BENEFITS VS. SHORT-TERM

Before concluding this chapter on the exaggerated health benefits of exercise, I should point out that the situation changes considerably—if the individual engaged in the exercise starts a regular program at age 18 and maintains it steadily thereafter.

In that situation, the dedicated exerciser will receive a definite cardiovascular benefit, while significantly reducing the odds of a heart attack or stroke. But in my experience, most dieters need to understand that "starting and stopping" exercise again and again over a period of years simply doesn't provide the same benefits that accrue to the dedicated and daily-performing exercise enthusiast.

When all is said and done, there are several very good reasons to work out regularly—even if you can't depend on exercise as a sure-fire way to lose weight.

Not the least of the arguments in favor of staying fit is the sheer sense of physical well-being that most people experience. After many years of studying this issue—and watching dieters struggle with it—I've come to realize that I can't separate the mental and physical benefits that come from exercising regularly while also engaging in the wonderfully exhilarating and self-affirming process of losing the weight you hate.

When patients ask me whether they should observe my 00-2-3 diet or "start up an exercise program" as a way to leave their obesity behind, I always answer them the same way:

"Why don't you try doing *both*?"

SPORTS NUTRITION

An esteemed nephrologist, Dan Gandy, used to tell me that the solution to any war was simple. Bring the leaders of the opposing forces together in one room and make them stay awake and listen to a two-hour lecture on calcium metabolism. At the one-hour break, the leaders would do anything to go home early, including signing peace accords.

Dr. Gandy could have said "sports nutrition" instead of calcium for the lecture topic. Have you ever seen the hype in a body builder's magazine? Even worse, listen to the trainer for the local high school who talks about carbohydrate loading, with amino acids, vitamins and minerals as a garnish. "Casting our false knowledge" hasn't made it to the locker room nutrition discussions yet.

Athletes are notoriously difficult nutrition patients. Like doctors and nurses, athletes not only know what to eat, but will gladly tell you what to eat. As an old jock, I guess I'm no different. Here goes ... sports nutrition.

Glycogen stores: you will hear that buzz phrase over and over again and with good reason. Proper function of muscle cells demands maintenance of intracellular glycogen stores.

As glycogen is burned (broken down into glucose), the body must replenish glycogen. Accomplishing that task all at once is impossible. Even if adequate glucose were available in the diet, glycogen replenishment tops out at about 6% of the glucose debt per hour. Replacing glycogen takes so long that most athletes try to avoid excessive glycogen burn during competition. One look at marathon runners will convince you. They are drinking sugar- or maltodextrin-enriched beverages frequently during a long road race. Look at the kayaker with that silly looking water bottle and siphon on his head. No, it isn't silly. He, too, is drinking sugar-enriched liquids to prevent excessive glycogen depletion.

Remember the dramatic Olympic moments of the distance runner staggering toward the finish line, refusing to give in to total glycogen depletion. He crosses the finish line and collapses. Everyone rushes to help; an intravenous sugar solution is quickly placed. Without glycogen, bad things always can happen and the runner could die.

If you exercise strenuously for two hours and burn, say, 600 calories, your body can replenish about 6% of that total per hour. Assuming you burned some small amount of fat and assuming you are a normal insulin individual, you can replace the glycogen stores in about 16 hours. Trained athletes can burn fat directly, sparing glycogen loss. They will recover in only about five hours.

High insulin patients will take up to 32 hours to replace the same glycogen stores. If they exercise again during this 32–hour time period, they will become further glycogen depleted, despite adequate supplies of glucose. The insulin just doesn't work well enough to get sugar into muscle or liver quickly. All of the extra glucose is shunted into the futile cycle or is being stored as fat.

My first rule of exercise nutrition—do not create a state of negative glycogen balance during exercise.

My second rule: treat negative glycogen balance with a burst of high glycemic index food following exercise but no more than 100 grams (less than four ounces). Fix the glycogen debt with low glycemic index foods beyond that.

The low glycemic index foods eaten for breakfast after an over-night fast will replenish your body protein, repair glycogen store depletion and prepare you for athletic endeavors slowly, but effi-ciently.

One hour before activity you need to eat 40–50 grams of high glycemic index foods, but not any more, if your exercise time is 45 minutes or less. Within one hour after your exercise you need to eat 100 grams of high glycemic index foods. Going beyond the 50 grams before and 100 grams after ceilings usually means you just make fat and burn protein. Going under the 50-gram and 100 gram ceiling levels means you will not maintain glycogen stores. Guess what, protein burning occurs again. Because each individual is different, the 50 before and 100 after ceiling levels are guidelines that change with exercise intensity and duration. Monitor recovery time as an indicator of successful eating.

The highly trained athletes burn fatty acids directly, but the overweight patient is trapped by his insulin preservation of fat if he eats amylose. He must maintain glycogen stores without activating fat storage. Do it with the low glycemic index diet.

The weekend warrior has more problems than anyone as far as glycogen stores go. He needs to avoid eating too much sugar, which would cause conservation of fat stores by insulin, at the same time he must eat enough other foods to enable his liver to keep producing sugar without burning protein. Breakfast consists of low glycemic index foods, coinciding with maximal liver production of glucose. He follows the low glycemic index diet to keep glycogen stores saturated throughout the day, avoiding fat synthesis and protein burn.

The diet principles I use for competitive athletes follow. The choice of foods is more important than the amount of foods.

I have used this diet with weight lifters, football players, runners, tennis players, baseball, basketball and soccer players. It works consistently. You may need to rearrange the time of eating, based on your workout schedule.

Avoiding burning protein is the first step to building an efficient athletic body. Avoiding amylose is the first step to avoiding protein burn.

SPORTS DIET

SPORTS NUTRITION DIET

Stretching 30 minutes in morning (moderate workout following if desired). In afternoon, stretching followed by high intensity training. Don't overtrain if your body fat is too high (20% for men and 25% for women).

1) Drink enough water. Do not lose more than 2% of body weight from day to day.

2) Take an all B with C vitamin.

3) Do not use ergogenic aids including ginseng, anabolic steroids, amino acids, bee pollen, high dose BCP (one a day is enough for women), andro or ephedrine.

4) Eat 50g high glycemic index foods three times a day.

5) Eat 100g high glycemic index foods within one hour following activity.

6) Drink 12–16 oz sugar-enriched or maltodextrin containing liquids (most "sports drinks") after activity (as part of #5 if desired).

7) Breakfast is unlimited fruit and protein (no bananas, cook the fat out of fatty meats). No more than twenty grams of amylose!

8) Mid-morning snack: protein, yogurt, nuts. Liquid supplements are okay, but Medifast® is a far superior supplement

235

if protein–based weight gain is desired.

9) Lunch is multi-vegetable salad with commercial dressing (source of corn syrup and maltodextrins); protein on the side with legumes, pasta and juices. This is a 50g, high glycemic index meal.

10) Afternoon workout is followed by 100g high glycemic foods. More pasta, for example, or Italian bread or bagels are acceptable *(see #'s 5 & 6)*.

11) One hour later have your protein supplement, nuts, marinated vegetables, dried fruit and a protein source.

12) Supper includes meat, 2 vegetables that grow above the ground, including one legume, cheese, oil and vinegar dressing, fruit, hot bread with butter, dairy dessert is ok (no restrictions).

13) Night time snack, preparing for fasting (sleep) eat nuts, dried fruit or popcorn. High glycemic index dessert okay, but only if you increase amount of low glycemic index breakfast the next day.

14) In training, alcohol is restricted to no more than 6 oz of wine or 2 real beers a day, if it is legal.

15) This training table is full! If you are trying to lose weight by exercising, do so before you try to condition your muscles for glycogen sparing performance!

16) Did you get enough to eat?

LOSE THE WEIGHT YOU HATE!
—Q&A WITH PARALEGAL LYNN BROWN

Q. Why did you decide to consult Dr. Shoemaker, and what took place when you did?

BROWN: Well, I just felt that I needed to do something, after having my child, and I was just not able to lose the weight. And I sat down with him. We went over his program and we discussed how he has helped people.

And this has been the only diet—even though it's not *really* a diet—that has ever worked for me. I just cannot have the glucose and amylose. But this approach really helped me, because I've now lost nearly 50 pounds. You know, I have a family history of diabetes and heart attacks, and I just felt that I needed to do something for my children.

I've been more than pleased with him as a physician. Any problems or concerns that I had, he was more than helpful. He certainly helped me to attain my goals. And I also take the medication that he believes in. It's called Avandia—and it has been a key part of my weight-loss strategy from the beginning. This medication gives you a sensation of warmth, as you're burning your fat.

Q. Please tell us a little more about yourself and your weight-problems.

BROWN: I'm now 47. And I had my first child at 38, and my

second child at 42. So I'm one of those "old mommies." But after I had Holden, my second child, I really had a problem getting the weight off. I was about 50 pounds overweight— and I simply could not lose it.

This was about four years ago, 1996, when I gained all the weight. And one day I realized that I wasn't pregnant any more —it was time to do something about my weight. I knew that in order to slim down, you really do have to make some choices. And I just decided that I was going to do it.

Q. How heavy did you get, after the birth of Holden?

BROWN: I had gotten up to around 175. And I'm about 5-5, with a medium frame. So by my reckoning, I was least 40 pounds overweight.

I tried various kinds of diets, and I might lose, maybe, five pounds or so. Maybe eight pounds at the most. The low-fat diets I went on simply didn't work. I tried everything! And nothing else worked like this [the Shoemaker 00-2-3 diet] has worked for me. I really believe that I'm one of those people who cannot have the special carbohydrates, the amylose foods.

Still, the maintenance diet I'm on now does allow me an occasional sandwich or ice cream cone. It's more a way of life. I think Dr. Shoemaker really teaches you to use common sense about your eating habits. It's a lifestyle, that's all. There's no magic pill, and no magic cure. You have to use your own intelligence and you have to say "no" at times. You have to push the food away from you.

My thing now is, I'm very, very good during the week. But when I'm with the kids on the weekends, I *will* have a couple of things I'm not supposed to. I think you need to reward yourself. But I'm very disciplined during the week. And Dr. Shoemaker will tell you that it's all right to reward yourself now and then. He'll tell you that if you have a craving, or you really feel that you want fried chicken—whatever—go ahead and have it. Don't deny yourself. And I think that's true.

Q. When did you first consult Dr. Shoemaker?

BROWN: Back about two and a half years ago, in 1999. And I didn't really understand his concepts at first … you know, the stuff about triggering your insulin with glucose and amylose, and why that causes your body to store fat. And believe me, it wasn't easy staying away from the breads and the pastas.

Believe me, I come from a long line of people that love to eat. And they're good cooks! And so yes, bread and spaghetti and pasta and pizza—I love all of them! But you know, you just have to do it. In my case, I think it was mainly because I would like to be around for my children.

I think I needed to do a reality check. And I had once been at the correct weight, back before I had children. So … to gain all that weight was kind of depressing for me, and I felt that I just didn't want to look that way anymore.

Having kids is a real motivator for weight-loss, believe me! I want to live to see them married, and I want to be around for all the moments in their lives. They're going to need me … but I wouldn't have been here for them if I'd kept on eating the way I was and gaining weight. I mean, it was ridiculous.

Anyway, Dr. Shoemaker is a very down-to-earth person. And that's very encouraging. I think a lot of him, because he's been very helpful to me.

Q. Did you take Avandia right from the very start of your 00-2-3 diet?

BROWN: In the beginning, I did not use the Avandia. But then I started using it later on—and I lost up to two and a half pounds

239

a week. I think I added an extra pound a week to my weight loss total by going to the Avandia.

For me, the diet experience was almost like a cleansing. Because I was drinking a lot of water and eating a lot of fruits and vegetables. I think I was going through a whole period of cleansing my body. I didn't eat any chocolate or starches or any sugar—and it was amazing how much weight I was losing by really following that.

Another important part of this is to write down everything you eat. And I was. And the weight just kept coming off of me—no soft drinks, no candy, no cookies. It's amazing what you can lose in a month.

But with the help of the Avandia, I lost two and half pounds a week for seven or eight weeks, and then it leveled off.

Q. Were there any unpleasant side-effects from the Avandia?

BROWN: No, absolutely none. Nothing. And I usually had plenty of energy. But if I felt that I needed a momentary boost, I would eat something. I'd have some peanut butter, or maybe some sherbet—which is about half the calories of regular ice cream. And today my weight is still way down around 155.

I go back to Dr. Shoemaker's office every month and get weighed. And that gives me additional motivation, so that I don't start slipping.

Q. What's the most important thing that people need to know about Dr. Shoemaker's diet, if they're going to use it successfully—both for weight-loss and maintenance?

BROWN: Two things are especially important. First, people who are struggling with either diabetes or obesity need to understand that they have a genetic problem ... and that this problem interferes with the way insulin works to manage their intake of sugars such as glucose and amylose.

The second important thing is to understand that Dr. Shoe-maker's diet is part of an entire *lifestyle*. It's a matter of thinking about the food you put into your mouth. What I really like about Dr. Shoemaker's approach is that he really wants you to *enjoy* the food you eat each day. He gave me dozens of delicious recipes, and I've used every one of them in recent months.

Dr. Shoemaker's philosophy of dieting is that it involves a broad, integrated approach to nutrition, exercise and enjoying every meal you put on the table. You can't "separate out" the parts of his program; you need to take full advantage of every part of it, if you're going to be successful. For example, you can't take the Avandia medication he recommends without observing the rest of the diet—that strategy simply won't work, and you will not achieve your weight-loss goals.

The point is that the diet and the medicine provide a one-two punch that basically compensates for the genetic imbalance that causes obesity in the first place.

13

AVANDIA: LADIES, GO RIGHT AHEAD AND BURN YOUR HIPS!

BULLETIN FROM THE FEDBUZZ NATIONAL NEWS SERVICE, WRITTEN BY CORRESPONDENT TOM NUGENT:

With the recent announcement that the Human Genome Project has finally succeeded in mapping most of the genetic code, medical researchers are poised to launch a revolutionary new approach to curing such chronic diseases as diabetes ... by simply "turning off" the flawed genes that cause the ailment.

BULLETIN NO. 2 FROM THE FEDBUZZ NATIONAL NEWS SERVICE:

Although gene-based therapies are still in their infancy for most chronic diseases, this approach is now fully operational—and completely safe— as a way to overcome chronic obesity in most patients.

It's true.

If you're one of the tens of millions of people who now suffer from chronic obesity, there's some very good news waiting for you right now at your corner drugstore—even if some doctors and pharmacists may not be aware of it yet!

Quite simply, the news is this: Thanks to some recent and extraordinary breakthroughs in pharmaceutical research, it is now possible to combine a gene-targeted drug (rosiglitazone, or "Avandia") with my "00-2-3" No Amylose diet ... and then to watch in amazement as you lose an average of 1.5 pounds per *week* of the weight you hate!

In this chapter, I'm going to tell you about an astonishing research study I recently conducted, the results of which were presented June 20, 2001, at a Denver, Colo., meeting of the prestigious Endocrine Society. The Endocrine Society has long enjoyed a reputation as one of the most authoritative medical research organizations in the world.

Entitled "Use of Rosiglitazone in Treatment of Hyperinsulinemic Obesity" *(see Appendix 4)*, my recent study followed 40 chronic obesity patients (with a follow-up of 100 patients now pending publication) through a 12-week trial period in which they used a brand-new kind of drug in combination with the diet described in this book.

The results weren't just remarkable—they were absolutely off the charts!

The bottom line: By linking a safe daily dosage of GlaxoSmithKline's new "Avandia"—a "thiazolidinedione-family" wonder drug that reduces insulin resistance—with my 00-2-3 regimen for controlling the same resistance through dietary reduction of glucose and amylose, I was able to achieve the following, certified results:

○ Although these patients were among my most "difficult dieters" (all had failed to lose weight over and over again), the women who took the drug and carefully observed the diet regimen lost an average of 1.5 pounds per week for 12 straight weeks. The best they had done with any of my diet programs was 0.5 pounds per week.

○ Even more remarkably, these women succeeded in removing an *average* of 2.4 inches from their hips during the same period! None of these patients had ever burned their hips like this before. The waist circumference, measured at the navel, also fell, but at a lower rate of 1.9 inches, on average, in 12 weeks.

○ The men involved in the study did even better—losing an average of 1.7 pounds weekly and even more inches off their waists.

○ Men and women alike enjoyed several other significant health benefits during the course of the study, including the following:

None of them developed the swelling (edema) that may accompany use of rosiglitazone when used for treatment of diabetes.

Most of the study-subjects experienced significant lowering of total cholesterol and LDL cholesterol, along with an accompanying rise in the level of healthier HDL. Precisely the reverse cholesterol-sequence occurs in most diabetics who take the thiazolidinedione medications.

You can read the results of my study, co-authored with Dr. Alexander Cobitz, in the proceedings of the Endocrine Society at your leisure.

And if you're struggling with obesity—along with 90 million other Americans in 2001, according to the CDC—you can also rejoice in the certain knowledge that help is on the way!

○ ○ ○

GENETICS AND WEIGHT LOSS: A PRIMER

The easiest way to understand the relationship between genetic programming and weight reduction is to take a quick look at the Endocrine Society study I conducted in order to determine if GlaxoSmithKline's diabetes medication—Avandia—might help my overweight patients to shed their flab.

In order to answer that question, among others, I gave 40 patients a 4 mg tablet of rosiglitazone (Avandia) twice a day, then asked them to strictly follow the no-amylose and low-glucose restrictions of my 00-2-3 diet.

One of the key questions I wanted to answer was this: Would the drug cause easily noticed elevations in cholesterol, especially LDL, and development of edema, as may happen when Avandia is used to combat adult onset diabetes? (Like so many other physicians, I'd often heard patients complain: "Yes, doctor, that Avandia sure helps control my blood sugar—too bad it also makes my cholesterol go up, along with my weight, too!")

For some time, however, I'd been trying to tell the manufacturers of Avandia that whenever patients used it in concert with my no-amylose diet, they didn't *experience* these negative side effects. Indeed, for several years during the late 1990s, I'd been using a forerunner of Avandia—troglitazone—as a tool that helped many insulin-resistant (but not diabetic) patients achieve startling weight-reductions.

As it turned out, troglitazone was eventually withdrawn from the market, after the U.S. Food and Drug Administration (FDA) began to question its safety. The FDA regulators were concerned, and quite rightly, by reports of "abnormal effects" on the liver —some of which had resulted in liver transplants, and a few of which were even implicated in the deaths of patients. According to some reports, as many as 200 of the several million people who took troglitazone may have been adversely affected by side effects from the drug.

Soon after the problems developed with troglitazone, two

different manufacturers almost simultaneously brought out two second-generation forms of the thiazolidinedione drug family. The first near-cousin of troglitazone was pioglitazone—and it was soon followed by the rosiglitazone compound that provides the key ingredient in Avandia. The creators of these new diabetes-fighting drugs were making some very hopeful predictions for them ... but like many other front-line physicians, I remained dubious.

Were these new medications going to prove helpful to patients over the long haul—or were they going to quickly follow such former "miracle" drugs as Duract and Maxaquin into early retirement? These two medications, wonderfully effective at first, were yanked from the market after being blamed for causing liver and other blood chemistry problems.

Fortunately for all concerned, this negative scenario never occurred. Within a year or so, research showed conclusively that Avandia doesn't compromise liver function, and that drops in blood sugar occur only rarely. At first glance, of course, this fact seems difficult to understand. How could a diabetes medication *not* lower blood sugar?

The answer, of course, is that Avandia achieves its effect not by stimulating insulin release or dropping blood sugar in other ways ... but by enhancing the activity of the genes that actually control the process of sugar-digestion.

In order to understand the process, let's take a quick glance at the wonderfully intricate landscape of the "Genetic Code"—the biochemical "map," if you will, which the body uses to accomplish the endless variety of biological tasks that together make up the business of living.

Remember those color illustrations from your Biology 101 textbook of the "one billion nucleotides" that form the Genetic Code? Remember the snazzy-looking charts depicting the linked adenine-thymine (A-T) and the linked guanine-cytosine (G-C)? But those "nucleotide bases" (the pairs that form the "genetic alphabet") are only part of the basic structure of DNA. In fact,

247

each of those nucleotides is connected to the next one in the sequence by a five-carbon sugar known as a "ribose."

The sugar linkages work together to create the two twisted strands—the famous "Double Helix"—that are the physical signature of DNA. Tucked into the grooves along the sides of these strands are other proteins ... the "acid proteins," which provide the cement that gives the entire structure strength and solidity. Like the mortar between bricks, the acid proteins allow the delicate DNA strands to remain firmly anchored within their nucleotides. Of course the entire DNA package is also surrounded by *another* layer of proteins, the histones, that act like a cardboard mailing tube to protect the precious DNA "documents" contained inside.

One of the most intriguing questions about the structural dynamics of DNA is this: Protected as it is by so many layers of "cement," how does the code manage to copy ("transcribe") itself onto the organic courier, the mRNA, that will carry the message from the nucleus of the cell out to the cytoplasm, where the DNA "instructions" for biochemical interactions can then be put into play? (Don't forget that it's out here in the cytoplasm that the message is translated, so that it can direct the cell's protein factories in manufacturing and managing whatever organic products might be required to keep cells alive and healthy.)

Even more remarkable than the act of Xeroxing copies of itself, perhaps, is DNA's uncanny ability to target specific segments of its information for reproduction in this manner. If the entire structure is encased in a series of protective layers of proteins, how does a specific string of genes suddenly become activated—while all other nearby genes remain unaffected? In other words, how in the world can DNA achieve such "differential gene transcription," if the Double Helix at all times remains encased in its smothering layers of protective proteins and sugars?

The answer to this problem can be found in the structure of DNA, itself.

Remember: certain DNA sections "refuse" to allow the acid protein "cement" to fill in the spaces between pairs. Clever! Why? Because these gaps can then serve as nuclear receptors, or "docking stations" along the DNA.

Next step: Whenever a molecule (an "agonist") that is structurally capable of locking onto a receptor comes wandering by— or is biochemically escorted to the receptor—the latter responds by shaking itself like a wet dog. Described figuratively, the receptor begins to shake and shimmy, in order to shuck off the layers of protective protein. At the same time, the receptor chemically signals the mRNA copying machine to get to work.

So far, so good. As the process continues to unfold, all of the genes controlled by the nuclear receptor will become activated —and the gene products will come pouring out, provided only that the nuclear receptor continues its "wet dog routine." But remember: If you remove the agonist from the equation, the source of the stimulation evaporates and then entire process grinds to a halt. Restore the agonist and *bingo!*, the copier fires up again.

Now here's where the *real* fun begins.

Let's say you were able to go into the laboratory and synthesize a group of agonists that could help you alter the process described above.

What if you created, in short, a category of agonists (the thiazolidinediones) designed especially to serve as diabetes-fighters at the molecular level?

This is precisely what GlaxoSmithKline did, before launching its particular member of the thiazolidinedione family of molecular glucose-metabolizing drugs: rosiglitazone. (The other family-members, of course, include both troglitazone and pioglitazone.) Although there are some important differences in safety and benefits among these three thiazolidinediones, they all share one crucial similarity: They all turn on an important nuclear receptor called "PPAR," short for "peroxisome proliferator-activated receptor gamma."

249

The terminology sounds complicated, but the process isn't. The key point here is that PPAR controls many of the genes that protect our health, in numerous ways. At the same time, PPAR defends our cells from the destructive effects that follow, whenever a second kind of nuclear receptor (a counter-balancing receptor known as the "cytokine receptor") gets turned on. (For more detailed information about how PPAR and the cytokine receptor affect the physiology of chronic diseases such as Post-Lyme Syndrome, sick building syndrome, chronic fatigue and more, see my recently published book, *Desperation Medicine*, Gateway Press, Baltimore, or visit the Chronic Disease Website at www.chronicneurotoxins.com.)

Although the biochemical interactions between PPAR and the genes are enormously complex, their net effect on sugar storage (and hence on fat manufacture) is easy to describe. The important thing to remember here is that PPAR turns on production of two proteins that transport glucose inside the cell.

To understand why this process is so important, it might help to remember the "FedEx" metaphor we used in an earlier chapter to describe the movement of cholesterol through the bloodstream.

Ask yourself: What if—like the U.S. Post Office at Christmastime—the insulin receptors in human cells became swamped with arriving packages? Perhaps a clerk "called in sick" or got injured on the job? *(Please see the chapter on Environmental Acquisition of Diabetes and Obesity!)* In that case, the "packages" of glucose headed for the muscles and the liver would simply pile up, then get stored away as fat, instead of being properly delivered. This is precisely what happens when insulin resistance prevents glucose molecules from being transported efficiently across cell membranes by insulin.

Are we clear so far? All right: how can we help the swamped postal clerks get those packages delivered?

Our friend PPAR provides the answer—by manufacturing the

two transport-proteins described above. Suddenly, it's as if a whole new shift of FedEx workers has arrived to give the Post Office guys a hand and clear up the overflow of packages.

And when the glucose packages are properly delivered to their waiting cells … *presto!*, they no longer wind up being converted into fatty acids, which is the first step on the road to *fat*.

Once safely inside the cell, this sugar can be burned efficiently for fuel, avoiding fat storage and protecting us from both diabetes and obesity.

So how does the new wonder drug, Avandia, fit into all of this?

It's simple. Engineered to perfection, the new medication (generic name, rosiglitazone) works to enhance the delivery of sugar into the cells where it belongs—instead of allowing it to be transformed into fatty acids. The result is that Avandia controls diabetes *without* lowering blood sugar—simply by redirecting the glucose that crosses its path toward the proper destination, by preventing the excessive manufacture of fatty acids from glucose and making it easier for fat cells to remove fatty acids from the blood stream.

As you probably remember from the chapters on insulin and cholesterol, Avandia causes edema in some patients and changes in cholesterol among others because of its close linkage with the insulin response to amylose.

To show you how this works, I should point out that my adult onset diabetic patients are all asked to follow my 00-2-3 diet, and many do. Most tell me they'd rather skip the toast for breakfast (along with the sandwich for lunch and the rice with supper) than spend the rest of their lives giving themselves regular insulin shots or taking insulin-releasing medications, while also gaining more weight from insulin and possibly experiencing harmful low-sugar reactions that could potentially affect brain function.

Sounds like a winner, right?

As it turns out, however, PPAR directs several other biochemical processes, in addition to moving sugar into cells.

Example: this extraordinary substance knows how to turn on the gene that makes "uncoupling protein."

One sure sign that this is happening occurs when patients who take PPAR begin to notice a sensation of warmth.

The process depends on "uncoupling protein"—which is a molecule that interrupts the storage of sugar-energy in specialized cells known as "brown fat cells." What happens is that the brown fat cells normally convert fatty acids into energy-concentrating molecules, called "ATP," and then store the converted energy in this way. That conversion requires the "coupling" of a series of enzyme-steps—a process known as "oxidative phosphorylation."

The important thing to remember here is that these enzyme-steps are all coupled. In the presence of uncoupling protein, however, those same reactions are disrupted ... so that the fatty acids wind up being burned *directly*, in order to generate heat.

Do you remember being a kid and swimming in a mountain lake ... when all at once you became chilled and your body started to shiver? That shivering creates heat from involuntary muscle contractions—much like the emergency heat setting on your heat pump thermostat.

On the other hand, to follow our example of the swimmer, if you had climbed out of the water before the shivering set in, your body would have re-warmed itself by calling on your brown fat cells. When signaled by an adrenaline-like hormone, these fat cells can supply a short-lived burst of heat ... even if it's not enough to prevent prolonged hypothermia.

Unfortunately, however, this hormone mechanism (the B3 receptor) wasn't designed to maintain a constant level of uncoupling protein production ... so it can't be used effectively in a weight-loss program.

But here's where PPAR turns out to be worth its weight in gold—once we realize that it can give us the prolonged stimulation of brown fat cells necessary to keep on chewing up those fatty acids. (Remember: The more work we can get from that uncoupling protein, the greater demand there will be for fatty acids to be pulled from the "depots" along the hips and waist and then sent on to the energy-starved brown fat cells.)

Obviously, then, we can predict that giving Avandia to obese and insulin-resistant non-diabetics will trigger a sense of warmth in them—provided they don't short-circuit the process by eating bread and other starches and thus triggering the kind of "high in-sulin response" that shuts down brown fat cells. Such patients are usually quite pleased to learn that the "warm feeling" they get— each time uncoupling protein "turns on"—is sure sign they're burning off their fat depots!

This is just what happens, ladies and gentlemen.

Avandia *works* ... and it leaves most of my delighted patients telling me happily: "Oh, yes, my feet are warm at night—not ice-cold when I get into bed, like they used to be. They're not hot, mind you, and there are no sweats and no fever. It's just a nice, comfortable feeling!" (Of course, that warming sensation will disappear rapidly, if you nibble on a few amylose-loaded wheat crackers before bed!)

AVANDIA MEETS THE SHOEMAKER DIET: GOOD NEWS FOR PATIENTS!

After watching several hundred weight-loss patients achieve as-tonishing diet-breakthroughs in recent years by combining Avan-dia with my 00-2-3 approach to losing the weight they hate, I'm excited about the huge payoffs that are available to any dieter who participates in this program. These benefits include:

O Increasing your protein stores until they return to their proper, genetically controlled level, and then *keeping* them there.

O Typically, losing 1.5 pounds a week (1.7 pounds for most

men) ... with most of it coming from hips and waist.

o A weight-loss maintenance rate that exceeds 70 percent. (Compare *that* with the 1–2 percent maintenance success rate achieved by all other diets, and it's easy to see that my way works!)

Although the scientific principles that underlie the Avandia-and-no-amylose strategy for weight-loss are wonderfully complex, the basic steps in the program couldn't be easier to follow. They're as simple as ABC, and here they are:

A. Don't put fat on your fat cell receptor.

B. Mobilize your fatty acids for energy, while burning fat for heat instead of storing it.

C. Eat enough protein so that your body won't burn your own for fuel.

Could any dieting regimen be easier to follow?

Exciting Suggestion for Successful Dieters: The next time you read one of those misleading articles about weight-loss in a "mainstream newspaper" (the Philadelphia Inquirer comes readily to mind, for some reason!) ... just chuckle quietly, drop the paper back on the table, and get back to what you were doing. Don't be misled by the "leading obesity experts"—the Gurus of the Conventional Wisdom who prattle endlessly about "more exercise and fewer calories" as the secret to dieting success.

Remember, those Gurus have all failed to accomplish the weight-doctor's most rewarding and satisfying goal: teaching ladies how to burn their hips!

(And don't fret about allowing the newspaper "to go waste." Remember that it can always be used in a pinch ... to start a fire, housebreak a puppy, or maybe even line a canary's cage!)

Burn your hips safely with Avandia and 00-2-3 ... and welcome to the wide, wide, wonderful world of the perpetually *thin!*

CASE STUDY NO. 4:
SHERRAN NAHM'S ASTONISHING DIAGNOSIS

She was one of the bravest—and most determined—patients who ever walked into my office.

"Dr. Shoemaker, there's something wrong with me," said Sherran Nahm, back in May of 2000. "I'm terribly overweight, even though I work out for several hours each day and also watch what I eat.

"But obesity is only one of my problems. I'm tired all the time, and I keep forgetting stuff. The other day, I went out to buy a gallon of milk at the Safeway ... and wound up stumbling around in the drugstore. It was really scary, when I realized that I couldn't remember a simple thing like a gallon of milk!"

o   o   o

A 51-year-old computer programmer and a resident of the boooming Ocean Pines resort community near Ocean City, Md., Sherran Nahm had been struggling with obesity for many years.

When she dropped by my office that memorable day in 2000, she tipped the scales at 223 pounds ... with a Lean Body Mass calculated to be 133 pounds, making her ideal body weight 160 pounds.

Sherran was just plain fat, and she knew it. During the previous year, she'd gone from a size-5 dress ... to a size so large she refused to divulge it!

A hard-working career woman, this thoughtful and self-disciplined patient had been referred to me by a very knowledgeable family practice physician who admitted up front that he'd "tried everything" he knew, and that nothing had worked.

It didn't take Sherran long to blurt out the history of her long struggle with obesity. That history contained several harrowing chapters, including the following:

O Way back in 1979, she had become significantly overweight and had gone on the "Medifast" diet program. The program had worked well for her, and she'd managed to shed 30 pounds.

O About 20 years later, however, her weight surged back up to the "obesity" level and she again turned to Medifast. But this time, nothing happened. The diet failed completely, and she remained overweight.

O Increasingly alarmed by now, she quickly tried several "fad" diets ... including Sugar Busters, the sibutramine program, Xenical and the Dr. Atkins' program.

Nothing helped.

Sherran couldn't figure it out.

A physical fitness nut, she was exercising for more than two hours each day. Nor had her eating habits changed significantly over the years. If Medifast had worked like a charm 20 years before, why wasn't it helping her now?

Sherran Nahm was a medical enigma wrapped in a metabolic mystery!

But the key to solving the puzzle would be found—as always —by listening carefully to each and every one of her *symptoms*.

In addition to her obesity, Sherran was experiencing the following:

O occasional headaches;

O muscle aches;

O chronic fatigue;

O delayed recovery following heavy exercise compared to previous years;

O sensitivity to bright light, but without red eyes or tearing;

O impaired short-term memory;

O difficulty in concentrating;

O daily diarrhea that sometimes kept her up at night;

O abdominal pain with cramping and tingling in her left hand;

O shortness of breath, but no cough;

O vertigo

As I reviewed this long list of symptoms with Ms. Nahm, two words kept jumping out at me:

Neurotoxic illness.

Could she perhaps be suffering from chronic Lyme disease? No … she'd had no exposure to ticks that she was aware of, and no other key Lyme symptoms, such as a "bull's eye" rash.

How about sick building syndrome? No … she didn't work in a sealed, "climate-controlled" building, and nobody else at her workplace had gotten sick.

But what was her exposure? It if this was neurotoxic illness, what was the pathogen? There has to be some organism that makes a neurotoxin that one acquires to have an acquired neurotoxic illness.

And then it hit me.

Her neighborhood!

Sherran Nahm lived in a resort community located between a Chesapeake Bay estuary and the Atlantic Ocean, not far from Ocean City, Md.

That community—Ocean Pines—had been the site of several recent invasions of two neurotoxin-forming microorganisms (*Pfiesteria* and *Chattonella*) which had been making people sick all along the water's edge. These dinoflagellate organisms were living and breeding in the estuaries along Maryland's Eastern Shore ... and they were vectors for both neurotoxin-related illness *and* obesity! (For more information on these subjects, see *Pfiesteria: Crossing Dark Water* and *Desperation Medicine*, by the author.)

With growing excitement, I asked Ms. Nahm to take my five-minute Contrast Sensitivity test, designed to pinpoint deficits in the brain's ability to distinguish visual patterns.

When her scores were tallied, I wasn't surprised. With so many new kinds of neurotoxin producers around, each of which can disrupt normal functioning of insulin receptors, why would anyone be surprised to find our environment making us sick and tired, with becoming fat an extra unwanted garnish.

The CS test results showed beyond a reasonable doubt that Sherran Nahm was suffering from a neurotoxin-mediated illness ... and based on what I knew about how neurotoxins hurt us, that these *organic poisons had also triggered her obesity!*

A few days after making this diagnosis, I started Sherran on some medications designed to shut down the symptoms of neurotoxic illness by binding the toxins out of the body. She began to improve within a week. After most of her symptoms had dissipated (in about six weeks), I prescribed Avandia, along with my standard 00-2-3 No-Amylose weight-loss program.

Sherran lost 10 pounds during the first month ... even though she was now exercising far less than before. She hadn't been able to do that before, even with more stringent calorie restriction.

During the first four weeks of my program, Ms. Nahm burned two inches from her hips and two *more* inches from her waist.

It took three more months to bring her weight down to 198. But that number was quite deceiving, since her Lean Body Mass (she was repaying the protein deficit her dysfunctional dieting had caused) had gone from 133 to 143 pounds ... which meant that her actual weight loss was much greater than 25 pounds.

When Sherran ended my weight-loss program at 20% fat and 172 pounds, her waist was 31.5 inches and her hips were 42 inches. (That represented a net loss of 4.5 inches from the waist and 4 inches from the hips.)

Thrilled and delighted, she shook my hand over and over again, as she described how her zestful energy—and her memory—had returned to her in recent weeks. I saluted her, of course. But I also warned her about the continuing threat from neurotoxin-mediated illness, which is definitely here to stay, as the human habitat becomes increasingly polluted by industrial chemicals and agricultural pesticides.

Because she intends to continue living in Ocean Pines, Sherran will have to remain on her daily medications. They are her only line of defense against the neurotoxins that are making more and more of her neighbors ill—with the distinctive groups of symptoms that most physicians do not yet understand. Try telling Sherran that her weight problem was caused by eating too many monster burgers and tubs of fried chicken!

In order to remain healthy (and *slim*), Sherran Nahm is going to have to follow the profound advice of the immortal Thomas Jefferson, who 225 years ago warned his fellow-countrymen:

"The price of freedom is eternal vigilance!"

14

ENVIRONMENTAL ACQUISITION OF DIABETES AND OBESITY

Pick up a daily newspaper, these days—almost *any* newspaper—and the odds are high that you'll soon find yourself reading a frightening story about the "soaring rates" of both Type II diabetes and obesity.

Ask yourself: How many times have you sat staring at the following headlines, as you slugged down your orange juice at the breakfast table?

ONE-THIRD OF AMERICANS NOW "OBESE,"
ACCORDING TO A RECENT STUDY BY CDC

BAFFLED RESEARCHERS SAY
THEY CAN'T EXPLAIN RECENT EXPLOSION
IN RATE OF ADULT DIABETES

If you're like most Americans today, you've probably been hearing about the "twin threat" from diabetes and obesity for some time now.

What you probably *haven't* heard, however, is the shocking story of how a few researchers have recently been uncovering a hidden connection between these two health scourges.

It's true. Although most of the "Medical Establishment"—including the CDC—remains blissfully unaware of the breakthrough, there's no doubt that *the recent discovery of this startling epidemiological link between obesity and diabetes to environmental exposure now promises to become one of the major scientific stories of our time.*

The story of how the increasingly polluted human environment has triggered a whole new family of diseases—"neurotoxic" illnesses that are the direct result of this pollution—was told in detail in my most recent book, *Desperation Medicine* (now available from Gateway Press, Baltimore, Md. and Amazon.com).

As I pointed out in *Desperation Medicine*, the toxins that are now being generated by our increasingly tainted environment also have a major impact on the body's system for storing and metabolizing sugar.

That impact has now begun to make itself known—via the rapidly accelerating (and highly alarming) incidence-rates for both diabetes and obesity.

But let's back up for a moment.

In order to understand how the toxic microorganisms that increasingly feed on our society's chemical and agricultural "waste products" are interfering with our ability to process sugar, let's pause for a quick look at some of the biochemical processes involved.

ENVIRONMENTAL TOXINS AND HUMAN HEALTH: A PRIMER

Remember that wonderful book by Rachel Carson, *Silent Spring*?

Remember how she warned us—way back in 1962, when her book spent more than a year as a huge bestseller—that the day would come when the birds no longer sang to us, because their young had all been wiped out by our agricultural pesticides?

Carson was a true visionary, a supremely prescient biologist whose once-dramatic predictions now strike most of us as routinely accurate. But the one phenomenon that *Silent Spring* did *not* predict was the emergence of new families of human diseases that would be spawned by genetically altered microorganisms thriving in new habitats altered by our chemicals and our own rapidly changing lifestyles.

The impact of these radical lifestyle-changes on human disease can be seen quite clearly in the epidemic of chronic Lyme Disease that is now spreading across the United States. Although there are several factors at work in the recent surge of Lyme, none is more important than the rapid growth in blood meal sources for hungry ticks, including deer and mice. As more and more farmland and forest is converted to shopping malls and suburban housing tracts replete with new boundary lines featuring succulent young trees, bushes and shrubs, the populations of "undergrowth, edge-dwelling animals," including deer and mice, have exploded. The readily available food and cover provides a fertile habitat for the animals that play a vital role in the life cycle of the ticks that carry the Borrelia burgdorferi spirochetes that cause Lyme disease.

As the deer invade the nation's backyards and vegetable gardens, they bring with them, and to us, the ticks that harbor Lyme disease and other vector-borne illnesses. In a recent "drag" survey of ticks in Hunterdon County, New Jersey, for example, the startling results showed that fully 63 percent of 1,000 analyzed ticks were carrying the Lyme spirochete. (About nine percent were infected with *Babesia*-causing bacteria, by the way, and two percent were carrying a related disease bacteria, *Ehrlichia*.)

The New Jersey study—sent to me by Dr. John Dowling— provided compelling evidence for the fact that changing lifestyles and changing demographics are now having a profound effect on many different human diseases.

263

Equally threatening, however, is a new epidemiological phenomenon in which entire families of disease-causing bacteria and fungi are now undergoing genetic adaptations that allow them to survive in an increasingly polluted world, while also manufacturing toxins of their own that make people sick.

These altered bugs—let's call them the "Mutants"—have recently become a major factor in the etiology of a dozen threatening diseases ... including sick building syndrome, chronic fatigue syndrome, estuarine-related illness syndrome and the endlessly misdiagnosed "fibromyalgia"—which usually turns out to be a toxin-mediated disorder, like the others listed above, that is caused by organic poisons made by living organisms.

How did all of this happen? What is the secret link between ecology-altering chemicals, including pesticides, and habitat alterations that leave perpetually-sick patients suffering from excruciating headaches, constant fatigue, muscle cramps and debilitating diarrhea? Is there a so-far-uncovered relationship between our alterations of habitat—both indoors and outdoors—and the unfolding epidemic of toxin-linked illnesses?

The search for answers to those question must begin with a single word: *Neurotoxins.*

NEUROTOXIN-MEDIATED ILLNESS: A GROWING MENACE

You don't have to be a rocket scientist to understand that as our environment becomes more industrialized by the minute, the 70,000 different industrial and agricultural chemicals we now use daily are triggering massive ecological changes on a scale unprecedented in human history.

What are these noxious substances that are having such a negative effect on the air we all breathe and water we all drink? Among the major offenders are the following:

O   pesticides

O volatile organic compounds

O food additives

O polymerizing agents (cyanonitriles and more)

O hydrocarbons from burned fossil fuels

O nitrogen and sulfur compounds (the source of acid rain)

Question: How have these environmental poisons helped to trigger the explosive growth of toxin-bearing disease organisms?

Answer: Because those microorganisms that were vulnerable to the toxic chemicals soon died out, those which were resistant gained a "selective advantage" in the struggle for survival—and rapidly began to flourish. Ironically enough, by choosing to kill such pests as fungus and insects with poisons of the Chemical Age, we actually *encouraged* the growth of survivor microscopic organisms, many species of which manufacture their *own* neurotoxins as part of their basic makeup.

What is chronic Lyme disease? Simply the sum of the physiologic effects caused by the neurotoxins that poison cells as they are released, from minute to minute, by Lyme bacteria in a human host. Even if antibiotics kill the causative Borrelia spirochetes, the biotoxins circulate endlessly, causing chronic illness symptoms.

What is sick building syndrome? Simply a group of symptoms (headaches, aching muscles, memory loss, impaired vision, joint-pain, etc.) that occur when cell tissues are poisoned by toxins ... and in this case, by toxins from many different species of fungi which have moved into new environmental niches created by closed-air circulation systems in newer buildings.

I first became aware of this growing family of "neurotoxin-mediated" human illnesses about five years ago, while doing research on a waterborne disease carried by a toxic organism (*Pfiesteria*) that was resistant to copper-based pesticides and fungicides routinely used on land that drains into Maryland's Chesapeake Bay estuaries. The surge in human illness from *Pfiesteria* eventually triggered more than $26 million in research grants focusing

265

on the toxin(s) and the environmental conditions related to it. This public attention led to the recognition by the U.S. Centers for Disease Control and Prevention (CDC), in 1998, of a "Possible Estuary-Associated Syndrome [PEAS]." The CDC stopped short of declaring the syndrome a "treatable disease," however.

Unfortunately, the CDC's official declaration came after the huge federal health agency had spent several years insisting that this voracious dinoflagellate rarely made people sick. And indeed, an important CDC study concluded—in October of 2000—that no patients with PEAS had been identified during the preceding two years. This finding directly contradicted the research I had done earlier with Dr. Ken Hudnell of the U.S. EPA National Health and Environmental Effects Research Laboratory.

Our study, published immediately after the CDC finding of "no PEAS cases," identified 37 patients with PEAS.

Still, it wasn't until 2001 that the CDC finally confirmed our extensively detailed findings—and published our study showing that the syndrome could be recognized in the absence of fish kill *and* treated successfully.

While performing the exhaustive research that became the basis for my 1998 book, *Pfiesteria: Crossing Dark Water* (Gateway Press, Baltimore), I learned that many of the toxins manufactured by these emerging disease agents are in fact low-molecular-weight compounds with the cunning ability to move from one cell to another *without necessarily traveling through the blood vessels.*

Collectively called "neurotoxins," these organic poisons typically cause a cluster of symptoms that include:

O   deep, persistent fatigue

O   weakness

O   chronic muscle aches

O   cramping

O   memory impairment

266

○ impaired cognitive function

○ difficulty assimilating new knowledge

○ disorientation

○ confusion

○ chronic cough that mimics asthma

○ sinus congestion

○ shortness of breath

○ headaches

○ sensitivity to bright lights

○ red eyes

○ blurred vision

○ tearing

○ numbness

○ tingling

○ vertigo

○ abdominal pain (no, it's not really "irritable bowel syndrome" or gall bladder disease!)

○ diarrhea

Although these biotoxins vary widely in terms of their biochemistry and their geographical distribution, the end result for patients is always the same. These patients are among the sickest I've ever treated … and yet most physicians refuse to take their complaints seriously, since the medical world does not yet recognize neurotoxin-mediated illness as a treatable disease!

Even a brief look at the current lineup up of fast-spreading neurotoxin-mediated pathogens is enough to frighten a trained epidemiologist. Among the most troubling recent outbreaks are the following:

In Maryland, Delaware, Virginia and North Carolina, mini-epidemics of *Pfiesteria*-related human illness syndrome have felled hundreds of local residents and possibly killed several people who contracted the disease and went untreated;

In the Inland Bays of Delaware, a toxic dinoflagellate called "chattonella" has been growing at an unprecedented rate, while fouling waterways and killing fish;

Along tropical reefs throughout the world, the highly toxic ciguatera microorganism has flourished in recent years, leaving thousands of tourists who unwisely ate large, predator reef-dwelling fish struggling with chronic symptoms for years at a time;

Throughout the U.S. and increasingly in Europe, new forms of toxin-spewing Lyme bacteria have contributed to the spread of chronic Lyme disease, leaving millions of permanently ill—with many of them completely disabled;

In the developed countries of the western world, fungi such as stachybotrys and aspergillus are blooming in "climate-control-led" buildings, while pumping their toxins throughout heating and cooling systems to cause sick building syndrome;

In the once-pristine lakes of Central Florida, massive growths of blue-green algae (also known as "cylindrospermopsis") have triggered numerous fish- and bird-kills and left local residents wondering how long their drinking water will continue to be safe.

SO HOW DO DIABETES AND OBESITY FIT IN?

Alarming in themselves, these recent outbreaks of toxin-linked illnesses around the world often display one other characteristic that deeply concerns health researchers.

In situation after situation, these toxin-diseases also appear to be causing inexplicable weight-gain *and* increasing diabetes among their victims, along with the other symptoms listed above.

So here's the $64,000 question, ready or not:

> What is the link between the neurotoxin-mediated illnesses that increasingly threaten our world and these other weight-related diseases?

Unfortunately, we can't look to the "experts" at the CDC for an answer to this pressing question … since the Atlanta-based science bureaucrats continue to duck the issue by blaming the "changing American diet" for the surge in obesity and diabetes. According to the federal scientists, we're simply eating too many "double cheeseburgers" and "super-size French fries" at the fast-food carryout joints, these days.

As anyone who watches the CBS Evening News can tell you, the CDC has spent the past decade insisting that our expanding waistlines are actually the result of ingesting too many "fat grams," while engaging in far too little exercise.

They couldn't be more wrong.

To understand why, let's return for a few moments to our "FedEx" model of how sugar gets distributed throughout the human body.

Let's ask ourselves: If the problem is increasing diabetes and obesity, *could there be something wrong with the delivery truck (insulin molecules), or with the receiving clerk (the cell receptors) which move the glucose "packages" from the truck into the cells?*

What if the environmental toxins described above are actually engaged in "shooting out the tires" of the FedEx trucks before they can get their precious cargo to the waiting clerks at the cell membranes?

In order to examine the evidence at the cellular level, we must first step back and question the definitions of both diabetes and obesity … by pointing out that the recently established diagnostic measurement for being overweight—the "Lean Body Mass" (a ratio based on kilograms of weight divided by meters squared of body surface area)—is utterly inaccurate as a method for

269

determining what a healthy person's weight should be.

Unreliable and difficult to employ, this arcane standard of measurement also raises a disturbing question: What medical facility in the U.S. today routinely measures the "meters squared" of a patient's "body surface area?"

In the same way, the standard diagnostic for diabetes (fasting glucose over 110) has recently been set at a much lower level than physicians used only a few years ago (140, then 125).

(Is it really surprising to discover that diabetes is "surging," when the definition has been made so much more stringent in recent years?)

The BMI, for its part, is an entirely useless measuring tool—yet its status as "the gold standard for obesity" goes unchallenged year after year. Although most experts in bariatrics (the branch of medicine dedicated to treating obesity) acknowledge that the BMI has major flaws, they argue that it's better to have *some* yardstick for determining "ideal weight" than no yardstick at all!

This "logic" bothers me to no end. To show you what I mean, let's go back to that rosiglitazone study I told you about in Chapter 13 ... and to the case history involving a patient who had been burning her protein needlessly through years of dysfunctional, low-fat dieting. Based on the BMI method for determining lean body mass and percent of body fat, this patient began her 00-2-3 program with a ten-pound deficit in lean body mass, which she rapidly regained. She then lost four percent of her body fat, which amounted to 22 pounds. Interestingly enough, however, her net loss in BMI was only *one point*—since her net weight loss came out to only 12 pounds.

Had I used the BMI as a tool of statistical analysis in this patient's dieting program, her weight-loss numbers would have appeared trivial. Yet she managed to burn three inches of fat from her hips, and two inches from her waist. At the same time, she restored her Lean Body Mass to its genetically programmed level —and wound up "feeling great and looking terrific."

Nonetheless, the BMI standard of measurement would have required any epidemiologist who used it to conclude that her 12-week diet had been a failure!

Truth time here: the BMI cannot be used for comparison when deficits in lean body mass (which usually occur in diets where high-insulin patients are allowed to eat amylose) are not calculated before the program begins!

So far, so good. If we agree that a fasting blood sugar of 110 is simply too low to support a diagnosis of diabetes—and that the BMI is unreliable as a measure of body fat—then what yardstick *does* make sense for these two conditions?

Answer: For many years now in my own practice, I have used physiologic diagnosis of glucose intolerance for my Type II or adult onset diabetics. Remember, these are *not* Type I diabetics, and they are *not* insulin-deficient patients who cannot produce enough insulin to meet the needs of sugar metabolism.

Fortunately for 10 million insulin-deficient patients, the marvelous advances in stem cell research of the last few years have permitted researchers to produce insulin-generating cells by manipulating undifferentiated primordial cells. And although this emerging technology holds out enormous hope for the Type I patients, it won't help the much larger group of Type IIs, whose problem isn't lack of insulin, but *resistance* to their own insulin!

So what values are required for an accurate diagnosis of diabetes? As far as I'm concerned, the diagnosis requires several key factors:

○ The patient must have a close family member with diabetes;

○ The patient's fasting insulin must exceed 10ng/ml and the patient must have produced three random blood sugars over 200—within a six-week time span—after ingesting an amylose-free meal. (I suspect that I'll soon be accused of "under-diagnosing" diabetes, of course. But I've been

271

using this yardstick for many years, and I intend to go right *on* using it!)

○ ○ ○

MEASURING OBESITY: FINDING THE RIGHT CRITERIA

Before we get down to answering the complex and controversial question, "What is obesity," I should point out that my diagnostic criteria for this ailment are rarely used by other physicians. (Which is fine with me—because I want to be *right*, rather than merely validated by the conventional wisdom of the day.) As a matter of fact, I don't even *like* the word obesity. All too often, the term amounts to little more than a slur among physicians, who seem to use it without any feelings at all for the patient whom they're describing. Every time I read a patient work-up by a health care provider who describes a patient as "morbidly obese," I find myself wondering: *Was the author of this document feeling even a shred of compassion for the overweight patient?*

My own approach to defining obesity calls for a functional diagnosis of the condition based on percentage of body fat. In my scheme, women are classified as normal if 20 percent of their body-mass consists of fat (as measured by the nomogram, *Appendix 3*). Men, on the other hand, should measure 15 percent body fat in order to fall within the normal range. Of course, I also allow women an extra ten pounds if they've given birth, along with an extra ten pounds after the age of 40. (Men are allowed 15 extra pounds after the age of 40.)

By subtracting the calculated "ideal body weight" from the patient's actual weight, we can come up with a reasonably accurate measurement of the number of pounds overweight.

Another approach I've used successfully in the past involves another yardstick: *Amount of Time Overweight.* Depending on the weight-loss program a patient chooses, it's a simple enough matter to calculate how long it will take to reach the "maintenance" segment of the diet, during which the restrictions on bread, pasta and other amyose-based goodies can be somewhat relaxed.

The trick here is to let the patient know that each time he or she "cheats" on the 00-2-3 weight-loss program, I will tack an additional three days onto the schedule for it. Then I tell the patient: The sooner you get to Maintenance, the sooner you can relax your program—so stop slowing yourself down by cheating! (I've found that this approach works especially well in patients who are in a big hurry to shed their flab.)

The good news for patients is that the physiology of weight-loss is uniformly consistent among high–insulin non–diabetics ... which means that if they follow my program carefully, they can usually count on losing at least half a pound per week.

DIABETES ... OR TOXIN-MEDIATED, ENVIRONMENTAL ILLNESS?

Soon after I began using contrast sensitivity (CS) testing as a biomarker for the presence of environmentally acquired, chronic, neurotoxin-mediated illnesses (the case definition includes exposure, symptoms and the absence of a confounding diagnosis), I began to notice that the pattern of illness among many of my high insulin patients simply "didn't fit the mold." Curiously enough, these patients often presented with multiple symptoms *and* a marked CS deficit. What was going on here? These patients looked more like neurotoxin patients than smorgasborg gluttons or Type II diabetics.

You can imagine the shock I felt, as it gradually became clear that neurotoxins were actually the basis of the illness affecting these patients! Of course, their health problems had been diagnosed routinely as "obesity" and "diabetes." All the lab tests confirmed insulin resistance. All the predictable metabolic problems tied to insulin resistance were there too. Of course, many *other* victims of these environmentally acquired illnesses had also been misdiagnosed, and wound up being told that they were suffering from one of the following ailments:

O fibromyalgia

O stress

O depression

O allergy

O asthma

O poor physical conditioning ("out of shape")

O memory loss due to aging

Could the large number of new patients who came to Poco-moke for help with weight loss be a marker for something other than sedentary, overeating lifestyles? Many of these patients gained the weight "overnight" and didn't respond to even the strictest of diets. They felt too bad to even think about 12 hours per week of exercise, much less 2 hours total. Some of the chronic Lyme Disease patients developed diabetes, despite no family history of the disease.

Could I add unexplained, new onset of diabetes and obesity to the growing list of commonly accepted medical misdiagnoses? The implications were enormous. If I could prove that societal change and resultant environmentally acquired illnesses associated with the change were the cause of the explosion of diabetes and obesity, then our entire Public Health Campaign Against Diabetes and Obesity was directed at the wrong enemy and was doomed to fail.

The answer came from a study that focused on 15 Type II diabetics who did not have a family history of the illness. I did symptom lists and CS testing in all of the patients. I repeated the drill with 30 patients who had a strong family history of diabetes.

The findings showed a marked difference in the number of

symptoms *and* CS deficits between the no-family history group and the others. The bottom line was that the subjects without the family history were actually suffering from neurotoxin-mediated illnesses: *They didn't have Type II diabetes at all!* (You can be sure that when I suggested treating their toxin-based illnesses as a way to attack their diabetes, these startled patients sent me more than one quizzical look!) Not all the patients were willing to try treatment of their supposed neurotoxin-mediated illness at first, but as the numbers of successfully treated, family history-negative diabetic patients grew, it became clear that the concept of environmentally acquired obesity and diabetes was well supported by clinical results.

After reviewing the study, I realized that I could use the symptom lists and CS tool effectively ... *by concentrating on diabetics without a family history.* Diabetics with a family history usually displayed (on average) a single symptom from the neurotoxin list, whereas most of the patients in the non-family history group displayed at least six or seven symptoms—all of which belonged to the constellation of health problems associated with neurotoxin-based illnesses. The best study results were that the "acquired" diabetics rarely needed to take any diabetes medications once the neurotoxins were cleared from their body.

The overall results of the diabetes study were nothing less than spectacular. Some of these patients had been sick for years, and had even sustained damage to such organs as eyes and kidneys, exactly as true diabetics (as opposed to "acquired" diabetics) often incur end-organ damage over time. The sole difference between them was the family history of diabetes, along with the CS deficit and the symptoms described above. And indeed, after treatment for neurotoxic illness, both the CS deficit and the blood sugar problems resolved. These patients had displayed the same A-1-C hemoglobin levels and the same elevated random sugar and insulin levels found in normal diabetics, but after neurotoxin treatment, the A-1-C hemoglobin, sugar and insulin levels returned to equal those of the control, non-diabetic patients.

275

The first-ever description and assessment of the neurotoxic symptoms in patients with neurotoxic illnesses was contained in the recently published paper (co-authors, Shoemaker and Dr. Hudnell) in the NIH/NIEHS journal, Environmental Health Perspectives, back in May of 2001. That study compared asymptomatic patients with estuarine exposure to those without such exposure in cases of *Pfiesteria*-related human illness syndrome and it established the importance of taking a neurotoxin history in the high-level, peer-reviewed medical literature.

While reflecting on these findings, I asked myself: If I can find 15 diabetics—in only six months—who don't actually have diabetes, but rather neurotoxin-mediated illness, how many Americans with misdiagnosed diabetes are *out there right now, suffering needlessly?*

I also found myself wondering: *Is the recent "explosion" of diabetes in the U.S. actually an "explosion" of neurotoxin-mediated illnesses?*

The bottom line on all of this is quite clear: Physicians who treat patients for obesity and diabetes need to ask about family history. They also need to ask about sensitivity to bright lights and the other neurotoxic symptoms. They should also conduct a Contrast Sensitivity test on each new patient, before making recommendations about diet.

Of course, the problem of neurotoxin-induced obesity is also growing daily in this country, even as the doctors continue to misdiagnose it. *(See the case study involving Sherran Nahm, for example.)* What are the sure signs that the overweight patient must actually be suffering from an environmentally acquired disorder?

O The patient doesn't lose weight successfully, no matter how carefully he or she observes the diet.

O Look for some of the symptoms on the long list of complaints (above) that are linked to neurotoxin-mediated illness.

O Take the CS test at your earliest opportunity (use www. chronicneurotoxins.com if your physician doesn't have the test yet), and learn in five minutes whether or not you've got the telltale (for neurotoxin illness) deficit of the ability to distinguish black from grey from white.

BIOTOXINS: THE ACTION IS ON THE MOLECULAR LEVEL

How many patients actually suffer from neurotoxin-mediated illnesses? While I have treated over 1000 patients with chronic Lyme Disease, there probably are many more patients who have their chronic illness related to exposure to buildings with resident mycotoxin forming fungal species. That said, let me qualify my comments by pointing out that these conclusions are based on patients I have treated, and not on scientific population-sampling techniques. But my experience with this kind of illness has been extensive … and it tells me that any organism that manufactures a biotoxin can potentially cause diabetes or obesity. Why? The answer will require a bit of explaining, but here it is in a phrase: The mechanism responsible for new onset of persistent insulin resistance probably does its destructive work by activating the endogenous manufacture of inappropriate amounts of a pro-inflammatory cytokine called "tumor necrosis factor alpha," or TNF.

In order to understand how the process works, let's start by remembering that the receptor-insulin-glucose interaction on the outer cell membrane is actually quite complex.

To get a feeling for just *how* complex the interaction is, let's follow a sugar molecule into the cell … where we will have a ringside seat from which to observe all of the reasons why the surge in diabetes/obesity is more likely to be the result of changes in the external environment.

277

DOWN AND DOWN WE GO,
ROUND AND ROUND WE GO ...

All set? Great! Let's take our journey through the Wonderful World of Molecular Sugar Metabolism in a series of small, easy-to-digest steps.

STEP 1: In most cases, a molecule of insulin must link up with a second, similar molecule—thus creating a two-piece hormonal entity known as a "dimer [pronounced die-mer]." The dimer's job is to turn on the receptor.

STEP 2: Now the receptor activates an enzyme, tyrosine kinase, which proceeds to drop a phosphate group on a specific amino acid—threonine—contained in the insulin.

STEP 3: Now an additional reaction kicks in, stimulating the receptor to pinch off a bit of membrane around the dimer-glucose-receptor complex.

STEP 4: Time now for a key maneuver: the shifting of the pinched-off membrane (in the form of a covered bubble, or endosome) to be moved into the cell.

STEP 5: Are you having fun yet? Stand by for a major thrill, as a positively charged hydrogen ion is pumped into the endosome ... which now opens up (de-granulates) and thus releases the glucose. The latter is then added to glycogen—if space permits —or else burned for fuel.

STEP 6: The insulin receptor is recycled to the membrane, and the insulin is sent back into the bloodstream as a single unit (monomer) in search of more glucose and insulin receptors.

INTRODUCING ... THE 1,000-POUND GORILLA ON THE SEESAW

Enormously complex, this labyrinth of biochemical reactions can easily go awry. One such breakdown can occur when TNF is tremendously over-produced in fat cells (and especially in the overweight) as a result of exposure to neurotoxins. Essentially, TNF disrupts the normal initiation of receptor activity by forcing the tyrosine kinase to drop the phosphate group on a *different* amino acid (serine), located directly adjacent to threonine. The phosphate groups are huge, on a molecular scale and completely alter the normal size/shape relationship of one molecule to the next in three dimensions.

The bottom line on all of this is that when the bulky phosphate group "gets in the way," the "lock and key" system of insulin attachment doesn't work, and the sugar never makes it into the cell. After that, the body responds—as we learned in Chapter 2—by either creating fatty acids from the sugar (and thus making you fat) or by allowing the sugar molecules to pile up in the bloodstream and tissues (and thus leaving you with diabetes). Is this insulin resistance? No! It's actually the effect of TNF on insulin receptors. To picture this effect, imagine the delicate balance between blood sugar and insulin receptors as a seesaw. Most of the time, the seesaw rides up and down smoothly. But when TNF arrives on the scene, it's as if a 1,000-pound gorilla had suddenly jumped on the seesaw, triggering wholesale havoc.

If you've followed our Bouncing Molecular Ball this far, you're probably asking yourself: "Okay, but if TNF does so much damage and the body is always making it to help fight off infections [along with monitoring cells for senescence—aka 'apoptosis,' or programmed cell death] ... then why don't *all* of us have diabetes or obesity?"

Well, many of us *do*—and for precisely this reason. But based on their genetic structure, many people will not develop insulin resistance or TNF-related problems.

(Question: How many of you out there—after your careful reading of the last chapter—have already figured out that gene-altering PPAR serves as a key factor in protecting us from the loose-cannon effects of TNF? You're right: Once again, it's PPAR to the rescue!)

To understand just how our pal PPAR provides the magic bullet to shoot down the effects of TNF, remember that both the glucose-transport protein gene and the uncoupling protein gene are activated by PPAR agonists (including Avandia, of course) which also interrupt the transcription of genes that leads to TNF production. (These genes, you will no doubt recall, are controlled by the opposing nuclear receptor: the *cytokine* nuclear receptor, which regulates the production of cytokines, including TNF in fat cells.)

Of course, the benefits of shutting down TNF production and its effects are only now beginning to be understood. Still, there's no denying the importance of this process—and more than once, I've found myself speculating that the powerful impact of Avandia on patients being treated for diabetes and obesity depends more on the control of TNF than it does on the manipulation of glucose transport proteins.

Avandia gets the job done effectively, because it works to restore the complicated balance to the molecular seesaw that is human sugar metabolism. In effect, this super-efficient medication "drives off the gorilla"—and restores a healthy balance (aka "homeostasis") to the metabolic process.

CAN YOU CATCH DIABETES FROM A SICK BUILDING?

It's a truism that we need cytokines for life; these vital substances enable cell-to-cell messaging. They also link hormone-messages to cells and to the immune system. But the cytokines were only recently discovered; the landmark scientific paper on the "superstar" of the cytokine family—TNF—was written way back in 1989! Still, the word is now getting out about this hugely important aspect of hormone management, with more than 10,000 references during the past five years to TNF in the "Medicine Key Word Directory" for academic articles. As you might imagine, there's a great deal of excitement in the academic community today about the wonders of TNF.

And why not? The fact is that we're just beginning to learn about the complex world of the cytokines. Already, we know that TNF directly disrupts the workings of insulin receptors. Example: If you want to prevent sugar from entering a muscle or liver cell, just add some TNF to the mix! It's also true that if TNF *is* present, the scant amount of receptor activity that *does* take place will be severely compromised by the cascades of biological effects that will ensue, thus poisoning the TNF. (Remember that the highest levels of TNF are always produced by fat cells in response to the effects of neurotoxins.)

There's no denying that we need TNF to accomplish its routine daily task of fighting off cancer and some infectious diseases. But too much of a good thing—too much TNF in the wrong place—can make us sick, fat or diabetic, depending on the specifics of our own genetic makeup.

Don't forget that certain biotoxins visit part of their destructive effects on us by activating the cytokine nuclear receptors—either directly or indirectly through activation of a compound called "Nuclear Factor" (NF-kB). Of course, the names and acronyms that describe these compounds aren't nearly as important as our key concept—the idea that biochemical balance is absolutely essential in the genetic control of insulin receptor effects.

Think about it. When your friend Joe in the next office (that's the building with the "sealed and climate-controlled" re-circulation of air system) starts putting on flab, while also becoming tired and short of breath all the time, don't blame his growing bulk on the Reuben sandwiches he eats at lunch. Not when that sealed building is home for all sorts of toxin-forming fungi that are thriving in the cooling system, and also activating TNF production in our poor friend Joe!

Nor should you assume that the members of your local Lyme support group are getting fat because they sit around eating bonbons all day. Instead, think about the fact that chronic Lyme Disease is the fastest growing, diagnosed (and *un*-diagnosed) vector-borne illness in the U.S. right now. Indeed, Lyme now provides the paradigm for chronic, biotoxin-mediated illnesses associated with infections.

The good news for the nation's 15 million Type II diabetics and the estimated 33–50 percent of all Americans now labeled as "obese" is that successful treatment of these neurotoxin-mediated illnesses stops the over-production of TNF, and also removes it from the insulin receptors. This healing step, of course, soon allows affected patients to return to their genetically programmed weights.

IMPLICATIONS FOR TREATMENT

One of the most exciting aspects of my job as a practicing family physician is directly related to these new discoveries. I can't tell you how rewarding it is to talk to my new diabetes patients … and to talk about something besides "diet and exercise!" Instead, I pepper these patients with questions about biotoxin-symptoms … including sensitivity to bright light, unusual pains, non-anatomic distribution of numbness and tingling, or unexplained vertigo.

My list of eminently discussable symptoms also includes metallic taste and earlier—if unverifiable—diagnoses, such as fibromyalgia, irritable bowel syndrome, stress, depression and poor physical conditioning.

As I recently told one patient whose new onset of diabetes was entirely due to exposure from a toxin-forming dinoflagellate (now appearing in an East Coast estuary near you) known as *Chattonella*: "The reason your doctor didn't understand your illness was that he hadn't learned the questions physicians must ask their patients in the Chemical Age!"

Let's face it: *Chattonella* hasn't even made it into the textbooks yet. Just try to find a physician in Indiana or Arizona who knows about estuarine-related exposures as causes of obesity! Yet I predict that within the decade, almost everyone will have heard about the accelerating growth of biotoxins and their huge impact on obesity and diabetes alike.

I don't want to pummel the CDC needlessly (the bloated federal agency is an easy target, after all), since some of the research scientists there are among the world's finest. Still, the CDC's widely discussed study of obesity (JAMA, 2000) failed to control its subjects for confounding variables such as dietary changes caused by eating low fat, cholesterol-lowering diets (a guaranteed source of weight gain!), cigarette smoking-cessation and neurotoxin exposure.

Although the CDC's frequent misstatements and inaccurate pronouncements are transparently obvious to most members of the scientific community, the agency continues to wear the Cloak of Infallibility when it comes to the news media.

And that's precisely why the All-Powerful Mandarins in Atlanta are still quoted everywhere, these days, as they sing their never-ending mantra about the virtues of "diet and exercise" … and as they continue to blame the twin epidemics of diabetes and obesity on fastfood French fries and couch-napping.

They're wrong, however—and the sooner the rest of us begin to wake up to the fact, the wiser (and the healthier) we're all going to be!

15

TAKING THE MYSTERY OUT OF FIBER

Isn't it amazing how the so-called "health experts" keep changing their minds from year to year?

Take that world-famous, five-letter word—"Fiber"—for example.

Back in the early 1960s, the experts all believed that "maintaining a low fiber-intake" was a key element in the successful dietary management of such chronic digestive ailments as diverticulosis and hiatal hernia. Their reasoning? According to the conventional dietary wisdom (CDW) of the day, it was essential to keep residual plant material out of the stool, in order to assure effective elimination.

By the 1990's, however, the Medical Establishment had decided that exactly the *reverse* was true: Eating lots of fiber actually enhanced the process of digestion-and-elimination, while also significantly reducing the fiber-eater's risk of developing certain kinds of bowel cancer. And now we find out that fiber doesn't really make any difference in the incidence of cancer of the colon after all.

Confusing, you say?

You bet it is. Just the other day, I received a visit from a new patient who'd already consulted a gastroenterologist and a general surgeon in the hope of discovering the source of his nagging abdominal pain. Unfortunately, this troubled soul had failed to observe Shoemaker's First Principle of Obtaining Good Medical Care: *Always consult a primary care physician first!*

It took me less than a minute to determine that my new patient had received the same advice from each of the specialists: "Be sure to include a lot of fiber in your diet!"

After paying the specialists' sky-high bills, the man with the gut-ache had begun eating cereal for breakfast, lunch and dinner. Two weeks later, when his abdominal pain showed no signs of abating, he wound up asking me the question he *should* have asked the two specialists:

"Dr. Shoemaker, what *is* fiber, anyway, and what effect does it have on the human digestive system?"

Answer: For starters, dietary fiber is not a single substance, but actually consists of many different plant materials ... all of which share one key characteristic: They are not subject to human digestion.

I should also point out that the fiber family consists of two major branches: soluble fibers, which dissolve in water, and insoluble fibers, which obviously *don't*.

The soluble branch of the fiber-clan includes the following elements:

O   The *pectins*, which are often used in the manufacture of jams and jellies, and as gels that hold sugar solutions in place;

O   The *gums*, which include guar, various mucilages, and a group of fractions of cellulose known collectively as "hemi-cellulose."

The important thing to remember about soluble fibers is that when you add them to water, they make the solution thick and viscous. And the same effect occurs in the human stomach: Add these fibers to your meal, and the result will usually be a pleasing sense of satiety. Obviously, the soluble fibers are capable of playing a major role in any weight-loss program. Even better, the soluble fibers help dissolve cholesterol, holding it in the intestine and preventing absorption.

How about the *insoluble* fibers? This group of plant elements consists mostly of cellulose and lignin, along with a few "breakdown products" from cellulose. Essentially, these insoluble particles form the structural foundation for plants, and typically include the membranes that make up plant gristle. Because these fibers aren't soluble, they don't trigger a sense of satiety. Still, they're quite useful in holding water in the large bowel— a scenario leading to larger, softer and squishier stools. Today's concepts suggest that by creating less pressure of stool against the lining of the bowel that the pressure problems associated with diverticulosis will be lessened.

Although these insoluble fibers can't help much with weight-loss, they do serve the valuable function of preventing complications of diverticulosis.

FIBER AND FOODS: SEPARATING FACT FROM FICTION

When it comes to protecting your digestive health, understanding the role played by dietary fiber is vitally important. And the good news here—especially for weight-loss patients—is that all of the no-amylose vegetables (those that grow above ground, remember) are full of soluble fiber. Cereals, on the other hand, usually contain a great deal of the insoluble kind. (That's an important distinction for diverticulosis patients, who need lots of the insolubles—and who receive them as dietary supplements, thereby avoiding contamination with amylose, whenever they decide to participate in my No-Amylose Diet.)

It should come as no surprise, of course, to discover that most news-media descriptions of dietary fiber are dead-wrong. Example: How many times have you read or heard that "Eating oats is a surefire way to dramatically lower cholesterol?"

Sorry, but that famous cliché is only partly true. The facts turn out to be a bit more complicated … starting with the reality that when you eat oats (including oat bran, by the way), you're actually taking in a mixture of soluble *and* insoluble fibers. The soluble stuff does, indeed, help to bind cholesterol and bile acids, so that they can be excreted in the stool. And this drainage effect will often trigger a reduction, however miniscule, in total serum cholesterol.

On the other hand, eating insoluble fiber has no effect whatsoever on cholesterol levels. And this fact is important … because about *97 percent of the fiber in oats consists of the insoluble variety.* Do you see now why I used the word "miniscule" in the above paragraph? Despite what you've heard on the CBS Evening News (or read in USA Today), the fact remains: Essentially, eating oats has no meaningful impact on blood cholesterol.

I take no pleasure in reporting this fact, but the fact remains: Eating all those "bran muffins" and all those bowls of oatmeal was to no avail (at least in terms of cholesterol-reduction)! Still, you *can* exploit the power of soluble oat fiber a bit—simply by purchasing a "pure" form of this plant substance in tablets sold at some health-food stores. Consuming two of these tablets per day will produce a few loose stools … but it will also result in lowering your total serum cholesterol by about ten percent. (You won't see a rise in HDL, however; the sole benefit here is a falloff in "harmful" LDL cholesterol.)

Another nice touch: these soluble oat fiber tablets cost only 15 cents per pair. And if your LDL cholesterol is sitting at 160, the tablets will allow you to yank it back to about 135—which is a health improvement worth having, in my view.

BUT WILL IT SAVE US FROM CANCER?

If you're like most Americans today, you've probably read your share of stories that trumpet high-fiber diets as "powerful weapons in the battle against colon cancer."

Once again, however, there's a very large fictional element in these supposedly "objective" news stories about the benefits of fiber.

According to the medical gurus of the news columns, plant fibers often work to "bind carcinogens in the bowel." But the gurus need to re-take Human Physiology 101,—where they would quickly be reminded of the fact that the large bowel functions primarily to reabsorb water, and thus to concentrate the fecal stream in order to manufacture stool. This process does not include the "binding" of any substance, let alone carcinogens. (The reality is that chemicals are actually bound in the small intestine.)

Although there is some uncertain scientific evidence that a high-fiber diet may slightly reduce the risk of large-bowel cancer, these findings actually raise more questions than they answer. Among the imponderables: which of the many *kinds* of intestinal cancer are affected? Also: How does your family history of these diseases relate to consumption of fiber? Also: Is there any way of determining whether fiber affects "right-side" bowel cancer, as opposed to "left side?" (The distinction is an important one, in terms of patient-outcomes.)

One of the great chapters in the unfolding saga of intestinal cancer research was written by a British researcher, Dr. Denis Burkitt, who made headlines back in the 1960s while studying the dietary habits of rural Africans. Among other findings, Dr. Burkitt's team came up with data showing that these isolated tribesmen had no significant coronary artery disease, gallstones, hiatal hernia, diverticulosis or cancer of the colon. Was their diet a factor? According to the Britishers, their diets were lacking in red meat, but contained lots of fruits, vegetables and whole grains.

During the next decade or so, as this population gradually became "westernized," however, the diseases listed above began to appear with increasing frequency. This provocative finding was only one of several scientific breakthroughs achieved by Dr. Burkitt & Co. Along with discovering some of the health-benefits to be obtained from fiber (later exaggerated, unfortunately, by the nutritional hype-artists), he successfully delineated the morphology and pathology of an important type of lymphoma, which now bears his name.

The tantalizing link between diet and disease, that at first glance seems so convincing to all of us that our Western diet makes us sick, has to be counter-balanced by the rest of the accoutrements of Western civilization. If someone did a study showing that the lead content of the pipes in Rome was a source for the fall of the Roman Empire, we would likely accept that idea. But if someone said that the health problems in Western societies were caused by electromagnetic fields generated by power lines, would we be so quick to agree? The problem of diet and disease can be studied by associations of diet and disease incidence, but only documenting all variables over a prolonged time period can provide us with any idea of causation and risk.

Conclusion: Does a Western diet cause bowel cancer? The answer has to be we don't know. So what should a reasonable, prudent person do to avoid bowel cancer? First, select your parents well. Second, eat lots of good food prepared lovingly and with style. Third, get checked regularly by your primary care doctor for possible colon problems and fix them as you find them.

GETTING BEYOND THE HYPE

In spite of the widespread mythology about fiber and cancer, its most significant contribution to human health is undoubtedly its usefulness in weight-loss, when soluble fibers work together to create a feeling of satiety in dieters.

The special importance of fiber as a dietary food has been acknowledged by the American Medical Association (AMA), which recently published a report on the subject. In that key study, the Chicago-based organization of 600,000 U.S. physicians officially defined fiber as "remnants of plant cells resistant to hydrolysis by the alimentary enzymes of man," and also as "a group of substances that remain in the ileum but are partly hydrolyzed by bacteria in the colon."

This definition highlights several features important for weight loss, including these:

O The "plant remnants" are carbohydrates.

O As such, the simple sugars (one ring), along with the disaccharides (two rings) and the three-ring sugars, are usually absorbed in the first part of the small intestine. We have already seen how some four-or-more ring sugars (including the complex carbohydrates, such as amylose) are digested in saliva.

O The key to understanding fiber and fat is to understand the importance of carbohydrates that are *not* absorbed during digestion.

Remember: If those carbohydrates *are* being absorbed, they will not appear in the large bowel—which contains huge amounts of bacteria. On the other hand, if these food materials are not digested, they will become an instant food-source for the waiting bacteria. And indeed, the manner in which the bowel bacteria metabolize this source of sugar is the key determinant in shaping the side effects of fiber digestion. Example: Many patients who eat oat bran (a good source of insoluble fiber) will later complain of abdominal bloating and cramping, followed by bulky stools. Such symptoms clearly suggest that the bacteria are not digesting the insoluble fiber efficiently. As a result, this stalled fiber captures a large amount of water in the stool—a phenomenon that distends the colon and thus triggers the abnormal peristalsis we call "cramps." This process also creates large, soft stools.

The side effects produced by the digestion of soluble fiber are somewhat different, however. Here the plant material dissolves in water and is thus dissolved in the large bowel. Less water will be retained inside the bowel as absorption increases—and the results will include both heightened peristalsis and more frequent stools.

WHAT REALLY HAPPENS IN A "GAS ATTACK"?

Although the subject can be a bit touchy, the production of intestinal gases actually represents one of nature's most interesting processes. Explanation: If a patient eats a type of sugar that can't be broken down and absorbed in the small intestine, then the sweet stuff will be sent on to the large bowel—usually triggering a feeding frenzy in the legions of bacteria that live there. As the bacteria enjoy the feast, they create the process known as "fermentation," in which a variety of often-pungent gases is created as the sugar is broken down. Simple examples of fermentation include making beer and wine in which yeasts release carbon dioxide as they digest the 6 carbon containing sugars into the 2 carbon compounds called alcohol. If bacteria contaminate the yeast populations, the wine is contaminated by the products of bacterial digestion which aren't alcohol. The result is spoiled or rancid wine.

In our bowel, the same kind of process is occurring too, with a variety of gases released. These aromatic freshets can include carbon dioxide, nitrogen, methane and also hydrogen sulfide. (The exact composition, of course, will be determined by the patient's own particular bowel bacteria and diet.)

Some of the most gaseous scenarios are those in which amylose is consumed by low-insulin level patients, or lactose (milk sugar) is ingested by subjects who lack the enzyme (lactase) that breaks it down. Alpha galactosidose (bean sugar) has also been known to set off fireworks displays, recorded forever in Blazing Saddles, involving large amounts of the *gaseosa* ... a fact of life which long ago inspired that beloved childhood refrain:

> *Beans, beans, the magical fruit—*
> *The more you eat, the more you toot!*

Let the record show clearly that most of the scientific credit for our understanding of gas produced by malabsorption of sugars belongs to Dr. Michael Levin, a University of Minnesota gastroenterologist who spent years collecting balloon-type sample-bags containing the results of human flatulence. One can only applaud his bravery—while hoping that his staff researchers did not become anosmic during their tireless efforts to lay bare the causes of excessive gas production.

MEETING THE "PIZZA CHALLENGE!"

In thinking about the relationship of fiber to weight loss, it's important to make the distinction between soluble and insoluble. And the next step is to chart the amount of fiber contained in some key foods *(Appendix 6)*. For example:

○ Total dietary fiber in white bread is less than 3 grams per 100;

○ The total for wheat bread is 8.5 grams per hundred;

○ All-bran will provide an impressive 18 grams per 100 of ingested material;

○ Puffed wheat checks in at 15 grams, while baked beans and peas supply 8 grams of fiber per 100 grams of food.

○ Most fruits are low on the scale—with peaches at about

2 grams, apples at 4. Many vegetables also get low scores: potatoes earn a 3 and carrots a 4.

Of course, the key differences among these different foods are best determined by examining the cellulose content of their different fibers. Peaches contain virtually no cellulose, for example, while peas contain less than 20 percent and beans even less than that. On the other hand, bran, puffed wheat and whole wheat are simply loaded with cellulose. These higher-fiber foods also contain more lignins.

These interesting fiber-facts make for some interesting anomalies, when it comes to weight loss. Example: Although it's certainly true that you'll find more fiber in any single serving of bran cereal than in three peaches, combined, the peaches are actually far more helpful in promoting weight loss! Another drawback for the fiber-containing cereals is the fact that they invariably contain large amounts of amylose. This fact underlines the importance of remembering my key dieting principle: "Amylose is usually digested very quickly in people with weight problems!"

But what about those physiologically lucky folks—usually tall and slender—who seem able to eat lots of amylose without ever gaining an ounce? What becomes of the amylose they do take in? Well, as we learned in an earlier chapter, what usually happens is that the body will break down this complex carbohydrate with saliva—thus setting off the "insulin response" and storing the extra sugar mostly as fat. But what happens to amylose that gets past the saliva and stomach? At that point, the fat-making substance gets hit with pancreatic amylase—the substance doctors measure in blood, when looking for damage to the pancreas or diseases thereof.

To test our hypothesis that tall, skinny individuals who can eat lots of calories with impunity are actually deficient at absorbing amylose, I recently asked a cohort of ten patients to go five days without consuming any of the stuff at all. They agreed. But then, as soon as the test was over, they all hurried off to a local pizza parlor—where each enjoyed an entire large pie and bread sticks at my expense.

Then the *real* fun began. Having already asked them to count the number of times they'd passed gas while observing my no-amylose diet, I requested that they repeat the process right after the Pizza Challenge. (Dr. Levin had already demonstrated, I might point out, that the average human male passes gas 13 times per day, regardless of diet. Females pass gas 8 times a day, also regardless of food intake.)

When the numbers came in, they were startling.

Although the test-subjects in the Pizza Challenge had eliminated *gaseosa* 10 times a day while on the no-amylose regimen, their emissions shot up to *22 per day during the 48 hours that followed the pizza experiment!* (By happy chance, the Pizza Challenge took place during the summertime, which meant that the subjects could drive around town with their car windows open.)

This anecdotal study demonstrated several important principles of human physiology, starting with the insight that one should not ride in an automobile with tall, slender people who have eaten pizza, unless said consumption occurred less than four hours before the car trip. Of course the study *also* demonstrated that amylose malabsorption is a significant factor in maintenance of the "slender state." And this finding gives powerful support to the notion that an amylose-restricted diet will usually help individuals whose bodies are genetically programmed to store amylose efficiently as fat.

I am particularly fond of relating this experiment to my colleagues who insist that weight loss only comes from reduced calorie intake, independent of calorie absorption.

When it comes to understanding the Wonderful World of Fiber, one fact seems absolutely essential: Although you can lower your cholesterol slightly by taking in a pure form of soluble fiber, the key importance of this natural substance is its usefulness in creating satiety among dieters.

Remember: Fiber can be a powerful ally—as each one of us struggles to LOSE THE WEIGHT WE HATE!

16

GOUT: THE INSIDE STORY
OR ...
HOW MEAT AND BURGUNDY WINE TOOK A REALLY BUM RAP!

Go ahead, don't be shy. Say the word out loud.

"Gout!"

And what image springs immediately to mind?

If you're like 99 percent of the rest of the English-speaking world, what springs to mind is this really heavyset guy wearing some sort of odd-looking purple pillow on his head, while grasping a leg of roasted mutton in one hand and a tankard of Portuguese red in the other.

And who *is* this aristocratic-looking plumpster with the scarlet nose-veins and the Leviathan-sized pot belly hanging over his gold-embroidered belt?

Step right up, Ladies and Gentlemen, and meet King Henry VIII of England (1509–47), who has an important message that he'd like to share with each and every one of you:

"Yowch! The grease from my mutton-bone dripped on my foot ... and my big toe is KILLING me!"

Poor devil.

As almost every schoolgirl can tell you, the hard-living Henry suffered from a disease—"The Gout"—brought on by wolfing down legs of mutton while slurping gallons of expensive *vino* and marrying another woman every few years (two died, two divorced and two beheaded).

According to the famous legend, the meat-loving Henry fell prey to a metabolic disorder in which excessive uric acid, derived from the purine content of protein, played havoc with his toe-joints.

It's a zany, colorful legend ... and I'm very sorry to have to report that it's completely false.

As a matter of fact, Henry's raging gout had very little to do with his wine-bibbing or his strange penchant for devouring entire sheep at a single sitting.

What actually happened—according to the best medical evidence—is that Henry was felled (or at least slowed way down) frequently by an acute attack of complications of high insulin. Just look at his pronounced "truncal obesity" and his ferocious consumption of such amylose-laden comestibles as freshly baked breads, potatoes from Ireland and double-crust pies jammed with four-and-twenty blackbirds. Anyone wonder what his cholesterol phenotype was? Who bets on Type IV?

In short: Henry's problem wasn't protein (or alcohol) ... it was *amylose*!

But let's back up a step. In order to understand the actual dynamics of gout, we need to remember how insulin is responsible for causing numerous problems in human metabolism. In past chapters, for example, I outlined how this important hormone contributes to low HDL and elevated triglycerides associated with a Type IV hyperlipidemia phenotype pattern. The pattern is a direct result of insulin's biochemical effect on lipoprotein lipase.

I also demonstrated how elevated insulin levels can contribute to both maintenance of fat stores *and* burning of protein.

In this chapter, however, I want to show you how insulin can also trigger a persistent elevation of uric acid levels in blood—a condition that frequently produces gout in amylose consuming, high-insulin patients.

SOME BACKGROUND ON GOUT

Because of the distinctive presentation linked to a disease—an acute, inflammatory arthritis that usually affects a single joint in sudden and dramatic fashion—that has been associated with gout throughout the ages, this disorder has been familiar to physicians almost since the beginning of medicine. And indeed, many esteemed scientists have labored over the centuries to lay bare the metabolic processes in which uric acid is manufactured and then employed by the human body. (Interestingly enough, the process seems to be similar in only one other species: Dalmatian dogs.)

As any medical textbook will quickly tell you, humans excrete uric acid into urine as a result of the last stage of nitrogen metabolism. Given that fact, it has always seemed logical to researchers that if you could reduce dietary nitrogen (and especially the large amounts of nitrogen contained in the "purine" compounds of most meats), then the amount of uric acid produced by the body would be similarly reduced. This line of thinking sounds logical and is well accepted by the Conventional Dietary Wisdom of today. Eat less red meat and drink less alcohol is the standard dietary advice for patients with gout. Wives and mothers all over the continent and the U.S. are pleased when their Henrys don't get sauced, making them care for Henry when he can't walk without assistance and can't stand the weight of a sheet on his foot while trying to sleep.

How about the meat proscription? This logical step makes some sense, but the benefit of limiting protein consumption and therefore, nitrogen ingestion, is limited by a key variable: the fact that gout and other disorders are far more affected by how the body manages uric acid in urine than by the nitrogen load.

To understand why, remember that the kidney filters uric acid out of the bloodstream and also dispatches it into the urine tubules by a process known as "secretion." Remember, also, that as the urine travels through the tubules, it can be reabsorbed by the kidney ... and that any uric acid which remains in the tubules will depart the kidney and enter the ureter for final excretion.

It's also helpful to recall that uric acid is a "weak organic acid" ... and that, like most other acids, it will lose a hydrogen ion in any solution more alkaline than acidic. In an acid solution, of course, the same ion will return to remake the uric acid.

Fortunately for all of us, the kidney owns an exquisite mechanism for controlling uric acid levels. And yet this secretion mechanism can sometimes be overwhelmed by other organic acids or by insulin. Dehydration can also slow down the all-important secretion of uric acid.

Don't forget that other organic acids—such as vinegar, vitamin C, aspirin, penicillin and the hippuric acid contained in cranberry juice—will also compete with uric acid for secretion. If you want to watch the process at work, give your Henry a high dose of vitamin C, with an aspirin or two, then wash it all down with "unsweetened" cranberry juice when you are trying to help him with his acute infection which is being treated with penicillin. You can rest assured that his resulting gout-attack has no association with wine *or* mutton! And if you really want the gout to be bad, just mix in 6 hours of work on a hot day in July when you are working in an attic in Worcester County, Md, eating only a peanut butter and jelly sandwich on rye for lunch.

As I've pointed out elsewhere in this book, insulin causes both salt and water retention. It also stores calories and nutrients. Is it really surprising, given these facts, that the same hormone blocks secretion of uric acid into urine? There are also some interesting recent data to suggest that insulin promotes uric acid reabsorption. This hormone conserves and stores everything, especially uric acid. High insulin people with gout must eliminate amylose. Try telling a gouty Irishman that his potato eating days are over … but save the day by telling him he can still have his two pints of hand pumped Guinness at the local pub. Potatoes or beer, gout or not?

WATER … THE BEST CURE FOR GOUT?

To understand exactly how the physiology of gout works, let's return to our bloated figure of royalty, Henry VIII. Is there any doubt that his high insulin caused his elevated uric acid … which in turn caused his gout? The triumvirate of insulin resistance: gout, obesity and Type IV hyperlipidemia are our focus.

While there are many patients whose gout depends on genetic abnormalities involving disordered uric acid metabolism, those who suffer—as Henry suffered—from high insulin are actually the victims of the breadstuffs (and other amylose-laden products) they eat, and not of roast beef. And indeed, research now shows clearly that restricting protein and proscribing alcohol are *not* the best treatments for high–insulin gout patients.

As a beer-lover, myself, I think it's most unfortunate that alcohol has been blamed so often for gout. Nonsense! If you recall, I permit my patients up to four glasses of beer (or three glasses of wine) per day on the 00-2-3 Diet. At the same time, I'm quite pleased by the fact that not a single one of my compliant diet-patients with elevated uric acid levels has ever experienced a flare up of the underlying disease. But let's be careful here: I am *not* suggesting that alcohol is protective against gout! I'm simply regretting the fact that its role in causing gout by inducing acid secretion by the kidneys has been overstated.

As an aside, I should also point out that the heart-health benefits of drinking red wine far outweigh the potentially deleterious effects of alcohol with regard to uric acid. Indeed, I'd greatly prefer that my patients enjoy a glass of red wine than a Manhattan, so that they could fully enjoy these benefits! Nonetheless, the fact remains: neither beverage, when consumed in moderation, will cause attacks of gout. (Try telling that to the Grandma who has suffered through a few of Grandpa's gout-bouts, however!)

Traditionally, managing this disease has involved three different treatments ... the most important of which calls for a high fluid intake. In most cases, simply asking a gout victim to drink three quarts of water per day is enough to prevent dehydration, while also shutting off the painful attacks caused by this disorder.

Another approach for those patients who produce excessive uric acid is to prescribe a medication, *allopurinol*, which often helps to reduce the amount of acid churned out into the bloodstream. A third strategy calls for a medicine known as *probenecid*, which stimulates the uric acid secretion mechanism in the kidney. Whether a physician decides to use one of these methods (or a combination) depends, as always, on the biochemistry of the particular patient.

So much for the standard medical practice. But there's another way to treat those forms of gout which result from high insulin —and it doesn't require taking medicines or drinking vast quantities of H2O. The strategy: Simply lay off Grandma's breads, biscuits and dumplings! Enjoy a leg of lamb with a glass of red wine, instead. Although many patients gape at me when they first hear this advice, the record shows that most of them leave their gout behind, and usually within a few weeks.

The biochemical principle at work here is easy to understand. By reducing the amount of amylose-intake, the patient shuts down the insulin surge that inevitably accompanies it. And when *that* happens, insulin's tendency to lower secretion and raise reabsorption of uric acid is greatly diminished. The beauty of this approach, of course, is that it depends not on medicines (and their side effects) … but on simply changing the patient's diet.

It's also true, however, that I can change the acid-percentage (as opposed to the alkaline-percentage) in a patient's uric acid, simply by prescribing a substance that will change the urine pH from acid to alkaline. If the uric acid is placed in an "alkaline environment," then most of it will be stripped of its accompanying hydrogen atom (and will thus become "urate"). On the other hand, if uric acid remains in a more acid solution, such as that found at normal urine pH, most of the acid will continue to hold onto to its associated hydrogen atom. This approach to the problem is called—rather colorfully—"ion trapping," and it's based on the fact that when we put a weak acid, like uric acid, into an alkaline environment, that acid will dissolve and be excreted efficiently in its unreabsorbable form as urate.

Question: How can an alkaline substance be added safely to the urine without, say, affecting blood pressure? One proposed solution has been to add bicarbonate (baking soda). This sounds like the perfect remedy, at first, because bicarbonate will, indeed, increase the alkalinity of the urine. Unfortunately, the sodium in the mixture will also set off a blood-pressure rise, however. A better alternative is to take a potassium citrate preparation that will shift urine into an alkaline environment via the citrate. (The potassium will not cause a blood pressure hike.)

There's no doubt that taking potassium citrate—whether in a liquid or a crystal form—will help maintain excretion of uric acid, and without any systemic side effects. I think it's a shame, however, that on about the last 25 occasions when I wrote prescriptions for potassium citrate, the patients had to wait up to four or five days in order to have them filled because the medication isn't routinely stocked in the local, small town drug stores. I'm always astonished to learn that other physicians aren't prescribing citrate as I do. Maybe if they could see the effect of citrate on my gout patients, they might change their prescribing habits!

Along with helping my patients control their uric acid reabsorption, potassium citrate offers another huge health advantage for those whose gout is caused by ingestion of amylose (as opposed to Blatz or Budweiser!). These patients can benefit by collecting some of their urine in a clear-glass container once a week, and then placing it in the refrigerator at ten degrees Centigrade or less. In cold urine, uric acid crystals will form if there is too much of a uric acid burden placed on the kidney. Gout, the silent kidney killer, announces itself to those who monitor cold urine.

After obtaining the urine (it should be a first-thing-in-the-morning specimen), patients should store it in the refrig until they get home from work in the evening. Next step: Examine the texture of the cold sample. If the urine has remained clear, your kidneys are handling the uric acid just fine and you probably won't have to worry about hidden uric acid loads and an imminent gout attack—or about the attack of gout that usually follows such a shift in your body's uric acid–balance.

If the urine looks cloudy, however (remember those glass-ball "Christmas scenes" that "snowed" when you shook them?), then you can be sure that crystals of uric acid are precipitating out of the sample ... which means that the aching, inflamed joints of a gout attack are probably headed your way, not to mention the potentially dangerous attack on your kidney function.

This test has proved so reliable over the years that most of my gout patients now willingly run this "refrigerator test" on their urine once a week. Why put yourself through the hassle—and the expense—of frequent blood tests for uric acid, when you can monitor yourself painlessly, and free of charge?

Remember: If you find a urine sample running "cloudy," the solution is simple. In order to prevent damage to kidneys as well as attacks of gout, patients should merely start taking regular doses of potassium citrate. About a day later, they should once again begin monitoring their cold urine. Once the crystals disappear (usually after about 48 hours), the patient can stop taking the citrate.

Of course, the same "cold urine" test nicely proves my point about the effect of amylose on uric acid-production. To see what I mean, study your cold urine before and after eating a heaping bowl of pasta. Make no mistake, those clouds in the urine after a feast of *fettucine alfredo* are compelling evidence of a key fact: the *alfredo*-eater has just experienced an insulin-surge, followed by a sharp boost in levels of uric acid!

While I'm at it, I should point out that one additional benefit from potassium citrate is that it acts as an inhibitor of aggregations of calcium oxalate salts around uric acid molecules in the urine. And that's extremely important—because the most common type of kidney stone emerges from these oxalates as they cluster around intact uric acid molecules. If the uric acid does not remain intact, however, it will not provide the nidus around which these crystals can coalesce and then launch the process of forming a stone.

Each time I send a patient to a urologist for treatment of calcium oxalate stones, the poor soul returns *not* with a prescription for potassium citrate but with a recommendation for a low-oxalate diet. What a waste of time (and a doctor's fee!).

The identified culprit in this scenario is usually oxalic acid ... which happens to be a substance I use in my part-time furniture refinishing business (it's a great bleaching agent!). I would prefer not to eat it, however. And most other people in the know seem to feel the same way. How many times have you been warned to keep kids and pets away from the "dumb cane" houseplant— precisely because it contains potentially dangerous amounts of oxalic acid in its leaves and resin?

The normal urology approach to calcium oxalate stones is to reduce the amount of oxalate in the diet, as if that really had anything to do with how the kidney stone forms. I've yet to treat a patient who was poisoned by eating too much rhubarb, which contains the greatest concentration of this acid. The list of other pungent foods that contain somewhat smaller amounts of oxalic acid includes horseradish, chocolate, cauliflower, cashews and spinach. Not to worry here, however: It would be pretty difficult —if not impossible—to eat enough oxalate to cause disease.

The best strategy for treating my calcium oxalate stone patients, I've discovered over time, is to determine whether they are over-producers of uric acid. If they make too much uric acid, they need to take *allopurinol* in order to prevent recurrent attacks of kidney stones. If not, on the other hand, I recommend the po-tassium citrate solution to prevent formation of calcium oxalate crystals in the cloud of urine.

One of the most interesting problems in my practice occurs when I confront the 47-year-old white male with the jumbo-sized beer belly. "What's the problem, sir?" Well ... the problem is that he just worked up a good sweat out there mowing weeds all afternoon ... and now he's suffering with an acute attack of gout. (One sure sign is that bulgy pouch on his elbow—or maybe he's got acute pain in his big toe-joint or his knee or ankle.) Regardless, my task is the same: I need to find out if he's hyper-insulinemic or not.

If he is, I tell him to forget the traditional "gout advice" for this situation, and not to worry about protein or alcohol. What he needs to avoid is amylose—which means breads, potatoes, rice, pasta, bananas and all the rest. On the other hand, if my beer-chugger is *not* a high-insulin patient, then I point out that he needs to avoid the protein, while perhaps taking one or more of the standard medications.

Either way, he *also* needs to start taking in large amounts of fluid each day.

Isn't human nature delightful? Every time I've offered this recommendation to one of my big-bellied friends, the response has been exactly the same.

"Say, doc ... will it be okay if I take that fluid in the form of *beer*?"

"You bet!" I tell them with a laugh. "Go ahead and enjoy yourself. But don't forget: If you start eating sandwiches with that Budweiser, you'll be back in this office within a week!"

17

COPING WITH CHILDHOOD OBESITY

We called him "the fat kid."

Do you remember him? Remember "Tubby" from the popular comic strip "Nancy?" Tubby had close-cropped, reddish hair and a belly that hung over his shorts like the Grand Coulee Dam. He wheezed when he breathed, and he inhaled an endless stream of marshmallow-topped cupcakes while barking loudly at one and all:

"Say, when do we *eat*?"

Tubby, the world owes you an apology.

Although your parents and teachers fretted over you and nagged you relentlessly about your eating habits, the simple fact is that you weren't to blame for your obesity.

You weren't fat because you willfully ate too much—or because you lacked "moral character."

Tubby, your *genes* were responsible for the fact that you weighed 180 pounds by the time you hit the sixth grade. They were responsible because they saddled you with a fairly common condition known as "insulin resistance" … a digestive anomaly in which the human body reacts to ingested sugar by manufacturing and storing fat with super-efficiency.

That's not to say, of course, that some children don't also suffer from metabolic illnesses—such as thyroid or adrenal or ovarian diseases, and maybe we will find out that leptin and leptin resistance belong on the shelf of known endocrine abnormalities causing obesity in kids.

But the percentage of kids who get hit with these "fat diseases" is actually quite small. In the vast majority of cases, you can be sure that if a child is carrying extra poundage, elevated insulin is the culprit.

Example: Not long ago, a medical professional visited my office for an urgent consultation regarding her 12-year-old son.

The distraught mother explained that the child had been "evaluated by every blood test known." Yet the doctors didn't seem to have a clue as to the true cause of the kid's obesity. His exam was normal. Nothing in his history gave an obvious answer.

Could I help?

Mom had brought a copy of the blood work, which contained only a few basic tests, including:

○ an 18-chemistry screening panel;

○ two thyroid tests;

○ a cortisol level, which indirectly measures the functions of the adrenal gland.

That wasn't enough, however, and I quickly suggested that we add both insulin and liver-function tests to the mix. Sure enough, the child's insulin level topped the charts at 27—and his GGTP, a test that reflected fat storage in the liver among other things, was way too high at 98. At the tender age of 12, the boy was already suffering from the metabolic consequences of elevated insulin. He was badly overweight—and he was storing fat in his stressed liver.

Like most mothers of overweight children, this one had nearly exhausted herself in the struggle to "restrict" her child's intake of sodas, junk food and candy. She'd also urged the kid to exercise. And he did. But nothing had worked. Meanwhile, the child went on suffering more than any slender individual can imagine.

I'm always amazed at just how cruel adolescent kids can be. "Johnny is a fatty! Johnny hasn't had a date in two years! Johnny needs *two* seats on the bus, each time the eighth-grade class goes on a field trip." Adolescence is tough on everyone ... but the assaults on an overweight kid's developing ego are often nothing less than brutal in a society that often seems pathologically obsessed with both weight and physical appearance.

The astonishing cruelty of today's social attitudes about kids and fat seemed especially evident, the other day, when I happened upon a magazine for teenagers. I could hardly believe my eyes, as I glanced at some photos of young women who were considered to be "sex symbols." And when I compared their images to those of some youthful concentration camp survivors in Bosnia, the similarities were striking—especially when it came to percentages of body fat.

Who decided that these starved 17-year-old models in the magazine (I renamed it: *Bizarre!*) should represent the essence of female glamour?

Childhood obesity is certainly a challenging diagnosis, and I've often found myself thinking that the *real* patient in these situations is the parent of the overweight child. I say that because I usually discover—quite early in the consultation—that the parent has never considered the possibility of including his or her obese child in the process of food shopping or food preparation.

But that situation can be remedied, and I insist on it. Children *can* learn how to cook, and they can also learn how to shop. And learning these skills is extremely important ... so that the young ones can begin to manage their food better. If they are high insulin at a young age, they need to be ready for being high insulin at an older age.

In short, these children badly need to understand that food is both the source of their obesity problem *and* the cure for it.

Along with educating these kids about food, I always recommend calculating the percentage body fat and determining lean body mass that are outlined in Appendix 3: *How Much Should You Weigh?*

I also request a blood analysis to measure such additional hormone functions as DHEA-S, androstenedione and testosterone. These three additional hormone tests give me essential information for determining androgen (male) hormone production that could be a confounding variable contributing to the extra weight of a patient. If the problem is delayed into puberty, be patient about the extra "baby fat."

If all of these factors turn out to be in the "normal" range (which is usually the case), I can then begin working intensively with parent and child on behavior modification. The child needs to keep a diet diary, and also to understand the consequences that will flow from eating various foods.

The child also needs to learn about foods in general—and this sort of teaching is best accomplished at the grocery store. Interestingly enough, I've learned over the years that teenagers can often spot the "hidden sugars" in prepared foods (the maltodextrins and the corn syrup, for example) faster than the adults can. On one illuminating occasion, for example, a razor-sharp teen informed me of the fact that the "best way to proceed is to shop the perimeter of the store" ... even before I could make the same speech to him!

DIETING FOR KIDS: HOW TO PROCEED?

In most situations where a child has an elevated insulin level and is also overweight, parents want to know one thing above all else: How can we find a diet that will allow our youngster to grow and develop normally, even while shedding fat?

The answer is wonderfully simple. Just put the child on a special version of the No–Amylose Diet.

But what about the overweight and prepubescent child who *doesn't* exhibit an elevated insulin level? The good news for these kids is that their weight problems almost never continue past puberty. What happens is that the naturally occurring hormones of adolescence, especially androgens, will "burn off" that baby fat, and the extra poundage will gradually disappear. Unfortunately, however it's often quite difficult to convince parents and grandparents that this scenario will occur!

So what can overweight children do to help themselves—and especially during social activities that involve food? Must visits to the local fastfood palace be placed "off limits" for these kids? No! Most teenagers will be delighted to hear that they can still drop by the Burger King or the Wendy's with their friends ... provided that they content themselves with only a few French fries, and a regular-sized hamburger. (And no "Apple Turnovers" for dessert!)

In my experience, most adolescents can handle the responsibility of eating less, once they discover that they'll still be permitted to visit McDonald's now and then.

Of course, the key problem with weight loss in adolescents is that their lean body mass is increasing as the child matures. For this reason, body-weight should never be used as the sole measuring-stick for determining how well the teenager is doing at controlling body fat. Instead, use my "Mirror, Mirror!" approach. Have the child stand in front of a body-length mirror, then jump up and down. If you see a lot of "jiggling," it's safe to say that the kid has a problem!

Although there are many rewards for practicing family medicine, nothing can top the marvelous experience of helping a troubled teenager overcome his or her obesity.

I don't think I'll ever forget the beautiful young Greek girl who was my patient back in the mid-1990s. Feisty and fun-loving, this young lady had been struggling with obesity throughout her childhood—and weighed more than 210 pounds by the age of 14. At that point, she began my No-Amylose Diet and worked very hard at it. I monitored her progress during the next few years, and was thrilled by her success. By her 18th birthday, her weight had declined to less than 160 pounds—even though she'd grown five inches taller during the intervening years! Even better, her body fat had declined from 57 to 26 percent.

I was delighted when this patient showed me the list of foods she'd served her parents on her 18th birthday. They were all low in amylose and glucose—the perfect foods for my Maintenance Diet! I was also delighted by the fact that she had bought the foods at her local supermarket, without adult supervision. And it was a joy to see the look of radiant happiness on her mother's face!

How should parents approach the problem of teenage obesity? As in every medical situation, the first rule of thumb must be: "Do no harm!" Parents should never insult their children by making unkind remarks about obesity. Remember: the condition is physiological (insulin-related) … and has nothing to do with gluttony!

Parents in this scenario should be fully supportive, while also remembering that the child is probably being made the unrelenting butt of jokes and mockery at school. Remember also that knowing how to manage food effectively starts with *learning* about food. Visit the supermarket with your child, and teach the kid how much food costs. Help the child to select the appropriate foods for his or her diet.

Also: Make sure you find a compassionate, knowledgeable physician who understands the relationship between insulin resistance

314

and amylose, along with the vital importance of protein-sparing in any weight-loss program.

After more than two decades as a family practice physician, I'm absolutely convinced that children who struggle with obesity need the no-amylose diet, just like their overweight parents! If little Johnny has a weight-problem, he cannot go to school every day with a peanut butter and jelly sandwich in his lunch box. He's going to be the one with the Tupperware container that contains the chicken salad, the corn chips and the fresh peach for dessert.

Unfortunately, children like Johnny are often penalized by public school lunch menus that include endless servings of high-amylose "Tater Tots" and roast-beef-with-gravy-on-bread ... followed by ice cream for dessert! Is it any wonder that the "Johnnies" of the world struggle to control their weight?

Still, there *are* ways that a parent can fight back. And the best way is to take your child into the kitchen and start teaching! You and your teenager can have a great time together, as you instruct your eager pupil on how to spice and serve food attractively. Remember that when kids *enjoy* the process of preparing and eating meals, the compulsion to over-eat will usually be reduced.

Give your child the benefit of the 00-2-3 Diet ... and you'll be giving the kid the most valuable gift in the entire world: inner freedom!

Recipes

The following recipes are a collection of original ideas from Ritchie, JoAnn, Sally and folks around the Pocomoke area. Each recipe, written in "local newspaper" style, contains one or two pertinent points for the 00-2-3 diet.

Recognize the amylose when it is used. The recipes are easily modified from the maintenance program to the weight loss program by eliminating amylose.

The glimpses of lifestyle in our area convey the idea that food, healthy food, is part of the pleasure of everyday life here. The individuals noted in the recipes live in and around Pocomoke, Maryland. Their ideas are not just locally applicable; they have meaning for everyone.

The common theme in the recipes is live well, eat well and maintain your weight loss. The recipes are placed in order according to when they were written, beginning with soup and ending with nuts.

Clam Chowder

Cold front! Wind from the northwest at 22 mph, and the overnight low will be 7 above zero. ...

It's the perfect day for a big bowl of hearty clam chowder.

Did you know that clams contain high-quality protein ... and that they're also low in saturated fat and cholesterol?

The only fat you'll find in this robust *entrée* is the relatively small amount contributed by the butter and the milk.

Yes, your arteries will definitely get a break today—since your side dish consists of a heaping spinach salad also containing fresh red bell peppers, a few florets of cauliflower, sliced mushrooms, avocado, Parmesan cheese, and Italian dressing made with canola oil.

You should be able to find a can of "Snow's Clam Chowder Concentrate" on the soup shelf at your local supermarket. If not, you'll have to shop around for a second best. Mix in a six-ounce tin of minced clams (include the juice), along with one can of milk, an eight-ounce can of evaporated milk and two tsp. of concentrated lemon juice and one dollop of dry sherry to smooth the texture and the taste. Heat on medium and do not boil. Stir frequently, there always is something sticking to the bottom of the pot. Add 1 tbsp. butter and two scallions, chopped fine. To season, add a dash of garlic, a twist of ground black pepper, two shakes of dry mustard, some ground coriander and a pinch of chervil (thyme is a poor second choice if you don't have chervil).

For a silky-smooth texture, try adding one additional tbsp. of dry sherry as the butter and milk blend. (You can substitute cooking wine, if need be—but remember that you will also be adding salt to the dish.)

As your soup warms on the stove, whip up your salad. A loaf of Italian bread provides a nice addition, if your hips can stand the amylose. Simmer your chowder for ten minutes or so, longer if you like it really thick. Be sure to stir frequently. This meal serves four, and should cost less than $7, including the bread.

Enjoy! And who cares if you catch Frosty the Snowman peeking in through the dining room window?

Live Dangerously—Eat an Omelet!

Do you remember that ghastly moment when Mr. Kurtz groaned from his deathbed, at the end of Joseph Conrad's classic story, *Heart of Darkness*:

"The horror! The horror!"

According to some literary scholars, Mr. Kurtz was reacting to the horrifying realization that he'd just eaten two fried eggs *with* the yolks ... and that the deadly cholesterol from these two time bombs was already racing toward his doomed heart!

Not true.

(I have it on good authority that Mr. Kurtz was *actually* reacting to the realization that he'd forgotten the mosquito repellent, as his boat started down the mighty Congo.)

o   o   o

I think it's a crying shame that poor old cholesterol continues to take such an undeserved rap.

As tried to point out in Chapter 11 of this book (*Why Do We Keep Feeding The Cholesterol Ogre?*), this naturally occurring substance is in fact essential to our own good health—since it helps the body repair and rebuild cell membranes, among several other key tasks.

Try telling that to the U.S. Medical Establishment, however, which long ago decided that cholesterol is the arch-culprit in coronary heart disease ... and that eating such high-cholesterol foods as egg yolks is tantamount to playing Russian Roulette.

Remarkably enough, however, the scientific basis for these scary reports has never really been established. Although few people (include medical doctors!) realize it, the five "landmark" studies on the alleged relationship between heart disease and elevated cholesterol left out women, children, Latin Americans, Native Americans and *everybody* over age 65! (Blacks were significantly under-represented, as well.)

Although there is some convincing evidence to show increased risk for coronary heart disease among high-cholesterol, middle-aged white men in America, the case is still far from closed.

As a physician and a lover of omelets, I simply don't believe that eating an occasional egg is as dangerous as it's cracked up to be. (*Ouch!* Sorry.)

If you're willing to take the risk, why not sample my Thrill-A-Minute Morning Omelet? To get started, find yourself a good omelet pan (mine is five and a half inches in diameter), coated with a non-stick surface. After melting a pat of butter in the pan, add some chopped scallions, sliced mushrooms, pimentos and marinated artichoke hearts. Saute these ingredients until cooked to a pleasing texture.

Next, whip four eggs in a glass or stainless steel mixing bowl (be sure to compost the egg shells), using approximately 20 strokes. Add the eggs to the pan and stir to mix well. Cook on high heat. When the egg is done on one side, sprinkle it with shredded cheese. Cook it for an additional 20 seconds. Now gently tilt the pan so that one half of the omelet slips onto a plate held beside it. Next step: flip the pan—so that the omelet folds over on itself and rests on the plate. At this point, the heat in the mixture will both melt the cheese and finish cooking the omelet.

In deference to the cholesterol content of the egg yolk, why not avoid saturated fat (other than the butter) in the rest of your meal? Try some fresh slices of cantaloupe or other melon, and these will provide a pleasing visual grace-note to your meal, even as they fill you up.

Now settle back and enjoy that omelet ... secure in the knowledge that your arteries will live to tell the tale, long after you've mopped up that last tasty morsel of egg yolk!

Introducing ... The Greatest Steak I Ever Ate!

Remember that hilarious moment during the old Saturday morning cartoons when Droopy the Dog smelled the sizzling hot dog links?

Remember how that mesmerized canine followed the shimmering stream of *hot dawg!* vapor all the way ... into a head-on collision with a dog twice his size?

Raarrrgghh! ... poor Droopy bites the dust again, as the *Looney Tunes* theme song blares from the TV screen: "THAT'S ALL, FOLKS!"

Guess what?

That same scenario—*Follow Your Nose Straight Into Trouble!*—has been known to take a bite out of more than a few humans, along with the cartoon canines.

Let me tell you about our recent trip to Phoenix ... and about our thrilling Quest for the Ultimate Porterhouse Steak.

The Quest began after I was tapped to give a speech at a national medical conference. The location? Phoenix, Arizona: one of America's warmest, driest, and largest (at 50 miles in diameter) cities. Perched in the heart of the "Valley of the Sun," Phoenix is a jewel of the desert—a shimmering, blue-sky metropolis that now ranks as one of the country's top retirement havens.

But when I told a few friends and neighbors who'd already visited Phoenix about our upcoming trip, they gave me some surprising advice: "Don't miss your chance to eat in one of those great steak houses—and make sure you order the porterhouse!"

All at once, the Quest for the Perfect Steak had begun in earnest.

Imagine our frustration, however, when our jet flight took an unexpected left turn to Memphis … then sat cooling its wings on the tarmac for three unscheduled hours.

When we finally reached Phoenix, we were told that that they'd given our rental car to someone else. *Sorry … but you're shockingly late!*

So much for our planned tour of the Ruins of the Cliff Dwellers.

At the hotel a few minutes later, things went from frustrating to *infuriating*.

"Sir … we don't seem to have you in the computer. Are you sure you're at the right hotel?"

Nor did it matter that I was giving the big speech the next day. If you aren't in the computer, you don't exist.

It took us nearly an hour to discover that these fumbling *hoteliers* had created a new, Sanskrit-based spelling of my name. I mean, how tough is it to get "Shoemaker" right?

Famished and exhausted by now, we consoled ourselves with the knowledge that we were about to sample a great steak—even if we had to *walk* to the restaurant from our hotel.

In the end, our noses found the place. Like radar homing devices, they locked in on the scent of mesquite and char-broiled cow meat. How fresh was the steak here? Listen … this Wild West Eatery actually had a long-horned steer tethered to the front parking lot!

And so what if the festivities began with an automatic 45-minute wait?

We settled into an alcove and ordered up some Nehi belly washers and a few appetizers. Half-starved by now, we went for it *all* and ordered the fried zucchini rings—along with the BBQ wings, the nachos and the fried mushrooms. Reheated or not, the zucchini hit the mark … and kept us from perishing until we could get our hands on the regular menu.

My eyes scanned the plastic … and jerked to a stop beside two words: TRAIL BOSS!

"Two pounds of Porterhouse from the best local beef," said the menu, before making us an offer we couldn't refuse: "If you can finish this huge steak, you can keep the knife!"

When that monster-porterhouse arrived, I could hardly believe my eyes. The huge steak was thick and perfectly cooked. And you can be sure that when the waitress set it down, the entire table leaned in that direction.

The fillet section was the first to go. Then it was on to the strip-steak side of the Porterhouse. It took me until ten o'clock Mountain Standard Time—but in the end, the Quest had been accomplished.

I'd eaten every morsel, and I could barely climb out of my chair.

But were they really going to give me the steak knife, as promised?

"Here, sir. Take home this clean one, gift-wrapped just for you!"

"But what about the knife I just used?"

"Oh no, that stays here. But don't worry: Yours is the same!"

It wasn't.

Like the other tourists, I had to content myself with a less elegant model—a thoroughly pedestrian steak knife that we now refer to as "The Bait-and-Switch Blade."

The steak house had bamboozled us a bit … but not over the food. To this day, that Phoenix Porterhouse ranks as the Greatest Steak I ever ate!

The "Rain in Spain" Never Falls On Those Who Can Cook Paella!

Ask the average American to name three delightful things about Spain, and the odds are high that the list will include:

○ *Flamenco*: With a rose clenched between her pearly teeth, the dancer in the stiletto high heels ignites the Barcelona nightclub.

○ *La Corrida de Toros*: Hemingway called it "The Moment of Truth"—that heart-stopping moment when the *matador* points his sword at the brave bull's neck.

○ *Paella*: A stunningly delicious *mélange* of shellfish, sausage, chicken, vegetables and saffron rice, this lavish feast is often described as "The National Dish of Spain."

Although the recipes for *paella* are endless (I've never made the same dish twice), the process of assembling a knockout *paella* (pronounced "pie-AY-ya") usually calls for the following steps.

First, build a charcoal fire with enough coals to heat a large pan for up to 40 minutes. (No, you *don't* have to buy a special pan to make *paella*.) Melt some butter in the pan and add pieces of chicken, preferably breasts. Saute them and turn them over, then sprinkle in plenty of rice, flavored with saffron, so that it covers the chicken and the butter. And now the *real* fun starts. With the help of your friends and family, start loading goodies into the pan!

Begin with small clams and distribute them evenly. Then add whole shrimp, scallops and one-inch–square chunks of the Polish sausage known as *kielbasa*. Throw in some Italian sausage, too, this feast isn't ethnically correct. Create a layer of each different food, and then begin dropping in the canned corn, the frozen peas, the mushrooms, the chickpeas and the cherry tomatoes.

Think we're done? Think again! Now it's time for the artichoke hearts, the black olives, the scallions, smoked oysters, broccoli and mandarin oranges.

As the juices bubble and simmer in the pan, this gorgeous *repast* smells better and better. It takes about an hour to cook the feast properly—which allows you and your helpers to enjoy a cold *cerveza* or two, while nibbling a few corn chips on the side.

After an hour or so, when the clams have opened, check the shrimp to see if they are fully cooked. (If they're done, so is your *paella*.) Let your guests help themselves—but be careful, because they tend to go after the shrimp, sausage and clams something fierce. Remember, also, that the saffron in the rice is the only seasoning you'll need for this astonishingly delicious feast. (You can substitute turmeric for color . . . but most Spanish chefs agree that nothing compares to that saffron taste.)

Serve this marvelous Spanish dish with an ice-cold jug of *Sangria* (the kids might enjoy a pitcher of cherry-flavored ginger ale), and everyone at the party will soon be calling you *amigo*!

Smart Squash

I've said it before and I'll say it again: The key to healthy, nutritious and economical eating is to *think about the food you're putting in your mouth.*

Acorn squash provides a terrific illustration of the Kitchen Thinker at work.

For starters: this tasty, yellow-gold vegetable is quite nutritious. As a matter of fact, acorn squash comes close to being the "perfect food," because it's low in fat and cholesterol, but *high* in vitamins and bowel-protecting fiber.

Full of complex carbohydrates that don't break down quickly (no blood sugar surge tonight!), acorn squash is also easy on the checkbook. The good news is that tonight's savory side dish will cost us less than a buck.

But does this high-quality veggie have a downside? Yes ... it tends to dry out a bit during the lengthy baking process. Which is why most cooks end up stuffing it—or slathering it in brown sugar and butter. (We're going to stuff it in an interesting new way, however, after thinking about the cooking strategy for this meal.)

We're also going to serve up our golden squash-delight with a mouth-watering *entrée*—a famous American food known as "hamburger."

All right, shoppers: Shall we spend $2.49 a pound for the fancy "ground round"—or save considerably on our food budget by paying only $1.69 for the cheaper cut?

Let's *think*. Why pay more than we have to, when we can use our cooking-wits to percolate the fat out of the meat, then convert the remainder into succulent chopped steak?

I don't know about you, but I'm sick and tired of the way beef keeps taking a bum rap. *Eat a hamburger—and stand by for the heart attack hidden in the saturated fat!*

The truth, of course, is that *all* forms of meat contain saturated fat ... and that we need the stuff in order to live. Among other essentials, the saturated fat that you can't see in a cut of meat contains stearic acid, an essential nutrient. (As for the fat you *can* see —why not follow my strategy, and simply cut it away from the meat you're going to serve? This simple—thoughtful!—guideline will make it easy for you to lower the fat content in any meat-dish, so you never have to worry about fat again.)

Another helpful strategy, when preparing economical cuts of hamburger, is to cook the meat slowly and pour off the fat. Then brown your burgers, add water to the pan, lower the heat and cover the meat with a lid. After a few minutes, you can pour off the fat that has percolated into the water. Brown the meat again and ... *presto!*

You just created several low-cost *and* low-fat burgers.

Okay: time to get busy with the squash. Go ahead and halve each vegetable, then remove the pulp and seeds (the latter can be roasted, and they taste like pumpkin seeds).

326

Next step: Make the sauce for stuffing. Combine a can of low-salt cream of celery soup with four ounces of chick peas, one minced onion, four ounces of diced ham and some shredded cheddar cheese. Stir the sauce on medium heat to melt the cheese. (Do not boil.) Add a shake of garlic, a shake of cumin and some MSG—provided that your diners aren't MSG-sensitive. Now add two shakes of dill weed and two of ground ginger, along with a splash of soy sauce. Taste the mixture and add more dill if seems too bland. Finally, add two tbsp. of white and wine and cook slowly until thick.

Ladle the filling into the squash, then cook it for 60 minutes at 325 degrees. Baste the vegetable as needed to keep it moist and then serve it on a side plate with your Healthy Hamburger and a Romaine lettuce salad.

If you use two pounds of low-end hamburger, your Smart Squash will feed four hungry diners for less than $7.

And when they ask you how you pulled it off, simply announce: *Oh, I just used my head!*

Will the Real Sweet & Sour Chicken ... Please Stand Up?

Quiz Question For Food-Lovers Everywhere:

Q. You've just served your dinner guests a mouth-watering platter of sweet and sour chicken. Which country created the recipe for this delightful *entrée*?

A. Hawaii
B. Mexico
C. Cuba
D. China
E. All of the above

If you answered "E," go immediately to the head of the cooking class—and let's get started on today's assignment, which is to cook up four big servings of this universally popular dish.

According to research-experts at the International College of Sweet & Sour Knowledge, this delightful combination of chicken and pineapple has been enjoyed in *all* of the countries listed above, for as long as anybody can remember.

Regardless of who first dreamed it up, Sweet & Sour Chicken ranks high on the list of Most Beloved Foods in many countries around the world. That's because it provides plenty of nutrition, but little fat—and also because it's just plain delicious.

The first step on the road to preparation is to cut four chicken breasts into bite-sized chunks, then marinate them with similar-sized chunks of pineapple. Refrigerate the mixture overnight, after stirring the marinade occasionally during the first few hours of refrigeration, in order to make sure the chicken gets tenderized by the pineapple. (I use four cans of drained pineapple chunks, along with my chicken pieces—but you can substitute fresh pineapple, provided that it looks wholesome and unspoiled.)

Important Step: Make sure you wash the chicken carefully before marinating it; this dish should not end up as Sweet & Sour Salmonella!

The sauce is simple to prepare and will not spoil. Mix one cup of white vinegar, one cup of sugar, half a cup of orange juice concentrate, half a cup of pineapple juice (or syrup from the can), one tbsp. of salt and one-half cup of tomato paste. Simmer the mixture for 10–15 minutes. The secret behind this sauce lies in achieving a pleasing harmony of sweet, sour and salty tastes. (Go ahead and add another one-half tsp. of salt, if the dish tastes too bland ... *and* if you aren't struggling with high blood pressure.)

Next step: Add some arrowroot or corn starch to thicken the sauce until it reaches the consistency of a cream sauce.

When cooking-time arrives next day, season a skillet or wok with garlic and ginger. Heat some peanut oil and stir it to distribute the spices. Now drain the marinated chicken and pineapple and spoon it into the hot wok, stirring constantly. (Don't let the wok cool down—just go ahead and cook two portions, if necessary.)

Add some of the sauce when your chicken is nearly cooked. Each chunk should be smoothly coated, but not drowned. Now heat the mixture and serve it to a standing ovation—less than $8 for four large servings.

While you're enjoying this universally loved treat, why not spring your Sweet & Sour Geography Quiz on your dinners and see who wins the Gold Star?

$2 Tenderloin

As soon as I saw the price-tag, I knew this was an offer I couldn't refuse.

Beef tenderloin at $2 a pound!

I didn't hesitate. Nor should you. The next time you run across a supermarket sale featuring this easy-to-prepare cut of beef, go for it. Then tie on your apron for some *real* outdoor grilling fun, as follows:

Step 1: Slice the loin into two-inch-thick pieces, while carefully trimming off the sinews.

Step 2: Marinade the meat for two hours in a zestful blend that includes the following:

O One cup of soy

O One-half cup of lemon juice

O Two tablespoons of safflower oil

O Pinches to taste of ground ginger, garlic, black pepper, cumin, and fresh basil.

Step 3: Time the lighting of your coals so that the fire is just right when the marinating is completed.

Step 4: Sear the meat, while turning it with a spatula. (You'll find that it cuts with a fork!)

329

Step 5: Butter a pan, add mushroom caps, then sizzle these on the side of the grill. At high heat, the mushrooms cook fast.

Step 6: Use a meat thermometer to tell you when the loin is done. (I like mine at about 130 degrees, but I find that many people—including my family—prefer 140–145 degrees.)

Step 7: Serve your "Loin and 'Shrooms" on a platter, surrounded by fresh, sliced peaches and strawberries.

o   o   o

Delicious? You bet. And here's a footnote that will make your *el cheapo* tenderloin taste even better.

Only a few days ago, while dining at the Ritz in Boston, I ordered a similar cut of tenderloin. They gave me a dinky, eight-ounce filet, but no fresh mushrooms, peaches or strawberries. Instead, I was presented with a few slices of tasty bread, and a pre-packaged salad (Sysco strikes again!). An elegantly clad waiter stood nearby, intent on grinding and sprinkling Parmesan and black pepper wherever he could.

And the cost? Only $37.50!

Zucchini and Sausage, JoAnn's Way

We're in luck tonight at the *Maison de Shoemaker.* My lively and lovely spouse JoAnn has decided to do the cooking.

And there's more good news: She's going to treat us to one of her *haute cuisine* specialties—zucchini and sausage casserole!

(How good in this steaming, savory *entrée* from the kitchen of Chef JoAnn? *This* good: Even our resident teenager, the effervescent Sally, can't get enough of her mother's gourmet concoction.)

Armed with fresh yellow squash and zucchini from the Farmer's Market, here's how JoAnn creates a feast for both the eye *and* the palate.

First ... she browns a pound of sweet Italian sausage and cuts it into small chunks.

Next ... she simmers the meat for a few minutes in order to drain off the fat, then pats it dry and with a paper towel and tosses it with one tablespoon of flour.

After that ... she combines six cups of thinly sliced zucchini and one cup of chopped onions. She sautés this mixture in butter until it's tender (do *not* brown it). Removing the vegetables from the heat, she coats them with three tbsp. of flour containing four twists of black pepper.

Now ... it's time to prepare the casserole by mixing 16 ounces of cottage cheese with one-quarter of a cup of parmesan. JoAnn stirs in two well beaten eggs and bakes the mixture for 30 minutes at 325 degrees.

When ... the casserole begins to bubble and the zucchini feels tender, she removes the dish from the oven and sprinkles it with four ounces of cheddar cheese.

Two minutes later, she serves it up.

Are we pleased? Are we clamoring for seconds? This recipe will serve 4 the first time you make it and 3 the next.

Unforgettable BBQ Sauce

Question for grilled chicken- and sparerib-lovers of the world:

Is there any joy on earth quite like the joy you get from whipping up the perfect barbecue sauce and then basting it onto your char-grilled supper?

Of course not.

Marcel Proust can have his skimpy little cookie (the *Madeleine*) dipped in steaming tea.

When it comes to summoning up "remembrances of things past," I prefer the savory aroma of barbecued chicken legs sizzling into tenderness on an outdoor grill. For reasons that I don't fully understand, this marvelous, multi-dimensional fragrance never fails to remind me of my years as a medical student in North Carolina—the barbecue headquarters for the entire Western Hemisphere.

I've tried the commercial barbecue sauces—everything from Cattleman's to Heinz 57—and I can tell you flat-out: They just don't get the job done. Either the sauce is so hot that you don't need a grill ... or it's so sweet and cloying that you wind up eating mouthful after mouthful of "Cotton Candy Chicken" and wishing you'd grilled the ruined bird *without* any sauce!

But it doesn't have to be that way. Try my homemade BBQ Sauce, as follows, and see if you don't end up quoting the immortal Harlan Sanders: "It's finger-lickin' good, folks!"

Start by combining four ounces of ketchup and one ounce of dark molasses with one tsp. of soy sauce, one tsp. of lemon juice, one of apple cider vinegar and a tsp. of dry sherry. Heat this mixture but don't boil it. Now add a pinch each of black pepper, garlic powder, fennel seed and marjoram, along with plenty of paprika. (The good news here is that the molasses will provide the "glue" that holds the sauce on the meat.)

Make sure that you prepare the sauce well in advance, so that the fennel and paprika will "mature" fully and thus join the strong, early tastes of lemon and vinegar to form a resonant, full-bodied flavor.

Now pour your sauce into a large pot and dunk the chicken legs, thighs and breasts in it. Save the wings for a different taste treat another day. Place the sauce-dripping meat on a hot grill. Sear and turn it quickly, then baste again and turn. Without skin and just the sauce on the meat, this meal will cook fast.

Who needs to wait around for the corn-on-the-cob to finish steaming? Let's eat!

Ah, memory ...

The Art of Grilling Steaks, 101

Question for steak-lovers everywhere:

Why do America's "backyard barbecuers" have so much trouble grilling a simple steak?

Think about it for a moment. How many times have you been asked to "drop by for steaks on the grill" ... and then wound up eating either a slab of raw, bleeding meat—or a charred, leathery beef-cut that looked as if it had just been rescued from the Chicago fire?

An all-too-familiar scenario, right?

But it doesn't have to be that way—not if you follow Dr. Shoe's easy-to-implement instructions for grilling the perfect steak.

First Instruction: *Marinate the meat in advance.* Brushing your top steak or your New York strip with lots of seasoned marinade before grilling will improve the flavor, and especially with thicker cuts of meat. (That tasty marinade will also help to keep your steak moist as it's sizzling on the grill.)

Next step: Build a small "chimney" of charcoal briquets inside a coffee can sleeve that will be placed in the grill pan. For best results, use crumpled newspaper and a small amount of lighter fluid to light the coals. Such prudence will reduce the threat of fire, even as it protects the environment.

Once your charcoal has ignited, you can get busy preparing a butter sauce. Melt a stick of low-salt butter in a sauce pan, after adding garlic, pepper, a whole thyme leaf, celery seed, dry mustard and one tbsp of concentrated lemon juice. Now cut a loaf of Italian bread into one-inch slices and baste each side thickly with the mixture.

To prepare a delicious meat marinade, combine pepper, garlic powder, basil leaf, ginger, ground cumin and soy sauce with a dash of sherry. Be sure to pierce thicker steaks with a fork in order to help the marinade do its job better. Remember, also, that the steaks should be seared quickly on the grill, to make sure they don't dry out during cooking.

Once your coals are hot, slap the bread on the grill and turn it quickly to avoid burning. (This crowd-pleaser will leave them *ooooooohhh*-ing in the aisles, trust me.) Set the bread aside and sear your steaks on both sides briefly. Then cover the grill with its lid in order to lower the fire. Let the meat smoke gently for 5–7 minutes on each side.

Now remove the lid and finish cooking the rest of the meat to taste. (I prefer to turn the steaks with tongs, by the way, rather than stabbing them with a fork.) You can tell when the meat is done by cutting off a small piece and sampling it.

Serve your steak-sizzlers with your garlic toast, and toss in a bowl of iced honeydew melon on the side. Then remember to bow graciously, as your dinner guests make like the audience at *La Scala*, with endless cries of *Bravo!*

Tomato Sauce

Although many amateur cooks don't realize it, all tomato sauces are not alike.

As a matter of fact, these aromatic and palate-pleasing sauces vary enormously when it comes to taste, texture, water content and consistency. And yet they're an essential in any dish where they appear. For that reason, I always like to emphasize Dr. Shoemaker's First Cooking Commandment: *If the meal includes tomato sauce, you gotta get it right!*

Formidable-sounding at first, the task of creating the Perfect

Tomato Sauce becomes a lot easier if you start with a basket of fresh Roma tomatoes. This smaller, juicier variety is just right for sauce-making ... which is why I'm so grateful to my good friend and neighbor, Bruce Nichols, whose backyard garden never seems to stop producing these delectable fruits.

Once I get my hands on a bushel of Romas (thanks, Bruce!), I reach for the Victorio juicer. This device employs a "worm" drive-gear that forces juice and fruit through a sieve, thus removing the skin and seeds from the pulp and liquid. Let freedom ring: No more blanching tomatoes to remove the skins!

Now it's time to begin "cooking down" the sauce. This step takes time and patience, and it should be done outdoors ... so try to schedule the cook-off for a lazy summer or early fall day. As the juice bubbles merrily in the pot, add fennel and oregano to taste. Your freshly cooked juice will be fragrant and vividly red —and you'll enjoy the added satisfaction of knowing that no "additives" have found their way into the pot.

After about four hours of leisurely cooking, I find that the bushel has produced four gallons of thick, hot sauce. Let it cool for a bit. Then take a quart of sauce and run it through the blender (on "high") for 30 seconds. Pour the resulting puree into a zipper-type plastic bag. Place your bags in a larger container and "square" them off neatly. At this point, your sauce is ready for the freezer.

Making homemade tomato sauces teaches us a good lesson about the economics of food preparation. Because there are so many steps involved—and because the cooking time extends over so many hours—manufacturing this savory sauce will never be a cottage industry.

But so what? How satisfying it feels—as you pour that first ladle-full of sauce over a bowl of piping-hot pasta—to appreciate a food-product not for its *cost* ... but for its quality and purity!

Dinner Time with the Iron Duke

I say, Guv, have you heard the story of how the Duke of Wellington bested the great French general Napoleon at Waterloo?

It happened on the 18th of June, 1815, and when the smoke cleared, the course of European history had been changed forever, in two very important ways:

First, the mighty French Empire had received a blow from which it would never fully recover;

Second, the eponymous Duke of Wellington would emerge as a major historical celebrity whose name would soon be linked to the following entities:

- an elegantly designed boot that became the rage of Europe;
- a zesty beef dish that still ranks as one of the world's most popular *entrees*;
- a Duke University fundraising organization, the Iron Dukes of Durham, that continues its relentless quest for the hard-earned dollars of Duke alumni to this very day!

Fascinating as it might be, European history won't help us much in the kitchen. So let's forget the military showdown in Belgium for minute, and talk about meat. Did you know, for example, that it's the fat deposits between muscle fibers in a cut of beef that determines just how tender the steak will be?

Broil a nicely "marbled" (lots of fat) steak, and the odds are high that the meat will emerge from the process with a high moisture-content. Leaner cuts of beef will be drier and tougher—and must be cooked more slowly (or under pressure) as a result. (Another canny strategy for the leaner cuts: Serve 'em drenched in a savory sauce.)

Definitely an "upper crust" dish, Beef Wellington is often served with a sauce made of goose pate mixed with Madeira. Typically, the sauce is rubbed into an expensive cut of tenderloin … which is then covered with a flaky crust. The best strategy here is to bake the dish slowly, which will allow both the meat and the crust to cook thoroughly.

Find a nice eye of round roast for about $2.50/lb. Marinate it overnight in plum sauce, vinegar, soy and olive oil. The marinade helps the nearly fat free cut of meat become succulent enough to pass as a Wellington for a fraction of the cost.

To prepare the sauce, pick up two tins of goose pate at the nearest supermarket (typical price: $1.49 per tin). Now add some finely minced scallions and ¼ of a cup of soy sauce, along with 2 tbsp of Madeira. (If you wish, you can substitute chicken livers for the pate and 2 tbsp of a tawny port for the wine.)

To make the pie crust, simply refer to the hot pie crust recipe in this section.

Next step: wash the eye of your round roast briefly in pickle brine. This quick bath will allow the brine's pungent dill-flavor to seep into the sauce and then into the meat. Now roll the round in the soy-pate mixture for 3–4 minutes. Wrap the roast in your pie crust, but don't pierce it. For a nice creative touch, place strips of dough along the top of the crust. (You can use the "Chippendale" strip pattern ... or simply dough-sculpt the images of Chip and Dale, themselves!)

Bake your Homage to the Duke for 25 minutes at 300 degrees, or until the internal meat temperature registers 145 degrees. Serve the Wellington with baked potatoes, and you should be able to feed ten people for about $18 ... which isn't bad for a gourmet dish that's still served in many of the world's finest restaurants.

Whoever said the British were the worst cooks on the planet? Was it the French? Hey, all *their* great general gave us was a decadent, high-calorie dessert! If you really want to know who won the Battle of the Kitchen, just ask yourself: When's the last time you enjoyed a *Napoleon*?

Upside-Down Turkey Breast

Gulliver was stumped!

If you've read that 18th-Century classic by the Irish writer Jonathan Swift ("Gulliver's Travels"), you probably recall the hilarious scene in which Our Hero was compelled to face the key question that had triggered an all-out war among the Lilliputians:

Should a soft-boiled egg be opened from the small end or the big end?

Tough question, right?

Yet it pales, when compared to the query that stands at the very heart of contemporary existential thought:

Should you slow-roast a turkey
breast-up ... or breast-*down*?

(That question becomes even more complex and challenging, of course, if you're cooking *only* the breast—and not the rest of the turkey!)

But not to fret.

Like Gulliver confronting the tiny folk, I refuse to run from this burning question, and I'll simply tell you flat-out:

Cook it breast-down at 290 degrees for five hours!

With a typical, seven-pound turkey, let's say, the above strategy will accomplish one very essential goal: making sure that the scant juices drain into the meat and not out of it.

So much for the Great Turkey Debate. And since you're already embroiled in a major controversy, why not startle your guest with another shocking approach to traditional baked turkey ... by building your stuffing around the *outside* of the turkey breast?

Shocking! And the surprises aren't over yet ... because I'm also going to recommend that you eliminate the insulin-surges that so often accompany the amylose in bread stuffings—by putting together a delicious stuffing that doesn't contain any bread.

Impossible, you say? Not really. Just grab a can of drained chick peas, a tin of patted smoked oysters (fresh are too wet), a can of drained mandarin oranges, some chopped mushrooms (same size as the chick peas), some pitted black olives sliced lengthwise and some coarsely sliced Spanish onions. Combine these goodies in a bowl, while adding sage, garlic, dill seed, black pepper and maybe even a dash of curry powder. Toss all of these ingredients gently … then throw in a few of your smallest red cherry tomatoes for a special touch of color.

Next step: mold the stuffing around your upside-down turkey breast. If the stuffing turns a bit crunchy on top, simply spray it with some cooking oil. Notice how the escaping turkey juices seep into the stuffing as it slowly bakes. Is it tasty? Do wild bears go bonkers when they spot a honey-dripping beehive?

Applause, applause! With this delicious, low-cal dish, you'll turn mealtime completely upside-down—even as you demonstrate your genius at answering the toughest philosophical questions.

SPICES: It's All a Matter of Strategy

Did you know that you can use common spices as a powerful tool in the preparation of flavorful meals—without having to rely on salt?

It's true. And the best part is, it doesn't take endless hours of study to begin discovering the subtle effects you can achieve—by blending spices in combinations that will usually bring out the best in food.

For simplicity's sake, I divide spices into several different categories including:

Leaf: This group includes thyme, oregano, savory, chervil, sage, basil, bay, marjoram, tarragon, dill, parsley and rosemary.

Root: Among the most savory of the root-based spices are ginger, garlic and onion. The root-spices are typically sharp and savory ... they usually require lots of toothpaste or mouthwash after ingestion, if you're planning a social evening.

Seed: This lively group of seasonings numbers among its ranks cumin, dill, coriander, celery, fennel, poppy, sesame, fenugreek and anise.

Another useful way to categorize spices is to label them as "early taste" or "late taste." The seasonings in the first group are sensed instantly, once they strike the palate, and they include mustard, vinegar, citrus and pepper.

"Late taste" spices just keep on happening, long after they've been swallowed. Among the most useful of these substances are fenugreek, paprika, turmeric and saffron.

Although many people don't realize it, you can teach yourself a lot about "Spiceology" by performing a few simple experiments. Example: Prepare a delicious salad dressing by combining a light salad oil (canola or safflower) with white vinegar. Shake the mixture—and then notice how quickly the taste of the vinegar leaps to your palate. Add a grinding of fenugreek or paprika, and you can see for yourself just how the "late taste" effect works. Now add any "leaf" spice of your choosing, followed by a "seed" spice, and shake the mixture again. Notice how these different tastes are "melding" into a symphony of flavors? Just for fun add a second leaf to your dressing. No real change, is there? In fact, the doubled spices seem to fight each other. Now with one seed, one leaf, one root, one early taste and one late taste, you've got it. Great tastes following a simple formula.

Like all great works of art, the dressing you just made will get even better as it matures. And here's the *really* good news for all of us spice-lovers: Delightful flavors and healthy cooking go together ... naturally!

Fried Rice: Making Haste Slowly

The Chinese are the masters of leftover cooking. Artists of the kitchen, they can take a leftover chicken breast, a green pepper, an onion and a handful of rice ... and transform it into a feast for the Emperor of Canton! From time immemorial, it seems, Chinese cooks have had a knack for weaving tastes, textures and colors into edible tapestries that delight their guests. (Just pause to eyeball the menu in any Chinese restaurant, and you'll marvel at the colorful variations they can spin from a bit or rice and a few vegetables.)

When it comes to preparing fried rice, these canny chefs also understand the importance of following that ancient Chinese dictum: "Make haste slowly."

Because this dish cooks rapidly, you need to take your time in gathering the ingredients ... and then to make sure they're close at hand before the oil starts to sizzle.

The best way to proceed is as follows.

First, when preparing white rice for a meal, double the portion and save the leftover cooked rice for a few days. Then, when you're ready for your frying extravaganza, wash the already cooked rice as carefully as possible—in order to remove the starch from it. Wash the rice *slowly* ... while using a whisk to help in the process, because the individual grains will not heat evenly if the starch glues them together. Now go ahead and store the rice in the refrigerator.

Next step: Prepare a delicious sauce for the fried rice by mixing 3 tbsp. of soy sauce, 1 tbsp. of dry sherry, ⅓ tsp. of MSG, 2 twists of black pepper, 1 tsp. of garlic, 2 tsp. of ground ginger and 1 tbsp. of cornstarch.

So much for the sauce. Now let's take a tour of the fridge in search of ... *leftovers*. Ah, yes—how about those chicken pieces, those scallions and that sweet red pepper on the second shelf? Grab 'em! Now slice everything as thinly as possible, so that your chicken or vegetable slices are no wider than the length of a grain of rice.

Time now to whip two whole eggs and reserve them.

Now remove the cold rice (approximately four cups) from the refrigerator and stir in two tbsp. of cold water. Lift and separate the grains. In a *wok* or large frying pan, heat 3 tbsp. of peanut oil (it won't smoke at high heat). Now add your scallions and stir them for 15 seconds. Add the rice next, stirring it so that the oil coats each and every grain. Add the egg and stir vigorously. Cook this mixture for two minutes, then add your sauce and stir for one more minute. Serve the savory dish hot and steaming.

When the applause begins, remember to bow *slowly* and gracefully, in the very best Chinese tradition!

(Medical footnote: Don't forget that fried rice can trigger a food-borne type of diarrhea, caused by a germ named *Bacillus cereus*, if the dish is allowed to spoil. So enjoy your fried rice … but be sure to throw away *these* leftovers!)

Lamb from Apollo's Kitchen

On the table: a dish of black olives, a slab of oil-drenched *feta* cheese, and a jug of ice-cold *retsina* …

Above the terrace café: the emerald slopes of Delphi, Apollo's grove, perched 2,000 feet above the foam-lapped Gulf of Corinth …

It's springtime, 25 years ago, and I've journeyed to Greece to recite my Oath of Hipprocrates.

My medical school classmates have already taken the Oath, during ceremonies at the Duke University Chapel. But I prefer the temple of the Sun God, and the mountainside hangout where he parks his famous Golden Chariot.

No hard feelings, I say; I hope the formal graduation went splendidly, back there in good old Durham. It's just that I have a different plan. Surrounded by pungent olive groves and basket-laden donkeys, I'm hoping to make my oath-taking the kind of experience you don't forget.

Relaxing at my wickerwork table above the groves, I sip the resin-scented wine and dream of tonight's supper: a leg of spring lamb with paprika-scented Greek-style potatoes on the side.

Is there any joy like it? Nibbling at a slice of savory *feta*, I watch a shaft of Aegean radiance break through the overcast. Apollo, god of light and wisdom, watch over me (and my patients) in all the years of arduous medical practice that lie ahead!

Now let the banquet begin ... starting with a fresh leg of lamb which has been de-boned by a skilled butcher—since cooking this delicate meat evenly can be a tricky challenge.

Next step: While honoring my sister-in-law Nancy's terrific lamb recipe, cut the meat into steak-sized chunks, then marinate it overnight in the refrigerator in a mixture containing half a cup of Dijon mustard, two tbsp. of soy sauce, one tsp. of fresh rosemary, one-half tsp. of ginger, one crushed garlic clove and two tbsp. of olive oil.

As with other marinated meats, be sure to sear the outside of the lamb on a hot grill. Then cover it with a lid and turn it intermittently. (Remember that you don't have to *over*-cook the lamb; it's just as safe as beef, and presents very little risk of causing a food-borne illness if thoroughly heated.)

Serve your lamb with a light salad, crusty bread and grapes.

And why not prepare a salad dressing that includes olive oil, vinegar with thyme, coriander, black olives and feta cheese ... all of which will bring back memories of Greece, while also winning the heart of the Ancient Sunlight God?

The Perfect Chicken Pot Pie: Build It, And They Will Come—To Dinner!

Here's a question for all you baseball fans who also enjoy hanging out in the kitchen.

Which renowned American baseball player—one of the greatest hitters in the history of the sport—insisted on eating a chicken dinner before each and every game?

The answer, of course, is: Wade Boggs, the recently retired, longtime third-baseman for the Boston Red Sox, who loved chicken so much that he always enjoyed a platter of it before taking the field.

Mr. Boggs, although I can't hit a curve ball like you, I *do* share your immense devotion to this ubiquitous American bird. I like my chicken fried ... and baked in the oven ... and blasted with barbecue sauce atop a smoking charcoal grill.

But most of all, I love the savory, soul-nourishing feast that goes by the name of "chicken pot pie."

What is it about pot pies that makes me feel so joyful and at peace ... especially on days (like today!) when the winter rain sloshes through the gutters and a frigid wind gnaws at the back of my neck?

As far as I'm concerned, there's no better way to shuck off the "winter blahs" than by baking up a succulent chicken pot pie ... even as I dream of that day in far-off April when the umpire will holler "Play ball!" and another season will begin.

The really neat thing about pot pies is the way you can make 'em from leftover chicken straight out of the refrigerator ... provided, of course, that you surround the meat with a mouthwatering ensemble of fragrant vegetables and chewy pie crust.

Building the perfect pie crust is a delicate art. But my strategy is actually quite simple. I like to use a frozen "pie shell" for both the bottom and the top of my crust. (If you line the two shells up evenly, they'll "seal" the contents nicely—so that your pie-innards don't end up on the bottom of the stove.)

344

Ready to get started? All right, your first move is to bone the leftover chicken, saving any sauce but discarding all of the skin. Next, cut the meat into one-inch-square chunks and slices. Then sauté (use butter) some leftover carrot rounds, fresh onion slices, some leftover steamed squash, a few fresh half-rounds of green pepper and some mushroom stems ... along with some frozen green peas and a few sliced pimentos (for color).

Happily, this is one of the few dishes I know that can stand the dense taste of tarragon, so go ahead and add a leaf—along with a bit of cumin seed, pepper, dry mustard, one tbsp. of dry sherry and a dash of Chinese plum sauce.

Next step: whip up a wild white sauce, using one tbsp. of butter, one tbsp. of flour and ¼ cup of warm milk mixed with ¼ cup of sour cream. Simmer this mixture until it's thick, then add the chicken chunks and slices to the sour cream sauce and stir until the chicken is warm. Pour the chicken and the wild cream sauce onto the vegetables and stir gently.

Now spray the pie shell with cooking oil and then add the filling. Settle the top shell on the inside of the bottom shell and pierce the top with a fork. Bake the pie at 375 degrees for about 40 minutes, or until it's done. (You'll find this pot pie filling so rich that you'll want to save *it* as your next leftover!)

Go ahead and cut this beauty into thick, steaming wedges and serve them up to your guest. And the next voice you hear will be that of the announcer:

A long drive to left ... it's going, going ... a home run!

Pie Crust

If you thought crab cakes could be made many ways, just try and make the best pie crust. My mother was an intuitive cook. Fresh biscuits, rolls, pies—just look at my dad. I tried to duplicate her pie crust. I think I rolled it too much (he shoots and scores!)

She took ¾ cup Crisco®, cut it into 2 cups of flour, leaving lumps, added cold water so it was damp, not wet or sticky (add egg if you want a golden glaze), rolled it out, leaving lumps, folded four times (only) and without handling much, made the crust.

Right, to get to California, go to Crisfield and turn left. You can't miss it.

Years ago, our neighbors, like me, also couldn't make dough right, either. They loved biscuits, though, and every morning we could hear whop! whop!; they were opening cardboard tubes to make biscuits. It sounded like a new-found war and let me tell you those biscuits weren't fit to eat.

The friendly grandmother from down the street tried to help me. Don't try so hard; less handling means better flakes. Her "never fail" crust was 1 cup lard, 3 cups flour, 1 tsp. salt mixed until crumbly, add beaten egg yolk, 5 tbsp. cold water, 1 tsp. vinegar. This can be rolled more than once without becoming puckish.

Ruth Hall doesn't agree that pie crust has to be made with cold water and minimal manipulation. She puts ¾ cup Crisco®, 1 tsp. milk and ¼ cup *boiling* water in a bowl and beats at medium speed with an electric mixer until light and fluffy (heresy!). She adds 2 cups of flour and 1 tsp. salt and beats at low speed until all ingredients are moist.

She divides the dough into two balls, wraps and warms for at least four hours. This is a great tasting dough!

All this pie crust is just chemistry. Water, salt and acid all change the interaction of saturated fat molecules and complex starch molecules. The heat of the reaction is controlled by cold water. Ruth breaks the large consolidated fat into individual molecules, each surrounded by water and starch. Cooling is accomplished by the large surface area created. Her recipe is like oil and vinegar salad dressing! Of *course* it has to be hot to mix evenly.

In the human body, all cells are surrounded by a membrane which has a structure analogous to Ruth's pie crust. Fat molecules are surrounded with a complex layer of starches and proteins. The organization of cells into functioning units or tissues is controlled by the amount of water, salt and acid too. Imagine that, a cell biology lesson from pie crust.

OYSTERS ROCKEFELLER
A Culinary Scandal in the Making?

Here's a puzzle worthy of the great English bard, himself. (I'm talking about The Spear, of course, who was the first to utter that immortal question: "What's in a name?")

Puzzle: How did a wealthy oil magnate named Rockefeller manage to get *his* name attached to a traditional Maryland oyster recipe?

Was the petroleum titan John D. Rockefeller a seafood chef *wannabe* on the side, or what?

Regardless of how it happened, there's no doubt that "Oysters Rockefeller" still ranks as one of the Old Line State's classiest seafood dishes.

Nor is there any doubt that the key to success in this particular enterprise is to cook the oysters slowly in a cream sauce that will penetrate the heavy bodies of the mollusk. Above all, making a good cream sauce requires patience. If you apply too much heat —or cook the ingredients too quickly—the result can easily become a culinary disaster.

To avoid such a catastrophe, take a lesson from my spouse Jo-Ann, who's a natural-born whiz at sauces. She recommends that you start by obtaining some fresh shucked oysters. Drain them and save the liquid. Then make a cream sauce consisting of two tbsp of flour, one-fourth stick of butter, and half a cup of cream. Add one-fourth of a cup of oyster liquid, but do not boil this mixture; merely simmer it for 5–10 minutes, while adding one ounce of dry sherry and two egg yolks. Keep stirring frequently, then remove the sauce and cool it. (If you followed these steps correctly, the sauce won't separate.)

The next part is easy. Slice enough scallions and mushroom caps (finely) to match the volume of sauce you made. Now sauté the scallions and mushrooms in butter until they're brown. Place some fresh shredded spinach in another bowl and pour the hot sautéed scallions and mushrooms on it. Toss the contents until the spinach is wilted but not flat.

Now take your cleaned oyster shells and place them on a broiling pan. Layer the bottom of each shell with the spinach mixture and place a fat oyster on it. Fill the shell with the cream sauce and cover it with parmesan cheese. Broil the shells until the oyster is cooked.

In recent years, of course, bacon seems to have crept into this recipe. I don't mind. Wrapping each oyster with partially cooked bacon before broiling does add an interesting flavor. I also like to sprinkle some sesame oil over the oysters before cooking—but not when bacon is along for the ride. I don't want to overpower the delicate flavor of those oysters!

Delicious! And I'm sure The Spear wouldn't mind a quick paraphrase:

> *This delectable oyster by any other name ...*
> *would taste exactly the same!*

HUEVOS RANCHCHEROS ... Or
Are You Daring Enough to Eat an Egg?

Here's a riddle perplexing enough to befuddle the Egyptian Sphinx.

Riddle: Why are Americans so terrified of the ordinary egg?

At first glance, the answer looks easy. It's the *cholesterol*, right?

After all, aren't chicken eggs full of cholesterol—and doesn't that waxy, fatty substance clog up human arteries faster than a rush-hour fender-bender in the heart of mid-town Manhattan?

Well, it's certainly true that eggs contain a bit of cholesterol ... about 100 mg per egg, as a matter of fact.

But did you know that the human liver, itself, manufactures more than *1,200* mg of cholesterol per day ... or more than 12 times the amount contained in a single egg?

It's an enigma, all right. If the human body produces this much cholesterol on its own, then why are we all running around like headless chickens (sorry!), while worrying about the impact of dietary cholesterol on our health?

The answer, of course, *(please see Chapter 11 of this book!)* is that we've all been deluded by the gurus of the U.S. Medical Establishment ... most of whom decided more than a decade ago that cholesterol ranks right up there with bubonic plague as one of the most dangerous health threats now confronting *homo sapiens.*

But the good news for egg-lovers everywhere is that you can enjoy an omelet or two for breakfast—several times a week, if you like—without significant harm to your health. As for the threat from "cholesterol" ... well, that subject remains exceedingly complex. According to the latest research, there are actually five different subtypes of HDL cholesterol—and some of them are actually quite good for you. (Some are not, however.) And of course, there's always the question of whether or not health-threatening "oxidation" of LDL cholesterol—aka known as "bad cholesterol"—really does raise your risk of heart disease.

While the Great Cholesterol Debate goes forward, however, one point seems perfectly clear: The risks associated with eating an occasional egg have been greatly exaggerated. So why not enjoy a zesty presentation of this great protein source—a Mexican version I call *huevos rancheros*, which simply means "ranch eggs" in Spanish?

To prepare this south-of-the-border breakfast, start by chopping up a Spanish onion with four scallions. Add two or three chopped Roma tomatoes. Now sauté the onions with one clove of garlic. Add the tomatoes and reduce to the liquid at low heat. Next step: Add one cup of mild *salsa* and toss in a few *jalapenos* (to taste). Finally, add even more zip by tossing a cup of shredded sharp cheddar cheese into the mixture.

Warm your breakfast plate and cover it with a corn *tortilla*. Then fry two eggs, sunny side up, and lay them on the warmed *tortilla*. Slather the eggs with your sauce and serve the dish with fresh fruit and freshly squeezed juice. Add a pot of strong coffee mellowed with some brown sugar and a two-inch cinnamon stick.

Now enjoy your breakfast, *ranchero* … secure in the knowledge that your cholesterol-level hasn't budged an inch, even though you dared to eat a couple of eggs!

Princess Anne Breakfast Goop

Invented right up the road in good old Princess Anne, Md., the dish you're about to enjoy still ranks as my all-time favorite breakfast experience.

The Goop!

I can't tell you how many times visitors to our rural home near Pocomoke have wolfed a platter of my Goop, then pushed away from the table with a contented sigh, followed by the urgent question:

"Ritch, what's the secret behind your Goop?"

The answer is actually *two* answers.

First, in order to assemble a truly memorable Goop, you need a bit of lemon *santolina*, which happens to be a very fragrant and yet subtle herb.

Second, in order to obtain the required *santolina*, you need to experience the unbridled joy of growing your own "kitchen garden."

Creating your own herb garden is a highly rewarding activity —on several levels at once. To get started, you need a patch of good, well-drained soil close to your house. Your proposed garden-plot should also include morning sun and afternoon shade. Here you will often be amazed by the number of different herbs that can flourish, year in and year out. Fennel … rosemary … sage … thyme … you name it, and there's a good chance that you can grow it, depending on geographic location and certain other soil-factors related to your particular corner of the world.

In addition to making food taste better, these delicate plants look pretty, smell good and produce some fascinating flowers. They also provide a nesting area for small insects and birds, including the ruby throated hummingbird, a personal favorite. By the way, backyard gardeners have long understood that planting basil among tomatoes—or chives among peppers—will greatly reduce the toll caused by insect damage each year. (Call your local library to learn more about the benefits of such "companion planting.")

But let's get back to the Goop. This breakfast delight was born a few years ago, when my spouse JoAnn happened to be growing a fragrant patch of lemon *santolina* in her kitchen garden. JoAnn broke off a leaf or two, took a deeply satisfying whiff, and immediately went to work as follows:

Slice a pound of *kielbasa* and sauté it with two pounds of diced red potatoes. Drain the fat, then reduce the heat to low. Now add one large minced onion, sliced black olives, green bell peppers, pimento, mandarin oranges and a few thinly sliced smoked oysters.

Spice the mixture with celery seed, pepper, a dash of plum sauce, some fresh red-hot chili garlic paste and your *santolina* (rosemary makes a good substitute, if you haven't planted that garden yet).

351

Serve the Goop piping-hot and stand by the $64 Question: "What *is* that tangy aftertaste?"

You guessed it: The *santolina*!

Razzle-Dazzle Garlic Bread

Do you know why I wrote this book, LOSE THE WEIGHT YOU HATE!?

I wrote it because—as a family physician who's been serving the same Maryland community for more than 20 years—I wanted to help people overcome one of the most painful and depressing health conditions known to modern medicine: obesity.

But I *also* wanted to share with my readers the joyful knowledge that you can eat well and take great pleasure in food, even as you carry out the steps necessary to keep your weight under control.

On my weight-maintenance diet *(see Chapter Eight, "Achieving Maintenance")*, patients who follow the daily schedule for controlling their intake of amylose and glucose are rewarded regularly for accomplishing this rewarding goal.

And I can't think of a more rewarding treat than "Razzle-Dazzle Garlic Bread"—a taste treat that will leave you and your guests cheering for the inventor of that wonderful herb we call "garlic." (And so what if nobody will come near you for 18 hours after you eat it?)

My dieters don't get to eat garlic bread very often. But when they do, I hit them with the philosophy that has sustained my entire medical practice since Day One.

Life is meant to be lived. Enjoyed! Embraced! Dig in and savor the glorious foods that are all around us, and savor the moments in which you can appreciate them.

To make my taste-terrific version of razzle-dazzle garlic bread, melt a stick of low-salt butter in a sauce pan. Then add to taste some garlic, some pepper, thyme, some celery seed, some dry mustard and one tbsp of concentrated lemon juice. Bring the spiced butter to a low boil, then reduce heat so your butter quarter isn't drawn.

Next step: Cut a loaf of fresh Italian bread into one-inch-thick slices, and baste each side thoroughly with the garlic sauce described above. Bake the bread in an oven for 20–25 minutes at 350 degrees, or simply place it in the broiler until crisp and toasty.

Serve the garlic bread with a flavor-bursting Caesar salad for lunch, or perhaps with a baked chicken or cheese-and-sausage dish for supper.

Settle back. Enjoy. Give thanks.

Break bread with those around you ... and celebrate!

Enchiladas Con Pollo

Looking for a change of pace—and geography—at tonight's supper table?

How about enjoying a *fiesta* of chicken-and-cheese *enchiladas*, fresh *guacamole*, and cooling tropical fruit?

Like millions of other Americans, I'm an enthusiastic fan of Mexican food. But I'm also a longstanding member of the Hiatal Hernia Self-Help Association ... which means that you won't find any of those red-hot *jalapeno* peppers in any of my *Latino* recipes!

But so what? Believe it or not, Mexican food doesn't have to be spicy in order to win a five-star rating. That's because rich texture and subtle, lingering flavors are actually the hallmarks of outstanding Latin cuisine—as you'll discover while preparing the following recipe for a mild and hearty version of *enchiladas*.

To get started, drop by the "imported foods" aisle of your local supermarket and pick up a jar of "moderate" *salsa*, along with a package of 8–10-inch wheat *tortillas*.

Soften the *tortillas* by steaming them for a few minutes. Then cut six uncooked chicken breasts into slices that are one-quarter-inch thick but four inches long. Saute these in butter until they're no longer pink. Meanwhile, add two containers of light cream cheese and two small diced Spanish onions to the cooking chicken. Stir frequently, adding garlic, fennel seed, cilantro, fenugreek (just one twist) and some ground black pepper.

Once the chicken becomes tender—but before it's thoroughly cooked—set is aside in order to allow the flavors to meld.

Next step: Prepare a *guacamole* surprise for your guests by mashing three fresh avocados, along with two dollops of mayonnaise some fresh lime juice. Mix these ingredients with a fork, while adding dashes of garlic, sage and cumin.

Now it's time to shape your stylish *tortillas* by rolling each one around a large spoonful of chicken and cream cheese mixture. Wrap each one twice. Then place the *tortillas* seam-down in a greased pan that has been sprayed with cooking oil. Cover the *tortillas* with shredded Swiss cheese and bake them at 350 degrees until done (15–25 minutes). Add salsa to the top of the enchiladas to taste.

When you're finished, the *tortilla* bottoms should be crisp. The tops should be coated with cheese and the innards should be piping hot.

Dip some *nacho* chips into your fresh *guacamole* … then follow up with a cooling dessert composed of mango slices, kiwi fruits, black seedless grapes and apple slices.

Savor your Mexican supper by eating it … slowly. Then kick back for the best part of this traditional feast: Your obligatory, 30-minute *siesta*!

Recipes
Shrimp Toast and Egg Rolls

Here's a delightful suggestion for a rainy day.

Instead of jumping in the car and slogging through the streets in search of some scintillating Chinese food, why not make your own—right there in the privacy of your kitchen?

How about a plate full of colorful shrimp toast and egg rolls to keep those rainy-day blahs at bay?

For starters, let's remember to deep-fry our Chinese goodies in peanut oil, which will keep our cholesterol intake low—even as it prevents scorching and smoking. Other oils—such as corn, vegetable and canola—boil at lower temperatures, and can thus leave fried foods soggy. And of course, it's never wise to use lard or other saturated fats for deep-frying.

All set? Great. Let's begin by trimming the crust from some whole wheat bread, and then cutting each slice into four equal triangles. Then mince one pound of shelled shrimp, one can of water chestnuts and one bunch of green onions. Coat these items with one tbsp of cornstarch and mix in one whole egg, whipped with 20 strokes. Add two tbsp of soy sauce (don't use the light variety), one tbsp of sherry, three shakes of garlic and two pinches of ginger powder. Stir until the texture evens. The mixture should be spread generously across the bread. Smooth the shrimp mix into a three-quarter-inch-high dome. Then brush the toast with a second beaten egg to create a glaze.

Once your oil is hot, use a slotted spoon and place the toast in the oil with the mixture-side facing down. If the mixture falls off, it means you didn't use enough egg! Deep fry your toasts until they're golden-brown ... and be sure to let all of your guests know just how much time and effort went into creating each one!

Luckily, spring rolls are much easier to make, now that many local supermarkets sell the pastry skins. You can use many different ingredients for your filling (just like the pizza-makers do). But I prefer to load in the same shrimp toast sauce I described above. Then I mix in strips of uncooked chicken, thin rounds of bok choy, bean sprouts, thinly cut mushrooms, scallions and left-over shrimp chunks.

Now you're ready to sauté the filling and add the sauce. Mix well and drain, then place the filling in the middle of the wrapper. Roll twice, being sure to fold in the edges and seal them with beaten egg. Now you can deep-fry them in hot oil (at least 360 degrees), and cook them a little longer than the shrimp toast.

Drain and serve ... and all at once you're looking out the window—

Bright sunshine!

Hamburgers on the Grill

Apple pie, baseball, Fourth of July fireworks and ...

Hamburgers on the grill!

If there's a more quintessentially American activity than "grilling a few burgers while nipping on a can of ice-cold Bud," I am yet to discover it.

Let's face the fact: There's something magical—maybe even *primitive*—about cooking meat over an open fire in your own backyard ... especially if you're holding a chilled *brewski* in one hand, while flipping the burgers with the other.

Still, there's a price to be paid (literally) for the pleasure of cooking ground beef outdoors. Unfortunately, grilling requires that you use a leaner grade of beef than cooking indoors ... simply in order to prevent flame-ups and burning meat caused by fat dripping into the flames. (Indoors, I can solve that problem nicely by cooking the meat very slowly for a long time on the stove.)

Although you'll pay a bit more for the leaner burger, most outdoor chefs don't seem to mind the extra tariff. And the best ones all understand the First Commandment of Successful Hamburger Preparation: A tasty burger depends on "balanced spicing."

Here's how it works. First, squeeze your supply of ground beef into a single, loose patty. Then add a bit of ground pepper, garlic powder, ground coriander or cumin, basil or thyme, a splash of soy sauce and two shakes of ground ginger. Then form the mixture into one-inch thick cooking patties. Work the meat with your hands to distribute the spices evenly, but also to take advantage of the thixotrophic properties of ground beef. The more you work it, the smoother the aggregate of meat, fat and spice becomes. As the meat texture softens, seal the edges of the burger so that there are no cracks in the patty.

Time now for the *real* fun. Go ahead and sizzle your burgers on a hot grill. Turn them quickly so that the outside meat is seared. (Don't use a fork for turning, or you'll end up with dry, tough burgers.) Next step: Close the lid on your grill to force smoke from your wood chunks into the spiced meat. You can alter the smoke-flavor by adding chunks of wood (previously dried but then submerged in liquid just before cooking) to your hot coals. Experiment with mesquite, apple, hickory, and cherry and see which taste you prefer. (My personal favorite is dried pecan shells —but not the hulls—soaked in red wine, lemon, water and bay leaf.)

Having a blast, aren't you? To achieve another delightful variation, try serving potato rolls or onion rolls instead of those bland hamburger buns. Baste the bread with a butter sauce, and toast it right on the grill. Add a slice of cheese to the burgers on your final turnover. (You can use bleu, Swiss, cheddar or Monterey Jack to taste.)

Serve these rascals smoking hot, and stand by for a booming chorus of *Yankee Doodle Dandy!*

Springtime Asparagus

If the first asparagus has arrived in the produce section, can summertime be far behind?

Delightful and delicious, these tender stems support spade-like leaves and closely bunched flower buds at the top ... making this strange-looking vegetable one of nature's oddest plant specimens.

But looks aren't everything, and the taste of fresh asparagus is exquisite. The best way to prepare the vegetable is to slowly steam it and then serve it with butter. No need for spices or sauces—provided that you've managed to obtain high-quality stems.

Apparently, such was never the case in France. Unsatisfied with their own varieties of the vegetable, the restless French decided—several generations ago—to create one of the world's most famous sauces specifically for asparagus.

(Or maybe the Frenchies simply snuck next door to steal the recipe for "Hollandaise Sauce?")

Whatever its origins, this stuff is fun and easy to make. And although I've experimented with it for years, I've never been able to improve on Betty Crocker's basic recipe, as follows:

Take two egg yolks (don't worry: asparagus usually *lowers* cholesterol) and mix them with three tbsp of lemon juice. Use a small sauce pan and a wooden spoon for this task. Turn the heat to "low" and add half a stick of hard butter. Stir until the butter is melted, then add the second half-stick. Keep the heat low and continue stirring, as the eggs slowly cook and thicken the sauce. If it tries to separate on you, add one tbsp of water, heat the mixture again and stir.

To show off your fresh asparagus to the max, serve it on a platter (accompanied by the Hollandaise) beside some cold snow-crab legs and sliced Florida strawberries. Garnish with a few mandarin orange sections and grate some zesty orange peel onto the Hollandaise.

Voila! French *or* Dutch, this savory sauce will leave them singing the cook's praises every time!

Shish-Ke-Bob

Tonight is a grill night again. The exceptional value on boneless chicken breast means chicken again! JoAnn gave me some official shish-ke-bob skewers not long ago, so I no longer have to use coat hangers to make bobs.

The idea of putting a hot piece of metal into food is not unique to shish-ke-bob. Baked potatoes cook faster with a skewer. The Greeks cook souvlaki using meat on a skewer too. Our grilled shisk-ke-bob gives all cooks a chance to create what they want. And you get the credit for a gourmet delight.

Just about any food can be used on a bob. Make sure that the size of fruit pieces, vegetables and meat are similar so that everything is cooked properly at the same time. I make different sauces for basting so guests can be creative in what they eat and how it tastes.

Cut 1½ inch chunks of beef, sausage, chicken and shrimp. Mushrooms (with stems), cherry tomatoes, Vidalia onions, jumbo black olives, cantaloupe and honeydew were on these bobs too. Make a butter and lemon sauce with fresh rosemary, garlic, celery seed and dried mustard. Add a "wood" sauce to the choices by melting one stick of butter and adding two tbsp of soy and one tsp ginger. Don't use this salty sauce if you have high blood pressure! The wood sauce gets its name from the intensity of its flavor, which is similar to the intensity of the smell of freshly worked walnut, cherry or oak. We used barbecue sauce for the third sauce.

The grill should be at medium high heat. Space the bobs on the grill so that they can be lifted and turned easily. Space your food choices on the skewer so that all sides of the food are cooked.

Baste each time you turn. These bobs cook quickly, so gather round to chow down.

Ice Cream

Special today, electric ice cream maker $49.95. Of all things, an electric ice cream maker! I guess I'm old fashioned (or as my friend down the street says "just old") but I like a hand operated ice cream maker. There is much wisdom in the saying "you don't get to lick the dasher if you don't turn the crank."

Our hand crank ice cream freezer is a little rusty. The metal canister that holds the mixture was dusty but the lip was clean. The wood bucket still holds water so we can use it. As soon as you place the filled canister in the bucket, surround with ice cubes and begin adding driveway salt (no, not inside the canister!). Keep adding more ice and salt as you turn the crank, which is connected to the dasher that stirs the mixture inside the canister.

Making ice cream is potentially easy. But consider these questions: How much salt in the brine? Will ice crystals in the ice cream form quickly if I crank too slowly and make the mixture grainy? Do I dare to eat a peach? Usually the finished product is so good, it doesn't matter how you make it!

Adding salt on top of ice melts the ice by lowering the freezing point of the solution. The ice water is colder than 32 degrees, causing water inside the canister, and therefore your cream mixture, to freeze. The more particles in the ice cream, the more salt must be added to the brine.

Today we are making mocha ice cream. Take one pound coarse ground coffee; mix in an open bowl with one-gallon water and store, covered, for two days in the refrigerator. Filter the coffee extract and save. The cold water extract gives no bitterness, no tannins; it is ideal for making instant coffee (just add hot water).

Take one cup cold extract coffee, one cup cocoa. Mix in one-tbs. vanilla extract, one cup sugar, one pint whipping cream and one pint half-and-half. Add a pinch of salt and stir well so that the sugar is dissolved and the powdery cocoa is blended. Fill the canister, secure the lid and you are ready for ice and salt.

Now the fun begins. Put on your best Tom Sawyer hat and convince your friends that it is great fun to turn the crank. Turn the crank until the resistance to turning increases and the mixture freezes. Frost will appear on the outside of the canister. Pull the canister from the brine and wipe off the salt. Let the fresh ice cream chill, still in the canister, 20 minutes in your freezer. Opening the canister is the reward for the weary crankers. Peel the fabulous ice cream off the wood blades of the dasher. Pass around the depleted dasher for all to sample, there are always just a few chunks of fresh ice cream that somebody missed. Now serve small portions. Ahh, this ice cream is so rich, but who can resist? Just this once, it's OK.

Warm Water Fish

Which tastes best: gray trout, speckled trout or yellowfin? Based on a local recipe, speckled trout wins.

Fresh fish is just about a perfect food. The meat is high quality protein. Any fat is usually polyunsaturated and full of beneficial omega-3 fatty acids. Fattening complex carbohydrates are missing. Just look, though, at a fish sandwich served at a fast food restaurant. A frozen piece of fish is coated with oil, breaded, deep fat fried, coated with synthetic mayonnaise and served on a roll with French fries!! Say goodbye to that fish sandwich as a healthy choice.

A better choice is to cook fish at home. Forget the breading and leave the frying pan on the rack. Fish from cold waters will have more unsaturated oils, including the beneficial EPA and

DHA fatty acid based oils, which help lower cholesterol, among other benefits. But, just how much mackerel, sardines, and blue-fish can you eat? We are fortunate in this area to have such easy access to fresh flounder, trout and drum, good sources of protein and beneficial oils. I hope that business of harvesting wild fish doesn't follow the way of harvesting oysters and crabs. The Chesa-peake Bay waterman's way of life is dying as the crabs, oysters and fish all become scarce. Don't get me started on environmental issues, especially toxic chemicals hurting aquatic ecosystems, it is time to cook.

Antoine's is a famous restaurant in the French Quarter in New Orleans. They serve red snapper cooked in a bag; a small portion costs a lot. Take six snapper (hold the ciguatera) or trout fillets, put them on aluminum foil. Sprinkle with lemon and butter and add black pepper. Wrap the foil loosely and put it over a medium charcoal fire, without turning, on an outdoor grill. Fish is easy to overcook (it gets tough), but this recipe was good at 10 minutes and not overdone at 15 minutes.

We served the fish with a spinach salad using an English dress-ing. In a blender, place ½ cup sugar, 2 tbs. sesame seed, 1 tbs. poppy seed, 1 medium onion–minced, ¼ tsp. Worcestershire, and a pinch of paprika. With blender running, add ½ cup of oil and ½ cup of vinegar. The spice theory says two seeds are redun-dant, but this dressing had a nice balance. Fresh strawberries fin-ish the meal.

This was such a good cardiovascular meal and we didn't have to go to New Orleans to enjoy it.

Potato Salad

Potatoes, like all root vegetables, store the plant's excess energy in a complex carbohydrate starch called amylose. Unlike other com-plex carbohydrates though, amylose is quickly broken down in saliva to sugar. Many people who have weight problems digest amylose efficiently and store the sugar from it as fat. While a potato doesn't have a lot of calories, it costs the body only a few calories to store the bulk of the potato starch calories. It isn't the calories you eat that count, it is the calories that you store that make the difference.

How many ways can potatoes be cooked? Like chicken and pizza, potatoes have been prepared with never ending creativity. Try potato salad a new way. In a 5-quart pot, bring the brine from two large pickle jars to boil with water, fennel seed, bay leaf and minced onions added. The pickle brine gives a dill flavor and cures the potatoes. I leave the potato skins on, but most people peel away the vitamin- and fiber-rich skin. Cut the potato into cubes no longer than ¾" in any dimension. Boil the potatoes in brine and spices until they are almost tender. Drain and set aside; the retained heat in the potatoes will finish the cooking.

Next, mince 1 Spanish or Vidalia onion and add to the potato pile. Dice 3 whole dill pickles and one red bell pepper. You can add anything else—radishes, pimentos, olives, artichoke hearts or hard-boiled eggs, but we didn't. Stir the additives in well. The salad had a harmony of taste and texture, with pleasing colors.

Next add a lot of oregano, celery seed, ground pepper, ½ tsp. of salt, if your blood pressure will stand it, and a dash of ground mustard. Mix in enough mayonnaise to coat the individual cubes and blend the spices. Chill at least two hours and serve to smiling faces.

Clams Monie

The secret to a good appetizer is that interesting light food, prepared cleverly, can be served quickly, look good and taste great before your taste buds get confused by the main course. It is even better if the appetizer for transition time can be eaten as finger food. This usually means that appetizers are more likely to be higher in calories and likely to have extra fat. Of course, fat adds taste. Just look at what goes first—the scallops wrapped in bacon, drizzled in sesame oil or the celery sticks with ranch dressing.

Clams Monie can be prepared well ahead of time (even frozen) and then microwaved or baked quickly. These spice and food tastes fulfill all my "well-balance spicing" criteria. Take 2-tsp. salt, 2-tsp. black pepper, 3-tbs. mayonnaise, 5 eggs, 1-tsp. garlic powder, 2 tbs. Worcestershire, 2 tsp. cumin, 2 tsp. ground thyme and beat together until smooth. Add 1 lb. grated bread crumbs (try different kinds!) 1½ lb. diced clams, 1 lb. claw crab meat. Mix together.

Hopefully the clam meat came from freshly shucked clams. Clean the shells and spray the inside with cooking oil. Fill each shell with the bountiful clam mixture, but don't pack down!! Top with ¼" strips of bacon. Sprinkle with paprika and chervil (parsley will do). Bake at 450 degrees for 8 minutes. Cool; wrap in ½ sheet foil and freeze.

Cobia

The omega-3 oils in fish have many beneficial effects. Cobia, a warm water fish, has less omega-3 oil than more northern fishes, but it gives significant health benefits to those lucky enough to eat it. Patients with high triglycerides, low HDL cholesterol and elevated apolipoprotein B are advised to ask their physicians about fish oils. Omega-3 oils are also beneficial for those with inflammation of joints (and they turn on PPAR gamma, chapter 13), though gastrointestinal side effects limit their use in rheumatoid arthritis.

A word of caution: vitamin E in doses over 400 IU a day reverses all the benefits of omega-3. I don't think that the proposed anti-oxidant benefits of vitamin E will outweigh its adverse effects on cholesterol, once patients understand that it does *not* prevent oxidation of LDL. Unfortunately, many inexpensive commercial sources of omega-3 oils are *contaminated* with vitamin E. It is okay to pay for purity, especially for omega-3 oils. Just don't swallow the Vitamin E, either in the oil or in the hype.

We had so much cobia; we ate it three different ways. Cooking it wrapped in foil, on the grill, with lemon and butter made the cobia taste oily. We all know to use this method only for fish like bass, trout and flounder. I marinated a slab of cobia steak in the refrigerator for three days, using lime juice and peel, sherry and pesto sauce. Wow! This cobia tasted like swordfish, with the oil taste gone. Be sure and turn the steaks at least three times a day while marinating, for best results. The pesto sauce was made with olive oil (another omega-3 source), crushed pistachios, basil leaf and coriander.

My favorite way to prepare cobia is smoking it, spiced with pomegranate sauce, fennel and cilantro. I used an artichoke heart-based vinaigrette to baste the slow cooking fish. No need to turn this fish; let it cook at 210° over pecan shells and hickory for four hours.

The next time you read about Pacific Coast salmon, smoked in alder for $40 a pound, just remember, Eastern Shore cobia and leftover pecan shells make for far better eating.

Lobster by the Pound

Who can forget the image of the rocky coast of Maine—waves crashing along the edges of the foggy spruce forests. A distant ship's horn sounds. Can't you just smell the lobster cooking with clams and mussels?

JoAnn had climbed Cadillac Mountain. Sally had finished her trail ride. Their goals for vacation were being fulfilled. I came to eat lobster, but no; Bar Harbor lobster restaurants with snooty waiters and big prices didn't suit me. We'll just drive a bit ...

There it is—Oak Point Lobster Pound (by the pound). Looking out at Western Bay into the Atlantic, full moon arising; this is going to be good. The steam pots are boiling, the worn wood tables are just waiting to hold our lobster feast.

"Yes, you can have a bigger lobster, but it's $5 more." The shoreman's dinner is a bowl of clam chowder, home made biscuits, coleslaw, two dozen Ipswich steamers, 1 dozen mussels, one 2½ lb. lobster for $24.95. Fresh blueberry pie is included.

There is no pretense in the place. Lots of good food and lots of laughs. This is what I wanted! Down home Pocomoke, meet Down East Maine!

I was only a little saddened that JoAnn couldn't finish her lobster tail; the claws were enough for her. I just had to eat her lobster too, no wasted food for us. Next week the diet starts!

The seafood here is steamed Down East style. It's plain; they don't use Old Bay or crab boil spices. The fresh lobster is so rich in flavor, coated with butter and lemon, who would ask for anything better?

JoAnn's lobster tail was just sitting there. I'm full—but I had just a little Old Bay in a baggie, with me. Mix the Old Bay in the butter and pour it all over the gorgeous lobster. Ahh, that's it, the missing piece! Now we're talking. The owner came over—"Mind if I try some?" The rest is in the eating.

Poached Salmon

When in Maine, eat lobster, mussels, clams and blueberry pie. When in New Brunswick, Canada, head for the local salmon house. The Miramichi River in New Brunswick is famous for its Atlantic salmon. Fresh caught salmon tastes very different from what arrives frozen in Pocomoke (and that usually comes from a commercial salmon fish farm).

Salmon can be prepared many ways. The difficulty in cooking salmon is that a 1-inch wide steak can be ½ inch thick on the sides and two inches thick on top. Broiling almost guarantees that some of the salmon will be either overcooked or undercooked. Baking can give the same result. Most of the restaurants we visited in New Brunswick offered poached salmon on the menu. At first I wondered if there were any legally harvested fish to be found.

Poaching is a cooking method similar to steaming except the water in your poacher is first brought to a boil, then the heat is reduced to simmer. After you place the fish on the rack, the moisture in the fish flesh is heated slowly; the meat cooks evenly. Steaming firm fleshed fish like salmon, boiling out the oils, would make the meat tough. Poaching gives a tender, juicy result.

Cut four 1-inch whole steaks perpendicular to the backbone. Do not fillet. Place the steaks on their sides, cover with slices of lemon, and poach slowly about 20 minutes.

Make a sauce by combining mayonnaise, sherry, tarragon, dry mustard and capers. Mix and place on top of the poacher lid to warm and let the flavors set up.

Go out into your backyard forest, (you are in New Brunswick now), and find the freshest ostrich fern patch that you can. Harvest only a few, 3-inch, young fern fronds, called fiddleheads. The spores have not developed and the fern is tender, like asparagus. Your fern patch is a renewable source of food, so use it wisely.

Sauté the fresh fiddlehead in butter with cilantro or chervil. Add to a thick white sauce *(see JoAnn's recipe)* with a dash of white wine and serve to a resounding silence. Fiddleheads? Ferns? After some brave soul says the soup tastes great you can finally relax. A 150-page fiddlehead cookbook was for sale in New Brunswick ($11.50). I didn't get it but I should have. The next time the same guests come over, serve them stringed fiddleheads. They will love them all over again.

Deli City Dinner

I have never had such a friend as Ed Fry and now he is gone. He was the first person I met in Pocomoke in 1979. "You're a doctor? You've got to be kidding." In 1981, he was my best man when JoAnn and I were married. In 1986 his heart "died" 36 times at a local hospital. At University of Pennsylvania, on the heart table, an experimental medicine corrected his conduction disturbance and kept his heart beating.

When he was paralyzed following back surgery, he told me he would beat me in a 25-foot walking race soon. True to his word, he later gave me first his wheel chair, then his crutches.

Did you ever eat at Ed's Deli City? His restaurant didn't have good ventilation, so we always smelled like fried onions and fried chicken after we left. His fried chicken was the best, but it was more fun to watch his staff make subs (no added charge for the extra protein), than it was even to eat the fried chicken. Ed, however, for all his knowledge of human behavior and his willingness to discuss philosophy, did not know how to make a good crab cake. If only he knew then what I have found out now about crab cakes (I wouldn't tell him my recipe even if he were still alive).

Ed laughed, years ago, at my request. "Please, Ed, sauté sweet red peppers, onions and tomato slices in butter." Remove from heat and mix in one pound of back fin crabmeat, shell removed. Add ground pepper, garlic, MSG, dill weed, cumin and toss with sesame oil. Put the loose mixture in a broiling pan and cover with Parmesan cheese. Spray lightly with olive oil. Broil 10 minutes or until done.

Tonight we had a Deli City dinner crab creation, French fries and all, in honor of Ed. The potatoes, skins on, soaked in vinegar, were cooked outside. These French fries take two paper towels to remove the extra oil. Around the outside of our house, it smells like Deli City.

Our Deli City meal, spiced with sadness and loss, brought back fond memories of Ed. JoAnn hugged me, wiped away my tears, and told me thoughts of Ed would remain with us; longer, I guess than the tastes of the delicious Deli City crab broil.

Eggplant Pocomoke

It has taken several years of composting and soil enrichment, but finally JoAnn's organic vegetable garden is producing well. She has found only a few harmful bugs including just one (tomato eating) hornworm. Organic gardeners have always said that insect pests are more attracted to stressed plants. Her care and the great soil ease everything's stress.

For my nickel, there are few tastes as good as a sun-warmed tomato, eaten right after picking. Eating a non-stressed tomato reduces my stress.

Eggplant isn't an easy vegetable to grow; bugs like it a lot. Poorly drained or too dry soils slow growth. It needs to be picked when it is small, just at the "high shine," as I thought I heard JoAnn call it.

Cooking eggplant follows the same rules as growing it: not too much liquid or too little either. I slice the eggplant ⅝-inch thick, too thin and the fruit falls apart and too thick the fruit soaks up too much oil and is soggy.

Coat slices with beaten egg, dip in seasoned flour and fry in safflower oil at medium high heat. Resist the temptation to turn the slices too soon; brown one side and then the other. When both sides are done, cover with homemade tomato sauce *(reviewed earlier)* or just use a commercial brand. Cover with Parmesan cheese, top with shredded mozzarella and simmer with the lid on. As the cheeses melt, remove from heat and let cool slightly. The cheese contains the only protein in this meal; add a little extra. This dish is only as good as the eggplant you use!

JoAnn's tomato basil salad, served on the side, is a summertime hit. Basil helps protect tomatoes, peppers and eggplant from insects and is, itself, a versatile spice. Pesto, made with basil, can keep for weeks refrigerated. Fresh basil, topped over sliced black olives and feta cheese bring both full early and late tastes to tomatoes cut into chunks. Make an Italian dressing to top this salad.

We served this meal with JoAnn's homemade French bread. This bread is full flavored and crusty; just dipping it in left over salad dressing made the meatless meal complete.

Okra and Improv Chicken

A long day in the office today—I don't have dinner planned. JoAnn is preparing for the new school year and Sally doesn't want to cook. She is afraid I'll write about it in my next newspaper column. When in doubt improvise, just like Jerry Garcia used to do.

OK, the boneless chicken breasts (remember $.99 a lb.) thaw quickly and will go well with fresh okra. Our ceramic broiling pan is ready. I see ads for expensive copper cookware, claiming without proof, to be better than ceramic. Our ceramic broiling pan will do well for this "Evening at the Improv."

Put four chicken breasts in the broiling pan and coat with melted butter. Bake with fresh rosemary for 10 minutes at 350 degrees. Remove from oven and surround the breasts with 1-inch cubes of leftover ham. Slice fresh Vidalia onions and yellow squash into 1½ inch by ½ inch long strips and place on the chicken, inside the ring of ham chunks. Spice with garlic, black pepper, marjoram and celery seed. Bake for 10 more minutes. Finally spread one can of cheddar cheese soup over the food, making a thick glaze. Bake for 40 minutes.

I used Vidalia onions, fresh from the garden. They are sweet, but when I ate one like an apple, JoAnn wouldn't kiss me for an hour.

While the surprise chicken is baking, cut the fruits of 3 garden rows of okra, beautiful, tender 4 inch-long fresh burgundy okra, into ½ inch-long pieces. This is a Carolina recipe; we would never use Clemson spineless (that's its name!) okra. Seal the okra pieces in a self-closing bag after adding a pinch of salt, black pepper, ground thyme and coriander. Add ¼ cup cornmeal and shake well. The cut ends of the okra should be dusted well with cornmeal. If not, add more cornmeal and shake again.

Heat corn oil in a 12-inch frying pan. Add the okra and sear the sweet-tasting vegetable so it doesn't turn to gummy gumbo. Taste the okra frequently while it is cooking in the pan "just to be sure it's edible." Usually there is very little okra left to serve after all the taste testing is done.

Even though Jerry Garcia wasn't around to enjoy this culinary riff, it tasted wonderful, for which we all were grateful.

Peking Duck

This crisp early morning sunrise is so invigorating. The first fall mist rises from the ponds as the air warms. The intense whiteness of the pekin ducks on the pond is cast as an almost perfect reflection.

How could anyone think of eating ducks such as these? Ducks have been domesticated as a food source since ancient times. Ducks are efficient predators of small insects, tiny toads, ticks and snails as well as being foragers of plants. They cost less to feed than chickens, but somehow chickens get the credit for being cheap to feed.

Because I love our pekins, our Peking duck dinner will be a duck fresh from the grocery freezer. The first time I made Peking duck, I was sure I would give everyone Salmonella food poisoning, but it didn't happen.

The Chinese use duck in many dishes, but Peking duck is a classic. This dish is usually served with thin pancakes and rich plum sauce. There is a great deal of time spent in preparation of the duck for such a small amount of meat to eat. Getting there is most of the fun in cooking.

Thaw the duck in the refrigerator, then remove the giblets and whatever else is stuffed in the duck. Rinse well; immerse in a large pot of boiling water. Turn frequently for 15 minutes to melt away most of the abundant duck fat. Remove from the pot, and truss up the duck with sturdy cord to drip-dry. Baste the drying duck with honey, inside and out. Let it drip dry again. Baste again and again.

I made a rack inside the refrigerator to catch the drippings from the duck. Always baste with fresh honey; don't recycle the old drippings! I did enjoy the creative comments made by those who opened the refrigerator, only to be greeted by the duck, which was hung securely where the meat should be.

After two days the duck should be glazed and dried properly. Preheat the oven to 375 degrees. Place the duck in a large roasting pan and bake until the skin is crackly crisp. In a Chinese restaurant, Peking duck is a truly elegant course in a large meal. Our meal was small but delicious. The dark duck meat had absorbed the honey flavor and didn't taste like bugs, snails or plants at all. Best of all, our pekins still looked pretty on the pond.

Raw Oysters, Sauces and All

What do you do on a cold, cabin fever day just like today? With snow on the way, my activity options are double digging the vegetable garden or staying warm in the kitchen, eating oysters. The garden will wait until later. The kitchen is inviting now.

Oysters are just about a perfect food. All non-moving shellfish, including scallops, clams and oysters, are low in cholesterol and saturated fat. The oyster protein is low in the particular amino acids thought by many experts to be harmful. Best of all, oysters can be eaten in so many ways.

The basic problem with oysters, though, is what to put on the formless creatures to give them interesting tastes. Let's face it, oysters don't have a lot of unique taste. If I could find true salt oysters (tasty, tasty) for sale, that would help, but the "salt" oysters for sale now, I suspect, grew up in the Chesapeake Bay and took a recent vacation to the saltier waters of Chincoteague.

You have to make good sauces to really enjoy raw oysters. Cocktail sauce, like barbecue sauce, comes in all degrees of heat. Take a full bodied ketchup and fill a cereal bowl half full. Add three heaping tsp. of a prepared hot horseradish (don't use the horseradish spread) and one tsp. of concentrated lemon juice. Add two pinches of paprika, one twist of black pepper, garlic and ground bay leaf. Stir well; the sauce needs time to chill and to set the flavors. I like Tabasco sauce in my sauce but many people don't, so it's optional.

Now make sauce #2 and #3. Start with one stick of butter, not margarine; melt without boiling. Add garlic, whole thyme, celery seed, black pepper and fenugreek in equal amounts. To make a lemon sauce add 3 tsp. lemon juice (adjust to your taste) and simmer 5 minutes.

To make a "wood" sauce (I have told you about this sauce before) use the above basic butter melt but add 3 tsp. soy sauce instead of lemon and add 2 tsp. ground ginger instead of fenugreek.

Dunk the drained, raw oysters into whichever sauce you want. After a few rounds, you'll begin to appreciate the subtle oyster taste. When that appreciation begins, who needs the sauces? Bring on another dozen fresh-shucked oysters!

By the way, save your oyster shells. You will need them to make Oysters Rockefeller.

Veal, the Crippled Calf

Every week I find some "special, low priced" items in the local grocery store. The secret in cost-effective shopping isn't collecting coupons—it's the old estate auction idea. "You can always find a bargain overlooked." Today, it was Portabella mushroom caps at $4 a pound. These large open gilled dark mushrooms are a gourmet's delight. Just a few caps give any meat dish a special, buttery, late taste.

These Portabellas will go great with the veal slices, which were also a bargain today. Veal is normally rather expensive. A local butcher said the price has gone up around here even more, in part, because local cardiologists now recommend veal as a meat that is low in fat as an alternative to beef. Does that mean that veal isn't beef?

The farmer next door used to raise veal. He would select the calf with the worst hips or back problems in the herd and would confine it in a stall where the crippled calf couldn't move. Calves, like people, have to be active to avoid constipation. The farmer found out not to plug up the poor calf using alfalfa as feed, and he did have plenty of extra milk to use as food. Maybe that's why veal now means a milk-fed, regular calf.

So many expensive dishes in restaurants feature veal. Veal cutlet, veal scallopini, and veal Marsala all call for coating this tender meat with flour or breading. I don't understand why cooks use so much breading, except to make us a fatted calf, too.

Veal doesn't have the same thickness of connective tissue outside the individual muscle groups because the poor calf isn't allowed to move enough to develop its sinews. Doesn't that idea bother you a little bit? What hormones are put into that baby cow to make it grow so quickly? If we eat it, will we get some bizarre hormone effects?

Maybe, but at least I'll die eating. Take one pound, inexpensive, thin sliced veal. Marinate 2 hours in the liquid from a jar of artichoke hearts or your own olive oil vinaigrette. Slice 8 ounces of Portabella mushrooms ⅜" thick and sauté one minute in butter with sliced artichoke hearts, coriander and a dash of garlic. Remove from your pan; add the marinated veal slices and ¼" thick green rounds of fresh leeks. Cook on medium heat, adding basil, black pepper, 2 tsp. concentrated lemon juice and a splash of white wine. Stir gently as the veal browns. Add back the mushrooms and toss in more artichoke hearts. Add powdered arrowroot, stirring well, to make a gravy. Veal Pocomoke without the breading. Delicious!

Hot Rod Baguettes

The origins of words, studied by etymologists, give us information about our past. Of course we need to remember the lessons of history but eating fresh baguettes, chewy French country bread loaves, with thick slices of sharp cheese, helps me forget the stresses of today. I'm going to ignore the fact that wheat flour is full of amylose, the plant starch that I wear too abundantly. What are a few pounds among friends?

Baguettes, tall and skinny crackle-crusted French loaves, get their name from "slender rod." I hope my recipe now doesn't result in bread that tastes like a slender piece of rebar!

What a wonder is bread. Just imagine, by simply mixing water, salt, yeast and yeast food (flour) we end up with dough. And then, when the dough is cooked, we have bread. JoAnn makes so many kinds of great tasting and great smelling bread. Don't you, too, have fond memories of the smell of freshly baking bread? Sally is getting her bread-smell memory banks filled now.

Baguette loaves have special baking requirements. You will need to use a baguette loaf pan. If you don't have one, just use your fish poacher or line a roasting pan in halves with foil. The baguette cooking idea becomes simpler if you can use a food processor to mix the dough. We don't have one so it was knead and knead;

anyone who helps out becomes a friend in knead indeed (Tom Sawyer—hat in hand).

Take 4 cups unbleached all-purpose flour, 2 tsp. salt, 2 tsp. SAF instant yeast, not rapid-rise (found in cake form in Poco-moke), and mix well. Slowly add 14 ounces ice water (not 15 oz., not 13 oz.) stirring frequently or with your processor running. After a minute, dough of even consistency will appear, almost by magic. Remember the piecrust idea and ice water? Let the yeast work five minutes, mix vigorously one more minute and set aside for at least six hours, in a warm place. Cover your dough with plastic wrap so the dog hair doesn't get into it.

Cooking the bread requires a plant mister, a 425-degree oven, parchment paper and an understanding spouse. You are doing what? The wet dough has risen immensely. Cut it into even pieces (3 or 4) and roll on a floured surface. Flatten and fold in half. Shape the dough into an evenly plump but slender rod shape. Use plenty of flour!

Now put the loaves onto parchment paper and into the hot oven. Quickly mist the sidewalls of the oven with water (not the bread) and close the door. Hurry, this sudden sauna blast of steam is the key to the baking technique and makes the crust crackly after it has baked 25 minutes. The inside is chewy and is just so good.

Happily, the oven didn't blow up with this experiment. The bread didn't last though; no leftovers. I'm sorry to say no puns on "bag it" were allowed today. After I lose my extra weight, I'm going to try this recipe again.

No-Amylose Breakfast

So what's for breakfast? If you eliminate amylose, the readily worn wheat starch, you also eliminate toast, biscuits, muffins, dough-nuts, bagels, popovers, cereals, pancakes, waffles and crumpets too. "But I like toast," you say. Of course you do and it looks good on you, right there on your hips.

My sister Ellen is visiting us this week. She can play anything on the piano (without sheet music!) and cook anything in the kitchen. Think about your friends who traveled to Mexico. What did they eat for breakfast? Fruit and protein usually, and lots of it. In Mexico, breakfasts are lavishly prepared and eaten at a leisurely pace. In the U.S., we are in such a hurry; a good breakfast is unusual.

Living in San Miguel, Mexico, means she has no big supermarkets nearby but fresh fruit is available year round. Living here, we think that eating fresh fruit, when visiting Mexico, will give us diarrhea, and it can if not washed. Guess what—the reverse is true, too. Be sure to wash your grapes from Chile, your strawberries from California and your avocados from Florida before serving your beloved sister from San Miguel. Please be sure to wash your hands wherever you are.

So what is for breakfast? New Zealand Kiwis are four for a dollar. Peel and slice ¼ thick to show off the green fruit with its distinctive black seeds. Slice fresh giant Fresno strawberries lengthwise saving the hearts (the cook gets to eat the edges!). Cut two fresh Arizona cantaloupes into ¼" boat-shaped slices. Next take a heart-shaped cookie cutter and trim a Mexican watermelon (yes, wash it too) into red Valentines. Next open and thaw a frozen container of North Carolina raspberries. Finally slice a Hawaiian pineapple into 2" strips. Ahh yes, fresh "local" fruit is pleasing to your eye.

Arrange the fruit, respecting color, shape, and thickness. Perhaps you will like pineapple slices inside of the cantaloupe boats, with an inner border of kiwi alternating with strawberries. Top with melon hearts and finally with raspberries.

This breakfast is so beautiful, but by the time you can take a picture, oops, its lunch time. Now what's for lunch?

First take some Florida avocados and ...

377

Oven Wedge Potatoes

With so many vegetables to choose from that grow above the ground, why do restaurants serve so many potatoes? French fries or baked potato with your chicken tonight? Before you answer, consider the alternatives—applesauce (an excellent vegetable choice?) or macaroni and cheese. I prefer the fresh macaroni myself. Unlike spaghetti squash, which has a typical squash vine, the macaroni plant has small white flowers, thrives in full sun and is drought hardy. Yes, the macaroni plant is valuable, if you can find one.

No wonder we eat potatoes with our restaurant meals.

Potatoes, like all roots, store sugar for the plant in the form of complex carbohydrate called amylose. While a beautiful fresh red potato doesn't have a lot of calories, the few calories in the potato often are stored nicely around belt lines, hips, ribs and chins. Potatoes sure taste good though. Do you know someone who is a meat and potato man? Is he too heavy? The problem isn't the meat—it is the potatoes.

Potatoes are so varied in size, shape, texture and use in cooking. Hands down, russet potatoes are the best for frying. New potatoes are the best for potato salad. Oversized, Idaho potatoes are best as baked potatoes. To cut down the baking time, most restaurants will parboil Idaho potatoes and then bake them, serving them in tin foil. I prefer to leave the tin foil in the box, bake the potato slowly and treasure the result of taking time to cook the fabulous potato properly.

Tonight, we are ready for oven baked potato slices. We will have marinated top round steak cooked on the grill (sliced thin), spinach salad and strawberries to accompany the prized oven baked potatoes. Take fresh red potatoes from the bin (don't pick up a bagful!). Wash well and dry. Cut lengthwise once and again into long quarters. Coat lightly with canola oil (safflower will do). Toss in an oven-roasting pan. Sprinkle with salt, just a little, add garlic powder and fresh ground black pepper. Turn frequently to make sure the spices are evenly spread and the wedges are oiled. Cook at 350 degrees for 60 minutes. Be sure to turn the cooking slices frequently so the wedges are browned on all sides.

Just before serving, remove the pan and turn the oven to broil. Spray the browned potatoes (not in the oven!) with cooking oil and sprinkle with fresh ground coriander and summer savory. Broil for three minutes and serve tongue-burning hot. These potatoes are so good that you can eat an extra portion tonight with a diet to follow tomorrow.

Nature Food

Today is the day. I'm shopping for lunch outside. I'm not Euell Gibbons, but I too have learned that nature provides a bounty of tasty vegetables for us in the form of flowers and petals. One caution: while it is true that the purple blossoms of the royal paulownia taste like toasted wild hickory nuts, leave them alone please. Eat your flowers but only if you know they are safe to eat and abundant.

The high bush blueberries have four spring spans of blooming. Jersey and Blueray are blooming now. Carefully pull off a blossom (before the fruit is set), and pull off the green leaves at the bottom. Ready? Taste it. It has a spicy blueberry flavor! Now, move on to the day lilies. Leave the Stella d'Oro alone. Find the fullest tiger lily you have along your wildlife border. Just before the lily opens, it is perfect for a quick sauté in butter. Even better, toss slices with your herbal vinegar, mung bean sprouts, fresh Brussels sprout slices and artichoke hearts. Your out-of-town guests won't forget this salad. They even will call you Euell Gibbons if they don't know better.

Dandelions and I don't get along. No, they grow beautifully for us, that's not it. I just don't like the taste of the greens. Let someone else say they are great in a salad but I'll take watercress any time as an alternative.

Violets are famous for their role in weight loss. An alkaloid in the fresh petal suppresses the hunger center in the brain. Perhaps this is where the shrinking violet idea got started. Don't eat the corms of the violet though. They are a powerful purgative and can cause severe diarrhea.

Find some fresh yellow squash plants. It is easy to identify the male and female flowers. The male flowers are longer, without any setting fruit. Look for a few days until you know which is which. Go ahead, try one. The male flower tastes like fresh squash without the seeds! Tired of all this fresh food? Make a tempura using male squash blossoms. Bet you can eat at least one!

Later this year, we will harvest nasturtium leaves and blossoms as well as calendula petals to garnish adventurous salads. These don't taste like wild hickory nuts!

No, don't eat the daisies, foxglove, Oriental poppies, jimson-weed, monkshood or morning glories. Like the Death Angel mushrooms, if you don't know for sure what they are, don't eat!

If you are really feeling adventurous, harvest some rugosa rose hips … on second thought, I'll buy the herbal tea in a store.

A special thanks to my mother, Sara Shoemaker, on this Mother's Day. She has written and illustrated her own book on edible and poisonous plants. She has encouraged me all of my life to learn more about our world, for which I will always be grateful.

Herbal Vinegar

Today, I think I've seen my best wine tasting. An oenophile carefully sniffed the bottom of a cork, swished his red wine in a handsome glass, smelled again and sipped. "Waiter, this wine tastes like vinegar!" The waiter replied, "Ah, yes, sir, but this vinegar has just a hint of vanilla, raspberries in June and a subtle oak aftertaste."

Louis Pasteur would have frowned. It was Pasteur who made vaccines for anthrax, rabies and Newcastle Disease, and showed how to kill bacteria by heating. For the wine lover, he is best remembered for defining fermentation and saving the wine industry from dastardly, vinegar-producing bacteria.

Yeast can use sugars of many kinds for fuel. The byproduct of yeast activity is carbon dioxide and ethyl alcohol. If the fermentation takes place without oxygen and if the yeasts have no competition for the sugar, all is well. Adding oxygen to the fermentation vat gives bacteria a chance to grow, despite the yeasts and results in the contaminating bacteria making vinegar.

Louis Pasteur simply told the French to put a cork on their vats of wine if they wanted wine and not vinegar. Good advice I'd say.

One of my octogenarian patients would rather have the vinegar than wine. He is adamant that vinegar purifies his body without creating a sour disposition. Vinegar is commonly used in our household for salad dressing. Mixed with oil and spices, our oil and vinegar dressings have no corn syrup and aren't fattening. Someone please find me a bottle of commercial salad dressing that doesn't have sugar, corn syrup or maltodextrin in it!

In Vermont, dairy farmers feed their cows (and themselves), a mixture of honey and apple cider vinegar called switzel. It heals mastitis, helps prevent cankers, and aids digestion. While another acid-based liquid, cranberry juice, has an undeservedly good reputation for helping to prevent urinary tract infections, vinegar delivers much more acid to the urine, giving a better bacterioprotective effect. Switzel helps many health problems.

Just for fun, wash an empty wine bottle well. Leave no soap! Heat a wine bottle volume of red wine vinegar to near boiling for 5 minutes. Heating will evaporate the minute amounts of acetone and butyric acid which always contaminate commercial vinegar. Put fresh, washed and dried rosemary, oregano or thyme leaves into the wine bottle with dill seed, whole mustard, and garlic powder. Fill the wine bottle nearly to the top with the hot

381

vinegar (a little air is OK), and stopper with the top of a wine cork down. Shake frequently while the herbal vinegar cools.

After two days, place on a cabinet shelf to age for two weeks. Purists will want their herbal vinegar drained; I like to hear "what are those little green things?" so I leave the herbs in the bottle. Just mix with oil and, "Voila! Instant Vinaigrette." This vinegar will not ferment; it is safe to use for months. It tastes so good though, it won't last very long.

Ice-Cold Beef Stew

If you live on the U.S. East Coast, when did you last have to turn on the heat in your house after Memorial Day? We did today. It is 53 degrees outside, with windblown rain that chased every picnic indoors.

We'll eat beef stew tonight in honor of my longtime friend, DNA paleobiochemist, Elmer Cogan. He died of exposure, not long ago when he was looking for frozen biologic specimens on Mount Everest. If only his favorite food had been there, he might be alive today.

We all know JoAnn's pressure-cooker beef stew is the best, but I wanted to try to cook stew tonight. Leftover roast beef, the last bit of grilled steak and one-week-old sliced London broil will have new life. Into a large pot they go, sliced into about 1 ¼" cubes. I could have used bottom round roast or chuck roast instead of leftovers.

Slice red potatoes into 1½" chunks along with 2" long slices of carrots. I just wash the root vegetables; peeling away the skins won't make me healthier. Just washing off the dirt is enough.

Slice two fresh onions and add to the pot, which now has two pounds of meat, 1 pound each of potatoes and carrots. Add 1 can of tomato sauce and three good squirts of ketchup. Add a six-inch sprig of rosemary from the garden along with 1 tsp. fennel, 1 tsp. dry mustard and four grinds of black pepper. Add three quarts of water and bring to a boil. Reduce heat and simmer, covered, for three hours. Stir frequently. Add water as needed.

While carrots, potatoes and onions all have amylose; the prolonged heating reduces the starch to a lower glycemic index food. Please don't ask me for details of why this is; it is true in the same sense that Mount Everest is and that Elmer Cogan isn't.

As the stew stewed, I was without astute observations. How did someone find out how to overcook tough meat with crunchy root vegetables, add a sauce and make a great, heart-warming supper for a chilly day? Sounds like desperation cooking to me.

No matter, a stew means a bubbling, boiling, turmoil and troubling ferment of juices. I often wanted to analyze a beef stew that had cooked long enough, just to see if it had elements of the primordial stew which evolutionists agree is the source of life. Any new DNA in the bottom of the pot?

For today, the rich tomato-based taste of soft carrots, potatoes and strings of meat will calm my turmoils and my bubblings as I ponder the meaning and origin of life.

I won't climb Mount Everest, but I will miss Elmer always.

Sesame Shrimp

Have you figured out why most of the employed chefs in the U.S. are men? In the average household, women do most of the cooking, no matter how many people there work for pay. Something doesn't seem right about the gender discrepancy of the paid labor force and the unpaid labor force.

In our home, everyday cooking duties are shared equally, depending on who gets home first. I would be curious to find out if everyday home-style restaurants had more women for cooks than so called elite, gourmet restaurants.

Who has time to cook these days? It seems that only someone who is paid to use the time to cook will do so. We use a lot of marinades to solve the problem of no time to cook and what to cook.

Marinades make the most sense for BBQ cooking. Any meat cooked at grill temperatures can easily be dried out. A marinade gives meat a unique flavor, in addition to maintaining moisture in meat either on a grill or in your oven.

Sesame shrimp is a great example of a marinade protecting and flavoring meat. Take two pounds of jumbo shrimp (yes, an oxymoron), peel and place in a container. Cover with 2 ounces sesame oil and add 2 tbs. of concentrated lemon juice. Add 2 tbs. ginger, 2 ounces soy sauce, 1 tsp. garlic, 1 tsp. of ground star anise and two ounces of dry sherry. Stir well.

Most marinades are either acid (lemon or vinegar) or have highly concentrated amounts of solute in the solvent. The chemistry of the marinade stops bacteria from growing, avoiding spoilage. Honey is a concentrated solution of glucose (not a waitress in a family restaurant). Honey will not spoil.

Put the marinating sesame shrimp in the refrigerator. Add 3 tbs. of sesame seed if you have them, but don't make a special trip to the grocery store if you don't.

Depending on who has time, two or three days later, heat a wok, cast iron pan, or curved frying pan to high temp. Add peanut oil and coat the cooking surface. Add a dash of garlic, ginger and scallions to season the pan.

Now put the drained shrimp in and stirfry as quickly as you can. The acidic, oil-based marinade coats the shrimp almost like a batter. Stirfry two or three minutes. Supper time!

As I grow older, time has become my most precious concern. This meal was prepared when I had time and served when we didn't. It didn't matter who cooked the sesame shrimp. Thanks to the marinade, we all had time to enjoy the great taste.

Mint Mango Heat Beater

So now it's fresh mangoes and tropical weather. Seasonal changes bring change in eating location (outside), eating methods (grilling), and foods eaten. The produce stands are full of southern speaking tomatoes and northern speaking tourists. Our tomatoes are still green.

When it's this hot, mashed potatoes become potato salad, and baked chicken becomes a bucket of fried (get two!) chicken. Let's go to the beach!

Jonathan Winters used to make jokes about the "hot sweaty women out in the kitchen." Here, it's hot enough. We will eat fresh fruit, vegetables and grilled food outside. It is time for sister Ellen's mint mango heat beater.

The mango tree is from Asia. The word has strikingly similar roots in the languages of subtropical India and the Malay Archipelago. Apparently the Portuguese brought the fruit to Florida. The fruit gets sweeter after it is picked; the tough rind protected the fruit on ocean voyages. It provides vitamin C too. If the English knew about mangoes, would they still have used limes to prevent scurvy? Limeys could have become mangeys.

Find a firm fruit with red in the rind. Set in a sunny window for a week, softening, the rind will soften. Peel and cut into the slippery fruit. Who knows where the seed begins? This fruit is not freestone at all.

To make a mint mango refresher, first work up a sweat outside. Take three fresh mint sprigs (any kind of mint will do), two green onions and one chilled tomato. Mince and mix with diced mango slices. Served chilled with corn chips or as a side dish. Cool!

To start off your 90 degree, 90% humidity day, have a mango breakfast freeze. Take two cups of yogurt, 1 tsp. vanilla, ¾ cup chilled orange juice (fresh squeezed is better), 1 mango, peeled and cubed, 1 tsp. lime juice, 1 tbs. honey and two cups ice. Put in a blender and run until smooth. Serve in a chilled glass.

It is so peaceful on this longest day of the year. The mint mango has taken the heat of the night away even before it arrives.

I hope my skin isn't allergic to mango juice. In this book of word origins, I just found out that mango means rash in Java!

Women's Cholesterol (Niacin and Garlic)

If a little is good, a little more is better, right? Give him an inch and he will take a mile. One per customer, not one handful.

The NCEP, a blue ribbon expert panel of physicians, reviewed what was known about cholesterol and heart attack in 1987. Cholesterol levels over 240 were well correlated with an increased risk of heart attack in the study populations.

The panel recommended however that to decrease risk, our cholesterol levels should be under 200! What? Even worse, the cholesterol recommendations were meant to apply to everybody even though the patients studied were white males ages 40 to 65 only. What should a 66 year old Asian woman's cholesterol be? Does anyone know for sure? Let's not guess now, cholesterol lowering medication can cost well over $250 a month.

It turns out the women's cholesterol treatment discussion, with one exception, is based on a physician's best guess. Where is the science? Let us not rush to judgment based on a policy that is founded on quicksand.

We know that ladies with high lipoprotein a, Lp(a), levels are at incredibly high risk for heart attack. Lp(a) is a bad actor with two arms that functionally link oxidized (bad) LDL cholesterol to platelets, forming a blockage in an artery. Estrogen lowers Lp(a). Maybe that is part of the reason why women have fewer heart attacks than men until menopause begins.

Niacin (vitamin B3) also lowers Lp(a), but only in mega doses. If a little is good, take a little more? You need to take a lot to prevent heart disease. A lot of niacin gives a lot of side effects like flushing, stomach pain, itchy skin and bad breath.

Take an aspirin to prevent most of the niacin side effects now and drop five crystalline niacin tablets into a glass of juice. You will drink this in 30 minutes. Your main dish will have some garlic, since garlic has chemicals in it that the body uses to make niacin.

Saute Vidalia onion slices in butter with two tablespoons of garlic. Add chopped green peppers, mushroom caps, chopped artichoke hearts, and small pitted black olives. Season with a little more garlic, black pepper, cilantro and just a pinch more of garlic. Stir well making sure that the garlic and onion tastes penetrate the interesting vegetable mixture. Reduce heat. Cook thirty minutes, long enough for everyone within a mile to smell your garlic. Top with red hot chili paste and serve to a group of niacin takers.

Now drink your crystalline niacin light and enjoy your marvelous garlic goop. You'll sleep better knowing that your blood vessels are clear, that the facial flushing is from the chili paste and your breath is just garlicky, nothing more.

But you will sleep alone.

Women's Cholesterol Week 2

Instead of trying to eat enough food to satisfy your daily requirements for vitamins and minerals, most people will take a pill, sometimes a lot of pills. Most people who take vitamins don't just take one of one kind. Vitamins seemingly like compnay in your stomach, so vitamins E and C are usually mixed with some combination of spartalina, gingko, garlic, bee pollen, zinc, vitamin B12 ... the possible combinations are endless.

The "if a little is good, a lot is better," idea doesn't always work for vitamins. Some become toxic at higher doses, others can cause constipation, kidney stones, headache and liver disease.

Niacin is a good guy for your cholesterol, remember it lowers Lp(a) in addition to lowering total cholesterol and raising HDL.

It is easy to pick out the mega-niacin doser though. He is the one with clean as a whistle arteries, and red, scratched skin, who is holding his stomach in pain while he sits all alone in a corner. His niacin makes his skin flush and itch terribly, burns small holes in his stomach and gives him the worst breath this side of elephant garlic. Halitosis is sweet baby's breath compared to the breath of the niacin man.

Niacin pill manufactures have tried just about everything to make the side effects of megadose therapy tolerable. Long acting pills, combo pills, enteric coated pills and now finally a crystalline form. Fortunately, observant patients have told their doctors that niacin is in a variety of foods including protein, grains, especially corn, and in some green leafy vegetables like spinach and zucchini. The highest levels of niacin, also called nicotinic acid, are found in tobacco. No, I'm not suggesting cooking with tobacco to avoid a heart attack.

Slice a fresh 6" zucchini lengthwise, sprinkle with fresh grated Parmesan cheese, top with ground black pepper and melted lemon butter. Bake at 350 degrees for 10 minutes. Yum. Now eat 15 more pounds of the great green taste of heart healthy, niacin-laced zucchini.

Of course you could take two pounds of tryptophan tables or eat ten pounds of meat to get the same amount of niacin.

So despite the possible benefits of niacin to help women's cholesterol and Lp(a) we just don't have much choice. Dietary sources of niacin and pills both aren't going to be a great idea.

I guess we will just have to keep on pushing estrogen to lower Lp(a), with bleeding problems and cancer fears as a garnish.

Now if we just had an estrogen pill that didn't have estrogen drawbacks ...

Avocado Dip

The secret to eating well starts with eating fresh. Yes, you can add sauces, flavors and unusual accompaniments to create a dish that sounds good, but making something taste good leaves no room for stale, flat, or soggy ingredients. I suggest you shop the perimeter of the grocery store. Fresh will usually be better than canned or frozen.

Even the big grocery stores around here often don't have affordable and attractive produce. There usually is some bargain though. JoAnn found California avocados at a great price recently. They have been sitting in the window where last week's mango was, softening, for JoAnn's acclaimed tortilla chip taco dip.

I have two prized T-shirts that now have salsa stains on them. If you stick a tortilla chip into salsa, how come it drips all over you before you can eat it? Maybe I need some salsa glue.

This avocado is just perfect. The skin almost jumps off it. The flesh pulls away from the seed but it sticks to everything. Not another T-shirt! Does avocado wash out? Maybe that is what guacamole means in Spanish. Salsa glue.

This avocado is now perfectly ripened, too. Cut in half, leaving the skin on. Flip out the seed and push the flesh onto a wire cookie rack. Rub back and forth. The avocado comes off easily, filling your bowl, not your shirt. Throw the cleaned skin into the compost. No mess, no hard clean up.

Blend in a mixer, 3 ripe, rubbed avocados, ¾ cup sour cream (not low fat), 8 ounces of real cream cheese and 2 tbs. lemon juice. Please, never use low fat cheese products if you want taste or weight loss. The manufacturer took out the milk fat, which sounds like a good idea. The idea was ruined, though, by substituting corn syrup for the fat. Instant sugar!! Believe it or not, the corn syrup is worse for a weight problem and for a cholesterol problem than the milk fat.

The avocado-cheese-sour cream mixture forms a 1" thick base for a large dish. Begin covering with cut-up vegies of your choice. JoAnn used shredded lettuce, minced mushroom caps, tomatoes, black olives, fresh Texas sweet onion from the garden (move over Vidalia), and small chunks of green pepper.

The whole dip was layered with shredded cheddar cheese and topped off with medium salsa.

Now the taste test. Ahh, exquisite fresh tastes. Now the T-shirt test. Dive a chip in from the side. Get a nice center of dip with goodies. Easy on the way up ... Victory! The T-shirt stays clean.

What a combination—great fresh eating and easy clean up.

Oat Bran Muffins

If you have eaten good food in Chincoteague lately, you probably have eaten something Mindy Howard made. She does specialty cooking, too, for diabetic patients, those with celiac disease and for those people who can't tolerate gluten. When it came time for Mindy to have a special diet, don't you know she started creating her own recipes right away.

Did you ever see what happens to a diabetic's blood sugar when he eats oatmeal? The sugar level skyrockets! Oats are supposed to be good for you! Just ask the American Diabetes Association.

Oat bran has a reputation for being healthy to eat, too. If what you want is insoluble fiber to help diverticulosis, oat bran fills the bill. Beyond that, there isn't a whole lot of what you need in oats. Unfortunately, by the time a commercial manufacturer gets done adding things to oat bran (such as sugar and starch), even the fiber benefits are reduced.

Fresh oat bran muffins sure taste good. Let's have some of Mindy's sugarless oat bran muffins knowing that the muffins are a good way to start eating healthy. Let's not give too much credit to oats though.

Recipes

Take two cups uncooked oat bran, mix in 2 tsp. baking powder, ½ tsp. salt, 1 cup skim milk, 2 eggs, 2 tbs. vegetable oil and 4–6 oz mixed fruit. Puree the fruit, skim milk and egg whites in food processor. Add fruit and 2 tbs. oil to the dry mix. Stir until all dry ingredients are moistened. Bake in muffin cups at 425 degrees for 15 minutes. Mindy says that the muffins stay soft on top, so taste one to see if it is done.

If oat bran had any significant amount of soluble fiber, it would help lower cholesterol at breakfast time. It doesn't, of course, but by eating Mindy's muffins you might avoid eating scrapple, fatty sausage or bacon on the side. That switch might lower your cholesterol.

Thanks Mindy! Congratulations on fixing a health problem by changing your diet.

Pecan Pie

George Washington Carver developed over 150 different foodstuffs made from peanuts. From peanut oil to peanut butter, the inexpensive, nutrient-rich peanut was made into just about anything by Dr. Carver. Peanuts have amylose, though, so I avoid them. What about cooking with nuts that grow on trees? They don't have any amylose.

Pistachios are now available in commercial quantities in the U.S. The pistachio nut is eaten whole or is ground into an additive for ice cream. Last year, I made a pesto sauce from pistachios but I don't see too many recipes calling for cooked pistachios. Shishkebob pistachios?

The same holds true for walnuts, cashews and pecans too. These nuts are all good for us, but aside from desserts, the nuts aren't used much in cooking.

Almonds are easier to work with. They slice, won't crumble easily, hold their texture well at high heat and provide a satisfying late taste.

I have made almond chicken as well as stir-fried pork with cashews in the past, hoping to obtain a nut flavor complementing a meat texture. More work is necessary; those recipes aren't ready for publication. Fresh green beans, steamed with mushrooms, served with sliced almonds and sesame oil is one of my favorite nut recipes.

The genius of Dr. Carver becomes clearer to me as I have tried different nut recipes. For now, rather than trying to be creative, let's blow any weight loss for this week and eat pecan pie. Both JoAnn and my mother make great pecan pie, their recipes are similar.

Beat together three whole eggs, ⅔ cup of sugar, ½ tsp. salt, ⅓ cup melted butter (not margarine), 1 cup corn syrup, whether light or dark your pie will change color but not taste. Add 1 cup pecan halves and mix lightly. Pour into pastry lined 9" pie pan. Bake at 375 degrees about 50 minutes. Yum! Cholesterol and sugar, take a hike.

Summary

One reviewer of the manuscript for this book looked at me with some concern saying that I had attacked about every sacred cow there is in nutrition. I am sure that my opinions and experiences will be greeted with skepticism by many, especially those who have accepted the popular misconceptions about weight loss, cholesterol, exercise, gout, high blood pressure, fiber and maintenance of weight loss without question and without fact.

I only ask that individuals interested in losing weight and maintaining weight loss, give this program a trial of two to three months. After an initial phase of trying ideas and eating without amylose, it is gratifying to see how many people come to recognize that eating lots of plant starch is not a good idea. Individuals who lose weight and then maintain weight loss usually will lower their cholesterol to genetically predetermined levels. Medication should be used only once an individual is at proper weight.

Exercise remains important for quality of life. Exercise is relaxing, refreshing, and mentally invigorating. It is not a panacea however; it is a part of daily hygiene. If you don't have time to exercise, you can still lose weight by using my No-Amylose Diet. Exercise is fun, don't be tortured by some machine or exercise program that hurts you, thinking you can lose weight by exercising.

One of my colleagues, a dietitian, looked at this manuscript and threw it down on my desk saying, "I don't believe this." I simply suggested that she try it. She commented that if my suggestions were as well accepted by patients who are not in my practice as they are in Pocomoke, that she would be out of a job. That's right. We would not need exchanges for a diabetic, low fat for a heart patient, amino acid supplementation for an athlete or ridiculous diets for the overweight. What we would need is common sense. Eat what tastes good, eat well, eat regularly and don't eat the foods that you wear.

The fundamental principle in this diet remains unchanged. The important feature is not the calories that you take in; it is the calories that you store. As Aldous Huxley has stated, the key to understanding is eliminating false knowledge. To that end my diet plan remains true.

Appendix #1

THE NO-AMYLOSE DIET (00-2-3)

No skipping meals, the starvation response burns protein

Adequate protein: 6–8 ounces final cooked weight

    Note: This diet is high carbohydrate and high protein

Lactose (milk) and fructose (fruit) [OK]

Learn the differences among carbohydrates

Artificial sweeteners [OK]

Avoid:

Glucose ... It may be disguised as dextrose and sucrose

Amylose ... You must learn this simple, short list, too
Bananas: the only forbidden fruit

Avoid all foods that grow beneath ground
(only onions and garlic [OK])

The cereal grains are the biggest problem foods: wheat, rice, oats, barley and rye (corn has a natural inhibitor of amylase—it's OK!)

No low-fat corn syrup or maltodextrin (hidden sugars)

Be careful with cheeses and yogurt: fat counts

Spices and condiments [OK]

Popcorn and baked corn chips [OK]; tortilla chips always safe corn chips may have sugar in spicy coating

No cereal, No chocolate, No fast foods, No regular soft drinks No commercial fruit juices; squeeze your own

Diet soft drinks [OK]

Caffeine drinks (coffee/tea) [OK]

Don't forget: moderation in eating includes eating good food, prepared well, presented pleasingly and eaten with gusto, not gluttony!

APPENDIX #2

The Glycemic Index

Puffed Rice	130
Rice Cakes	130
Glucose	100
White Bread	100
Whole Wheat Bread	100
Russet Potatoes	98
Grape Nuts	98
Carrots	92
Rolled Oats	90
Beets	88
Honey	88
White Rice	82
Brown Rice	82
Bananas	82
White Potatoes	81
Pasta	79
Whole Wheat Pasta	78
All Bran	74
Pinto Beans	60
Peas	49

Grapes	45
Oranges	40
Navy Beans	40
Apples	39
Tomato Soup	38
Chick Peas	36
Pears	36
Yogurt	34
Whole Milk	32
Skim Milk	32
Lentils	29
Peaches	29
Grapefruit	26
Plums	25
Fructose	20
Soy Beans	15

APPENDIX #3

HOW MUCH SHOULD YOU WEIGH?

How much should you weigh? Should you weigh what your mother did? How about your father? Your brothers, sisters, cousins? Will pinching an inch give you an idea? The answers to these questions are, simply stated, all of the above. You should weigh your genetic component of lean body mass, with about 20% extra weight as fat if you are female, and about 15% extra weight as fat if you are male.

Lean body mass is controlled genetically. It is the only set point that I acknowledge. If you lose lean body mass in a weight loss program, you will regain the weight. That is a guarantee.

So how much should you weigh? The gold standard, the best way to measure, for determining ideal body weight is immersion in a water tank. By calculating displacement of water according to a formula, specialized centers can determine exactly what the lean body mass of the patient is. This measurement is not readily available. A variety of alternative mechanisms have been devised, none of which are ideal.

The most popular method, based on cost, is the triceps skinfold thickness measure. Anything pinched more than an inch is a problem. Another measure is the body mass index (BMI) which is a contrived scale of height versus weight. Another measure has its roots in the Metropolitan Life Insurance Company, which rated patients' life expectancies based on their heights and weights.

Sure enough, the higher the weight, the earlier the death, and, therefore, the higher the premium. Metropolitan tables suggest that I should be seven feet tall!

I don't have any use for these methods. The triceps skinfold thickness varies tremendously. It is not reproducibly valid for individuals who have upper extremity obesity. The BMI does not correlate at all with what patients know their weight should be. There is no distinction between men and women in the BMI tables. These tables do not separate the powerfully built individual from the stout individual who happens to weigh the same amount. The life insurance tables are the worst. I can only imagine the profit margin that the life insurance companies realize by using these unbelievably distorted tables to tell us what we should weigh.

Please look at the tables that follow; I use these tables on a daily basis. Part of the initial new patient work up is finding out what the patient feels is a proper weight for himself. Believe it or not, almost invariably, patients know exactly what they should weigh and what they should look like when they finish the program, as determined by 20% body fat for women, and 15% for men. I look at someone who wants to lose 100 pounds from 230 to 130, and ask "is this a realistic goal?" Usually the answer is yes. I have learned to trust patients who tell me what they should weigh.

I am reminded of the folklore about Sir William Osler. Dr. Osler, from England, is widely credited as being the father of modern American medicine. He is renowned for his ability to take a history, do a bedside physical exam without touching the patient, and do a touching physical exam in proper order to reach a diagnosis. Dr. Osler is famous for so many things in medicine, but to me his most important direction to physicians who trained with him and those of us who followed, is simply to ask the patient what is wrong. Patients will tell you what is wrong in their own words. The physician needs to be able to listen to those words.

The weight loss tables that I recommend are easy to use. How can they possibly be valid? The simple nomogram for women is accurate almost without fail (within five pounds) between the patient's perceived goal and their actual realized goal. The tables are not quite as good for men. The tables use a man's circumference around the navel and his wrist circumference as the only two measures. Some men have large love handles, which makes their waist measurements high, and some do not. Almost all men have a wrist circumference of about 7 to 7.5 inches.

Take a minute using my tables to calculate your percentage of body fat. Multiply the percent of fat times your current weight. Subtract that number from your weight. This is your lean body mass. Add 20% (15% for men) of your lean body mass to reach your target weight.

Realistically, women should add 10 pounds for having had a child. Pregnancy can do that. Also, add 10 pounds for age more than 40.

Some men will want their final weight to be 10% fat. That is safe. Women will suffer predictable abnormalities in hormone function if they lose to below 20% body fat. Remember that calculated body fat is an external, artificial measure of what you should be.

The best measure of all is the mirror. Look in the mirror, see what the mirror sees. If you have too much fat, you will know. If you think you are in good shape, ask your friend, a spouse, loved one, whomever; they will tell you. Finally, if you need some external measure besides a scale, and I certainly hope you do not rely on a scale, put on a pair of pants. If the pants fit, good! If they are too tight, take note. If they are baggy, pat yourself on the back. When you look good in the mirror and your clothes fit, you are done.

So how much should you weigh? The tables that follow give all of us a good estimate of ideal body weight. Please don't be tied to someone else's standard of what is best for you. Throw away those old weight tables and those body mass index lists. You will know when your weight is proper for you.

PRACTICE

1. If you are a woman, scan Table 3.1 and Table 3.2 which follow; you will use these later to calculate your body's percentage of fat.

Table 3.1

Body Fat Computation for Women

Hips Average
(measure at greater
trochanter)
Measurement_____   Constant A_____
                                                (from Table 3.2)

Abdomen Average
(measure at the navel)
Meaurement_____   Constant B_____add A & B_____

Height in inches_____   Constant C_____minus C_____

                                Equals % Fat_____

Put the average of your measurements in the blank space on the computation form. Now look at the "hips" column in Table 3.2. Note that there is a number to the right side of each hip measurement. This number is a "constant" and is used in the computation of body fat from the measurements you have taken. Write down the constant for each measurement percentage on the computation form to the right of the measurement. Now add constant A to constant B and subtract constant C. The number you have left is percent fat.

An example may be helpful. If a lady had an average hip circumference of 42 inches, an average abdominal circumference of 28 and is 64 inches tall, we would get the following calculations:

Hips Average
(measure at greater trochanter)
Measurement_____ *42* _____   Constant A_____ *50.24* _____
                                                         (from Table 3.2)

Abdomen Average
(measure at the navel)
Meaurement_____ *28* _____   Constant B __*19.91*__ add A & B __*70.15*__

Height in inches____ *64* ____   Constant C __*39.00*__ minus C __*39.00*__

                                       Equals % Fat_____ *31.15*

According to these measurements, she is about 31 percent fat.

Table 3.2

Conversion Chart for Predicting Body Fat for Women

Hips		**Abdomen**		**Height**	
In.	**Constant A**	**In.**	**Constant B**	**In.**	**Constant C**
30	33.48	20	14.22	55	33.52
31	34.87	21	14.93	56	34.13
32	36.26	22	15.64	57	34.74
33	37.67	23	16.35	58	35.35
34	39.06	24	17.06	59	35.96
35	40.46	25	17.78	60	36.57
36	41.86	26	18.49	61	37.18
37	43.25	27	19.20	62	37.79
38	44.65	28	19.91	63	38.40
39	46.05	29	20.62	64	39.01
40	47.44	30	21.33	65	39.62
41	48.84	31	22.04	66	40.23

Hips		Abdomen		Height	
In.	**Constant A**	**In.**	**Constant B**	**In.**	**Constant C**
42	50.24	32	22.75	67	40.84
43	51.64	33	23.46	68	41.45
44	53.03	34	24.18	69	42.06
45	54.43	35	24.89	70	42.67
46	55.83	36	25.60	71	43.28
47	57.22	37	26.31	72	43.89
48	58.62	38	27.02	73	44.50
49	60.02	39	27.73	74	45.11
50	61.42	40	28.44	75	45.72
51	62.81	41	29.15	76	46.32
52	64.21	42	29.87	77	46.93
53	65.61	43	30.58	78	47.54
54	67.00	44	31.29	79	48.15
55	68.40	45	32.00	80	48.76
56	69.80	46	32.71	81	49.37
57	71.19	47	33.42	82	49.98
58	72.59	48	34.13	83	50.59
59	73.99	49	34.84	84	51.20
60	75.39	50	35.56	85	51.81

From *The Complete Book of Physical Fitness*, A. G. Fisher and R. K. Conlee.

PREDICTING BODY FAT FOR MEN

It is quite easy to get percent fat for men since only the wrist and waist are measured. First, measure your waist at the belly button and then have someone measure your wrist circumference just in front of the wrist bones where the wrist bends. Now subtract the wrist measurement from the waist measurement and reference Table 3.3 with this number and your weight.

Table 3.3

Body Fat Computation for Men

WT. (lbs.)	Abdominal Circumference Minus Wrist (inches 22–28.5)													
	22	22.5	23	23.5	24	24.5	25	25.5	26	26.5	27	27.5	28	28.5
120	4	6	8	10	12	14	16	18	20	21	23	25	27	29
125	4	6	7	9	11	13	15	17	19	20	22	24	26	28
130	3	5	7	9	11	12	14	16	18	20	21	23	25	27
135	3	5	7	8	10	12	13	15	17	19	20	22	24	26
140	3	5	6	8	10	11	13	15	16	18	19	21	23	24
145	3	4	6	7	9	11	12	14	15	17	19	20	22	23
150	2	4	6	7	9	10	12	13	15	16	18	19	21	23
155	2	4	5	7	8	10	11	13	14	16	17	19	20	22
160	2	4	5	6	8	9	11	12	14	15	17	18	19	21
165	2	3	5	6	8	9	10	12	13	15	16	17	19	20
170	2	3	4	6	7	9	10	11	13	14	15	17	18	19
175	2	3	4	6	7	8	10	11	12	13	15	16	17	19
180	1	3	4	5	7	8	9	10	12	13	14	16	17	18
185	1	3	4	5	6	8	9	10	11	13	14	15	16	18
190	1	2	4	5	6	7	8	10	11	12	13	15	16	17
195	1	2	3	5	6	7	8	9	11	12	13	14	15	16
200	1	2	3	4	6	7	8	9	10	11	12	14	15	16
205	1	2	3	4	5	6	8	9	10	11	12	13	14	15

WT. (lbs.)	Abdominal Circumference Minus Wrist (inches 22–28.5)													
	22	22.5	23	23.5	24	24.5	25	25.5	26	26.5	27	27.5	28	28.5
210	1	2	3	4	5	6	7	8	9	11	12	13	14	15
215	1	2	3	4	5	6	7	8	9	10	11	12	13	15
220	0	2	3	4	5	6	7	8	9	10	11	12	13	14
225	0	1	2	3	4	6	7	8	9	10	11	12	13	14
230	0	1	2	3	4	5	6	7	8	9	10	11	12	13
235	0	1	2	3	4	5	6	7	8	9	10	11	12	13
240	0	1	2	3	4	5	6	7	8	9	10	11	12	13
245	0	1	2	3	4	5	6	7	8	9	9	10	11	12
250	0	1	2	3	4	5	6	6	7	8	9	10	11	12
255	0	1	2	3	3	4	5	6	7	8	9	10	11	12
260	0	1	2	2	3	4	5	6	7	8	9	10	10	11
265	0	1	1	2	3	4	5	6	7	8	8	9	10	11
270	0	1	1	2	3	4	5	6	7	7	8	9	10	11
275	0	0	1	2	3	4	5	5	6	7	8	9	10	11
280	0	0	1	2	3	4	4	5	6	7	8	9	9	10
285	0	0	1	2	3	4	4	5	6	7	8	8	9	10
290	0	0	1	2	3	3	4	5	6	7	7	8	9	10
295	0	0	1	2	2	3	4	5	6	6	7	8	9	10
300	0	0	1	2	2	3	4	5	5	6	7	8	9	9

WT. (lbs.)	Abdominal Circumference Minus Wrist (inches 29–36)														
	29	29.5	30	30.5	31	31.5	32	32.5	33	33.5	34	34.5	35	35.5	36
120	31	33	35	37	39	41	43	45	47	49	50	52	54	56	58
125	30	32	33	35	37	39	41	43	45	46	48	50	52	54	56
130	28	30	32	34	36	37	39	41	43	44	46	48	50	52	53
135	27	29	31	32	34	36	38	39	41	43	44	46	48	50	51
140	26	28	29	31	33	34	36	38	39	41	43	44	46	48	49

Appendix #3

WT. (lbs.)	**Abdominal Circumference Minus Wrist (inches 29–36)**														
	29	**29.5**	**30**	**30.5**	**31**	**31.5**	**32**	**32.5**	**33**	**33.5**	**34**	**34.5**	**35**	**35.5**	**36**
145	25	27	28	30	31	33	35	36	38	39	41	43	44	46	47
150	24	26	27	29	30	32	33	35	36	38	40	41	43	44	46
155	23	25	26	28	29	31	32	34	35	37	38	40	41	43	44
160	22	24	25	27	28	30	31	33	34	35	37	38	40	41	43
165	22	23	24	26	27	29	30	31	33	34	36	37	38	40	41
170	21	22	24	25	26	28	29	30	32	33	34	36	37	39	40
175	20	21	23	24	25	27	28	29	31	32	33	35	36	37	39
180	19	21	22	23	25	26	27	28	30	31	32	34	35	36	37
185	19	20	21	23	24	25	26	28	29	30	31	33	34	35	36
190	18	19	21	22	23	24	26	27	28	29	30	32	33	34	35
195	18	19	20	21	22	24	25	26	27	28	30	31	32	33	34
200	17	18	19	21	22	23	24	25	26	28	29	30	31	32	33
205	17	18	19	20	21	22	23	25	26	27	28	29	30	31	32
210	16	17	18	19	21	22	23	24	25	26	27	28	29	30	32
215	16	17	18	19	20	21	22	23	24	25	26	28	29	30	31
220	15	16	17	18	19	20	22	23	24	25	26	27	28	29	30
225	15	16	17	18	19	20	21	22	23	24	25	26	27	28	29
230	14	15	16	17	18	19	20	21	22	23	24	25	26	27	28
235	14	15	16	17	18	19	20	21	22	23	24	25	26	27	28
240	14	15	16	17	17	18	19	20	21	22	23	24	25	26	27
245	13	14	15	16	17	18	19	20	21	22	23	24	25	26	27
250	13	14	15	16	17	18	18	19	20	21	22	23	24	25	26
255	13	14	14	15	16	17	18	19	20	21	22	23	24	24	25
260	12	13	14	15	16	17	18	19	19	20	21	22	23	24	25
265	12	13	14	15	15	16	17	18	19	20	21	22	22	23	24
270	12	13	13	14	15	16	17	18	19	19	20	21	22	23	24
275	11	12	13	14	15	16	16	17	18	19	20	21	22	22	23
280	11	12	13	14	14	15	16	17	18	19	19	20	21	22	23
285	11	12	12	13	14	15	16	17	17	18	19	20	21	21	22

407

290	11	11	12	13	14	15	15	16	17	18	19	19	20	21	22
295	10	11	12	13	14	14	15	16	17	17	18	19	20	21	21
300	10	11	12	12	13	14	15	16	16	17	18	19	19	20	21

WT. (lbs.)   **Abdominal Circumference Minus Wrist (inches 36.5–43)**

	36.5	37	37.5	38	38.5	39	39.5	40	40.5	41	41.5	42	42.5	43
120	60	62	64	66	68	70	72	74	76	77	79	81	83	85
125	58	59	61	63	65	67	69	71	72	74	76	78	80	82
130	55	57	59	61	62	64	66	68	69	71	73	75	77	78
135	53	55	56	58	60	62	63	65	67	68	70	72	74	75
140	51	53	54	56	58	59	61	63	64	66	68	69	71	72
145	49	51	52	54	55	57	59	60	62	63	65	67	68	70
150	47	49	50	52	53	55	57	58	60	61	63	64	66	67
155	46	47	49	50	52	53	55	56	58	59	61	62	64	65
160	44	46	47	48	50	51	53	54	56	57	59	60	61	63
165	43	44	45	47	48	50	51	52	54	55	57	58	60	61
170	41	43	44	45	47	48	49	51	52	54	55	56	58	59
175	40	41	43	44	45	47	48	49	51	52	53	55	56	57
180	39	40	41	43	44	45	47	48	49	50	52	53	54	56
185	38	39	40	41	43	44	45	46	48	49	50	51	53	54
190	37	38	39	40	41	43	44	45	46	48	49	50	51	52
195	35	37	38	39	40	41	43	44	45	46	47	49	50	51
200	35	36	37	38	39	40	41	43	44	45	46	47	48	50
205	34	35	36	37	38	39	40	41	43	44	45	46	47	48
210	33	34	35	36	37	38	39	40	42	43	44	45	46	47
215	32	33	34	35	36	37	38	39	40	42	43	44	45	46
220	31	32	33	34	35	36	37	38	39	41	42	43	44	45
225	30	31	32	33	34	35	36	37	38	40	41	42	43	44
230	30	31	32	33	34	35	36	37	38	39	40	41	42	43

WT. (lbs.)	Abdominal Circumference Minus Wrist (inches 36.5–43)													
	36.5	37	37.5	38	38.5	39	39.5	40	40.5	41	41.5	42	42.5	43
235	29	30	31	32	33	34	35	36	37	38	39	40	41	42
240	28	29	30	31	32	33	34	35	36	37	38	39	40	41
245	27	28	29	30	31	32	33	34	35	36	37	38	39	40
250	27	28	29	30	31	31	32	33	34	35	36	37	38	39
255	26	27	28	29	30	31	32	33	34	34	35	36	37	38
260	26	27	27	28	29	30	31	32	33	34	35	35	36	37
265	25	26	27	28	29	29	30	31	32	33	34	35	36	36
270	25	25	26	27	28	29	30	31	31	32	33	34	35	36
275	24	25	26	27	27	28	29	30	31	32	32	33	34	35
280	24	24	25	26	27	28	29	29	30	31	32	33	33	34
285	23	24	25	26	26	27	28	29	30	30	31	32	33	34
290	23	23	24	25	26	27	27	28	29	30	31	31	32	33
295	22	23	24	25	25	26	27	28	28	29	30	31	32	32
300	22	22	23	24	25	26	26	27	28	29	29	30	31	32

WT. (lbs.)	Abdominal Circumference Minus Wrist (inches 43.5–50)													
	43.5	44	44.5	45	45.5	46	46.5	47	47.5	48	48.5	49	49.5	50
120	87	89	91	93	95	97	99	99	99	99	99	99	99	99
125	84	85	87	89	91	93	95	96	98	99	99	99	99	99
130	80	82	84	86	87	89	91	93	94	96	98	99	99	99
135	77	79	80	82	84	86	87	89	91	92	94	96	98	99
140	74	76	77	79	81	82	84	86	87	89	91	92	94	96
145	71	73	75	76	78	79	81	83	84	86	87	89	91	92
150	69	70	72	74	75	77	78	80	81	83	84	86	87	89
155	67	68	70	71	73	74	76	77	79	80	82	83	85	86
160	64	66	67	69	70	72	73	75	76	77	79	80	82	83

WT. (lbs.)	Abdominal Circumference Minus Wrist (inches 43.5–50)													
	43.5	44	44.5	45	45.5	46	46.5	47	47.5	48	48.5	49	49.5	50
165	62	64	65	67	68	69	71	72	74	75	76	78	79	81
170	60	62	63	64	66	67	69	70	71	73	74	75	77	78
175	59	60	61	63	64	65	66	68	69	70	72	73	74	76
180	57	58	59	61	62	63	65	66	67	68	70	71	72	74
185	55	56	58	59	60	61	63	64	65	66	68	69	70	71
190	54	55	56	57	58	60	61	62	63	65	66	67	68	69
195	52	53	55	56	57	58	59	60	62	63	64	65	66	68
200	51	52	53	54	55	57	58	59	60	61	62	63	65	66
205	49	51	51	53	54	55	56	57	59	60	61	62	63	64
210	48	49	50	51	53	54	55	56	57	58	59	60	61	62
215	47	48	49	50	51	52	53	54	56	57	58	59	60	61
220	46	47	48	49	50	51	52	53	54	55	56	57	58	59
225	45	46	47	48	49	50	51	52	53	54	55	56	57	58
230	44	45	46	47	48	49	50	51	52	53	54	55	56	57
235	43	44	45	46	47	48	49	50	51	51	52	53	54	55
240	42	43	44	45	46	46	47	48	49	50	51	52	53	54
245	41	42	43	44	44	45	46	47	48	49	50	51	52	53
250	40	41	42	43	44	44	45	46	47	48	49	50	51	52
255	39	40	41	42	43	44	44	45	46	47	48	49	50	51
260	38	39	40	41	42	43	43	44	45	46	47	48	49	50
265	37	38	39	40	41	42	43	43	44	45	46	47	48	49
270	37	37	38	39	40	41	42	43	43	44	45	46	47	48
275	36	37	38	38	39	40	41	42	43	43	44	45	46	47
280	35	36	37	38	38	39	40	41	42	43	43	44	45	46
285	34	35	36	37	38	39	39	40	41	42	43	43	44	45
290	34	35	35	36	37	38	39	39	40	41	42	43	43	44
295	33	34	35	36	36	37	38	39	39	40	41	42	43	43
300	33	33	34	35	36	36	37	38	39	39	40	41	42	43

Appendix #3

Table 3.4

Computing Your Lean Body Mass

Although it is interesting to see how much of your body is fat, you need to compute lean body mass (LBM) to determine a realistic body weight.

There are two steps that must be taken to compute lean body mass.

Step one: Multiply your body weight in pounds by the percent fat. This will give pounds of fat on your body. For example, the lady in our example was 31 percent fat. If she weighed 160 pounds, she would have about 49.6 pounds of fat.

Total Weight x % Fat = lbs. of fat

160 x .31 (31%) = 49.6 lbs. of fat

Step two: To determine your LBM, simply subtract pounds of fat from your total body weight.

Total Weight-Pounds of Fat = LBM

160 lbs. total weight—49.6 lbs. of fat = 110.4 lbs. LBM

Table 3.5
Your Realistic Weight Goal

			Percent Fat			
LBM	10	13	16	19	22	25
90	100	103	107	111	115	120
95	105	109	113	117	121	126
100	111	114	119	123	128	133
105	116	120	125	129	134	140
110	122	126	130	135	141	146
115	127	132	136	141	147	153
120	133	137	142	148	153	160
125	138	143	148	154	160	166
130	144	149	154	160	166	173
135	150	155	160	166	173	180
140	155	160	166	172	179	186
145	161	166	172	179	185	193
150	166	172	178	185	192	200
155	172	178	184	191	198	206
160	177	183	190	197	205	213
165	183	189	196	203	211	220
170	188	195	202	209	217	226
175	194	201	208	216	224	233
180	200	106	214	222	230	240
185	205	212	220	228	237	246

APPENDIX #4

USE OF ROSIGLITAZONE IN TREATMENT OF HYPERINSULINEMIC OBESITY IN NON-DIABETICS

The Study

FDA approved, IRB approved

40 patients, all healthy, with no ongoing medical symptoms requiring acute care, who presented for elective management of weight loss and who provided informed consent, for a 12 week study on the effect of activation of PPAR gamma and a special, no–amylose, low glycemic index, insulin response sparing diet. All patients must have failed to lose weight previously with other dietary modalities (refractory obesity).

O Fasting insulin 10 ng/ml

O Fasting blood glucose less than 110

O No sustained success with any prior weight loss program (average number of attempts=4)

O Average weight loss using no–amylose diet previously, 0.5 lbs/week

O Rosiglitazone, 4 mg. taken twice daily, with the no–amylose diet

O Patients seen monthly, with monitoring of liver function tests and cholesterol studies to be compared to baseline studies. Presence or absence of edema, a sensation of warmth, calculation of lean body mass and percentage body fat by a standard nomogram recorded on each visit.

The Diet

O High carbohydrate:
   Three servings each of fresh fruit and vegetables that grow above the ground

O High protein:
   Minimum of 6 ounces of protein (final cooked weight) daily, not fried

O No food made from wheat, rice, oats, barley or rye (corn products OK; corn has a natural inhibitor of salivary amylose

O No bananas (the only "forbidden fruit")

O No vegetables that grow below the ground (including carrots, radishes and peanuts, as well as other, more obvious, amylose sources

O No extra table sugar, or foods with added sucrose

O No corn syrup enriched foods, no maltodextrins

O No obvious fat on protein sources (trim the fat, but marbling OK)

The diet specifically suggests that patients take the time previously used to no advantage by counting calories and measuring fat grams, to prepare foods that are pleasing to the eye and that taste great. Portion size is not controlled, but patients are requested not to overeat. No low-fat foods are permitted. No exercise prescription is given, "Don't do anything different."

Results:

Appendix #4

	30 patients compliant with diet	10 patients are not
Average weight	216 pounds	221 pounds
Insulin ng/ml	17.1	17.9 (fasting)
Age	44.6	45.8
Male	3	4
Female	27	6
Ave weight loss		
Women	1.5 lbs/wk	gain 0.3
Men	1.7 lbs/wk	0
Prior attempts with diet	0.5	0.5
Inches lost off hips, measured at the greater trochanter		
Women	2.4	0
Inches off waist, measured at the navel		
All patients	1.6	0
Lean body mass increase	3.1 lbs	0
% Body fat lost	4.6	0
Sensation of warmth	80%	0
New onset edema	0	20%
Total cholesterol		
Baseline	232	220
At 12 weeks	8.6% fall	6.6% rise
HDL cholesterol		
Baseline	43	49
At 12 weeks	4.6% rise	0.5% rise
LDL cholesterol		
Baseline	156	146
At 12 weeks	10.1% fall	4.8% rise
Side effects	none	none
Hypoglycemia	none	none
Elevated LFT	none	none

Note: BMI was NOT used, as that measure does not distinguish fat lost from protein regained.

415

Results that challenge "Accepted Practice Paradigms"

1. A successful weight loss program requires a low-fat, hypo-caloric diet, with regular exercise.

    Fact: Patients in this study did not count or reduce calories consumed, did not restrict fat consumption, and did not undertake any new exercise program.

2. A weight loss program is based on eating the food pyramid, with 6–11 servings a day of cereal grain products.

    Fact: Patients in this study were specifically prohibited from eating wheat, rice, oats, barley and rye, as the amylose in those foods is quickly hydrolyzed by salivary amylase to glucose. The rapid rate of rise of blood glucose, called by some "high glycemic index," that follows consumption of these cereal grains engenders a rapid insulin response that results in enhanced fat storage in hyperinsulinemic patients.

3. Rosiglitazone is reported to routinely cause weight gain, a rise in total and LDL cholesterol, and in some, the appearance of peripheral edema.

    Fact: Patients in this study who followed the no-amylose diet had none of the above and indeed lost a dramatic amount of weight and inches in a short period of time. In addition, total cholesterol and LDL cholesterol fell, and HDL cholesterol rose. Non-compliant patients did experience the unwanted side effects.

4. Thiazolidinedione drugs are too dangerous to be used in non-diabetics on an elective basis.

    Fact: Patients in this study suffered no adverse events in the short period of time (12 weeks) that they took the medication. Hypoglycemia and elevated LFT were not observed. Benefits accruing from use of rosiglitazone with the no-amylose diet included weight loss, especially in areas that are refractory to change with diet alone (hips), a global sense of well being, a pleasing sensation of warmth, and a regain of lean body mass, possibly due to protein-burning diets used by patients before beginning this weight loss program.

5. The rise in obesity and obesity seen in American society today is due to increased fat consumption, sedentary life style and "suburban activities" that include frequent fast food consumption.

Fact: Patients in this study were rarely binge eaters or frequenters of high fat, fast food establishments. These patients have a diagnosis of insulin resistance, they all had experienced failure of weight loss by using "standard" low calorie, low fat diets. With rosiglitazone and the avoidance of foods that cause the rapid rise of blood sugar, these patients achieved weight loss unmatched in their adult lives.

PPAR gamma and rosiglitazone use in obese non-diabetics: why did these patients lose weight while other patients taking rosiglitazone, but also eating amylose, suffer multiple undesirable effects, including weight gain, edema and dyslipidemia?

Known beneficial effects of activation of PPAR gamma by rosiglitazone on lipids, LPL, differentiation of preadipocytes, uncoupling proteins (UCP 1,2,3), free fatty fluxes in muscle and adipose tissue, TNF and TNF receptor transcription, 5'deiodinase activity (the key enzyme generating T3 from T4 inside cells), activation of the organic anion transport protein system in bile canicular cells, and downregulation of production of either (or both!) matrix metalloproteinases and plasminogen activator inhibitor-1, all could be the contributing factors.

Conclusions: A small study like this one raises intriguing questions about our current concepts regarding management of hyperinsulinemic obesity. These data suggest that manipulation of PPAR gamma and therefore the transcriptional regulation of its genes by selective agonists, in combination with a radically different diet prescription, may provide superior benefits for the dieters most refractory to standard treatment. This study may provide hope that these benefits will generalize to "less-difficult" dieters as well. With the emphasis in our society placed on cholesterol lowering diets, which include low-fat foods and an emphasis on cereal grains in the diet, it is possible that we have overlooked the far more important role of PPAR gamma in physiologic control of lipogenesis, fatty acid storage, thermogenesis and obesity. With safe, effective agonists of PPAR gamma available for use, clinicians need to continue to search for additional treatment approaches to obesity.

—Ritchie C. Shoemaker MD

APPENDIX #5

Physical Activity Calorie Chart

Activity	Calories burned per hour per kg body weight
Badminton	2.6
Bicycling, 10 mph	2.7
Dancing, ballroom	1.6
Dancing, modern	2.6
Gardening and yardwork	3.2
Golfing	2.3
Housecleaning	1.6
Hiking	3.6
Jogging, 6 mph	4.2
Jumping rope	3.8
Painting, outside	2.1
Racquetball	4.1
Rowing machine	3.1
Scrubbing floors	2.9
Skating, ice	2.6
Skiing, cross-country	3.7
Squash	4.3

Activity	Calories burned per hour per kg body weight
Swimming	3.5
Soccer	3.7
Table tennis	1.9
Tennis, singles	2.9
Tennis, doubles	1.8
Volleyball	2.2
Walking, 3.5 mph	2.4
Waterskiing	3.0
Weight training	1.9

How Long You Need to Exercise to Burn Excess Calories

Activity (in minutes)

Food Reclining	Calories	Walking	Cycling	Swim-ming	Running	
Apple, large	101	19	12	9	5	78
Bacon, 2 strips	96	18	12	9	5	74
Banana, small	88	17	11	8	4	68
Beans green, 1 cup	27	5	3	2	1	21
Beer, 1 glass	114	22	14	10	6	88
Bread and butter	78	15	10	7	4	60
Cake, ¹⁄₁₂, 2-layer	356	68	43	32	18	274
Carbonated beverage, 1 glass	106	20	13	9	5	82
Carrot, raw	42	8	5	4	2	32
Cereal, dry, ½ cup w/ milk and sugar	200	38	24	18	10	154
Cheese, cottage, 1 tablespoon	27	5	3	2	1	21
Cheese, cheddar, 1 ounce	111	21	14	10	6	85
Chicken, fried, ½ breast	232	45	28	21	12	178
Chicken, TV dinner	542	104	66	48	28	417
Cookie, plain	15	3	2	1	1	12
Cookie, chocolate chip	51	10	6	5	3	39
Doughnut	151	29	18	13	8	116
Egg, fried	110	21	13	10	6	85
Egg, boiled	77	15	9	7	4	59
French dressing, 1 tablespoon	59	11	7	5	3	45
Halibut steak, ¼ pound	205	39	25	18	11	158
Ham, 2 slices	167	32	20	15	9	128
Ice cream, ⅙ quart	193	37	24	17	10	148
Ice cream soda	255	49	31	23	13	196

421

Activity (in minutes)

Food Reclining	Calories	Walking	Cycling	Swim-ming	Running	
Ice milk, ⅙ quart	144	28	18	13	7	111
Gelatin, w/ cream	117	23	14	10	6	90
Malted milk shake	502	97	61	7	26	386
Mayonnaise, 1 tablespoon	92	18	11	8	5	71
Milk, 1 glass	166	32	20	15	9	128
Milk, skim, 1 glass	81	16	10	7	4	62
Milk shake	421	81	51	38	22	324
Orange, medium	68	13	8	6	4	52
Orange juice, 1 glass	120	23	15	11	6	92
Pancake w/ syrup	124	24	15	11	6	95
Peach, medium	46	9	6	4	2	35
Peas, green ½ cup	56	11	7	5	3	43
Pie, apple, ⅙	377	73	46	34	19	290
Pie, raisin, ⅙	437	84	53	39	23	336
Pizza, cheese ⅛	180	35	22	16	9	138
Pork chop, loin	314	60	38	28	16	242
Potato chips, 1 serving	108	21	13	10	6	83
Sandwiches:						
Club	590	113	72	53	30	454
Hamburger	350	67	43	31	18	289
Roast beef/gravy	430	83	52	38	22	331
Tuna fish salad	278	53	34	25	14	214
Sherbet, ⅙ quart	177	34	22	16	9	136
Shrimp, fried	180	35	22	16	9	138
Spaghetti, 1 serving	396	76	48	35	20	305
Steak, T-bone	235	45	29	21	12	181
Strawberry shortcake	400	77	49	36	21	308

APPENDIX #6

Composition of Whole and Refined Wheat Grain

Component	Whole	Refined
Bran, %	14.0	<0.1
Germ, %	2.5	<0.1
Total dietary fiber %	12.6	2.9
Insoluble fiber, %	11.5	1.9
Soluble fiber, %	1.1	1.0
Protein, %	14.2	13.5
Fat, %	2.7	1.4
Starch + sugar, %	69.9	82.8
Total minerals (ash), %	1.8	0.6
Ca, mg/g	0.44	0.25
P, Mg/g	3.8	1.3
Zn, ppm	29.	8
Cu, ppm	4.0	1.6
Fe, ppm	3.5	13.
Mn, ppm	24–37	2.1–3.5
Se, ppm	0.04–071	0.01–0.45
Vitamins		
Thiamine, mg/g	5.8	2.2
Riboflavin, mg/g	0.95	0.39

Component	Whole	Refined
Vitamin B6, mg/g	7.5	1.4
Folic acid, mg/g	0.57	0.11
Biotin, mg/g	116	46
Niacin, mg/g	25.2	5.2
Vitamin E, mg/100g	1.8–2.3	0.04–0.12
Pantothenic acid, mg/100g	0.37	0.18
Natural phenolics, ppm	831–1662	2.3–9.1
Ferulic acid, ppm	490–521	38–44
B-tocopherol, mg/g	32.8	5.7
Lignins, mg/100g	490	<490
Phytate P, mg/g	2.9	0.1

From *Contemporary Nutrition*, Vol.17 #6 1992

Dietary Fiber in Adults

Table 1: Total, insoluble, and soluble dietary fiber in commonly consumed foods (expressed in grams per serving)

Food	Serving Size	TDF	IDF	SDF
Fruits				
Apple, unpeeled	1 med	2.8	2.5	0.3
Banana	1 med	2.0	1.4	0.6
Orange, navel	1 med	2.2	1.8	0.4
Pear, canned	½ cup	2.1	1.7	0.4
Strawberries, fresh	½ cup	1.4	1.1	0.3
Vegetables				
Green beans, canned	½ cup	1.3	1.0	0.3
Broccoli, raw	1 cup	2.9	2.6	0.3
Carrots, raw	1 cup	2.5	2.3	0.2
Celery, raw	1 cup	1.8	1.7	0.1
Corn, canned	½ cup	1.6	1.5	0.1
Kidney beans, canned	½ cup	6.6	5.2	1.4
Peas, green, frozen	½ cup	2.8	2.6	0.2
Grains				
White bread	1 slice	0.7	0.5	0.2
Cereal, cornflakes	1 cup	1.0	0.9	0.1
Cereal, 100% bran	½ cup	13.0	11.9	1.1
Cereal, shredded wheat	2 biscuits	5.7	5.1	0.6
Cereal, oat bran	20 g	3.4	2.1	1.3
Cereal, 40% bran flakes	1 cup	6.5	5.8	0.7

Key: TDF=total dietary fiber; IDF=insoluble dietary fiber; SDF=soluble dietary fiber.

Adapted with permission from Martlett J. Content and composition of dietary fiber in 1177 frequently consumed foods. J Am Diet Assoc 1992; 92: 175–186.

Glossary

Affinity—The efficiency of receptor–insulin interaction. High affinity means rapid uptake of glucose or fatty acids into a cell.

Amylose—The complex carbohydrate found in many starchy vegetables and seeds. Amylose, like glycogen, is many glucose molecules linked together.

Anabolic Steroids—Synthetic muscle building adrenal hormones with many metabolic effects, some good and some bad.

Apo A1—The good stuff that links cholesterol to the enzyme that esterifies (inactivates) it.

Apo B—The bad stuff that helps oxidize LDL.

Bile Acid—Compounds made by liver, stored in bile, that aid in digesting fat.

Catabolic—Breaking down (protein).

Chylomicron—The carrier in blood of ingested cholesterol and triglycerides.

Cytokines—Cell to cell messengers with many effects. Include pro–inflammatory compounds such as TNF, IL–1, IL–1B and anti–inflammatory compounds. Links the immune cells in blood to genes located primarily in fat cells.

Diverticulosis—The medical name for a large bowel condition characterized by the presence of small balloon shaped out-pouchings of large bowel that can become inflamed, infected or begin to bleed.

Ergogenic—Muscle building

Fat Burn Direct—reversal of the process of fatty acid storage in which fatty acids become used for fuel.

Fat Burn Indirect—Conversion of fatty acids to glucose which is used by the body for fuel.

Fed State—The mechanisms by which the body stores calories and makes compounds necessary for life after a meal.

Fructose—A simple sugar with the same chemical formula as glucose but with a slightly different structure.

Genotype—The gene composition of an individual.

Glucose—A six carbon ring. A simple sugar. It is the most important carbohydrate in our body.

Glycemic Index—The number assigned to a type of food which reflects how quickly blood glucose rises after eating the food.

Glycogen—A complex carbohydrate composed of many glucose molecules linked together. It stores glucose inside a cell.

Hamstrings—The large group of muscles in the back of the thigh that flex the knee.

HDL—General name for 5 types of high-density lipoprotein.

Hypothalamus—An important gland in the brain which controls the master gland, the pituitary.

Insulin—A hormone released by cells in the pancreas in response to rising blood glucose levels.

Insulin Resistance—Presence of elevated levels of insulin in the blood but with normal blood levels of glucose.

Isomer—Two compounds with the same formula but a different structure.

Ketones—The break down product of fats and fatty acids found during direct fat burn.

Lactic Acid—The breakdown product of inefficient glucose burning within a cell. Most commonly found when oxygen delivery to the muscle cell is diminished.

LDL—General name for low-density lipoprotein.

Lp(a)—The factor that links oxidized LDL to a platelet, helping make a plaque.

LPL—Lipoprotein lipase, the enzyme that breaks apart chylomicrons.

Maltodextrin—Common food additive that is broken down quickly into glucose, found in many commercially prepared foods, especially salad dressings. Don't eat it.

Megadose—Use of vitamins in hundred of times the daily requirement.

Muscle Fibers—The individual muscle units within a muscle group.

Myofibrils—The individual muscle units within a muscle cell.

Phenotype—The observed expression of the genetic make up of an individual.

PPAR Gamma—The nuclear receptor that controls DNA replication of an important group of "helpful" genes. Counter balance to the cytokine nuclear receptor.

Protein Burning—The approach to weight loss that results in either fat storage or guaranteed regain of lost protein weight.

Protein Sparing Weight Loss—The approach to dieting that prevents the body from consuming its own lean body mass.

Set Point—A genetically determined amount of glycogen and lean body mass (protein).

Starvation Response—The increased efficiency of calorie absorption which occurs following a fast of six hours or more.

Thiazolidinediones—A group of medications that activate PPAR gamma.

TNF Alpha—Tumor necrosis factor alpha, an incredibly active cytokine that can disrupt normal insulin receptor functioning and activate immune responses.

Abbreviations/Acronyms

JAMA	Journal of the American Medical Association
NFkB	cytokine nuclear activating factor
A1C	measure of sugar on hemoglobin in diabetics
BMI	body mass index
CDC	Centers for Disease Control and Prevention
AHA	American Heart Association
FDA	Food and Drug Administration
TNF	tumor necrosis factor alpha
ASBP	American Society of Bariatric Medicine
ADA	American Diabetes Association
CDW	conventional dieting wisdom
SF	saturated fat
NIH	National Institute of Health
VLN	ventrolateral nucleus hypothalamus
VMN	ventromedial nucleus hypothalamus
GTT	glucose tolerance test (get to throw away)
VLCD	very low calorie diet
PDR	Physician's Desk Reference
HDL	high density lipoprotein cholesterol
LDL	low density lipoprotein cholesterol
Lp(a)	lipoprotein a
NCEP	National Cholesterol Education Program
SHEP	systolic hypertension in the elderly
PPAR	peroxisome proliferator activated receptor gamma
ATP	adenosine triphosphate (energy storage molecule)
PEAS	Possible Estuarine Associated Syndrome
EPA	Environmental Protection Agency
VCS	(CS) visual contrast sensitivity

430

*I*NDEX

Frequently Used Terms

Amylose

0023

Glycemic Index

No–Amylose Diet

Low–Glycemic Index diet

Glucose

Insulin

Protein sparing

Maintenance

Low fat diet

Calorie counting

Exercise

Cholesterol

Gout

Fatty acids

Corn syrup

Maltodextrins

Cholesterol

HDL

LDL

RNA

DNA

ABOUT THE AUTHOR

Ritchie C. Shoemaker, M.D., lives in Pocomoke City, Maryland, with his wife JoAnn and daughter Sally. He is board certified in Family Practice, with subspecialty interests in chronic illnesses caused by exposure to biotoxins, obesity and sports medicine. Ritchie is a naturalist, with an avocational interest in wetland ecology.

He graduated from Duke University in 1973, magna cum laude in molecular biology. He developed an awareness about the pivotal role played by insulin in obesity while working in a clinic providing access to care for the medically underserved.

At Duke Medical School, other interests solidified his answers to questions about treatment of obesity, especially a deep involvement in the "new" Family Practice movement. Ritchie started a national medical student primary care journal, *First Contact*. Concerns about the proper rehabilitation of sports injuries led to a thesis on the molecular biology of muscle injury and repair. He graduated in 1977.

While in Family Practice residency in Williamsport, Pennsylvania, Dr. Shoemaker designed a model for rural health care delivery systems. The result of this work was the establishment of a small clinic in Emporium, Pennsylvania, an area where there were more elk than people.

Working in Pocomoke City since 1980, Ritchie remained in solo practice until he affiliated with McCready Hospital, Crisfield,

Maryland, in 1997. The hospital shares his rural health care dream. He has previously authored three books, *Weight Loss and Maintenance, My Way Works; Pfiesteria: Crossing Dark Water;* and *Desperation Medicine.*

Ritchie was named the Maryland Family Practice Doctor of the Year 2000 and was one of the 5 finalists for the National Family Practice Doctor of the Year 2001.

As an independent and free thinker, Dr. Shoemaker challenges established ideas about diet, cholesterol, and exercise among others in this book. Using his training in molecular biology to support his ideas, his programs have been shown to help patients lose weight, reduce cholesterol and develop control over diabetes. He quotes Aldous Huxley, "the key to understanding is casting out false knowledge."

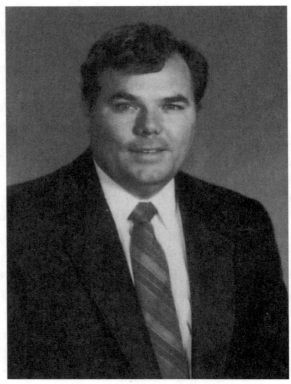